KETTERING COLLEGE
MEDICAL ARTS LIBRARY

DISCARDED

D1623068

ATLAS OF ROENTGENOGRAPHIC MEASUREMENT

Sixth Edition

Other books by Theodore E. Keats:

An Atlas of Normal Roentgen Variants That May Simulate Disease, Fourth Edition

An Atlas of Normal Developmental Roentgen Anatomy, Second Edition, with Thomas H. Smith, M.D.

Emergency Radiology, Second Edition

Radiology of Musculoskeletal Stress Injury

Atlas of Roentgenographic Measurement

SIXTH EDITION

Theodore E. Keats, M.D.

Professor and Chairman
Department of Radiology
University of Virginia School of Medicine
Charlottesville, Virginia

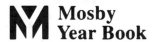
Mosby
Year Book

St. Louis   Baltimore   Boston   Chicago   London   Philadelphia   Sydney   Toronto

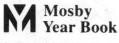

**Mosby
Year Book**

Dedicated to Publishing Excellence

Sponsoring Editor: James D. Ryan
Assistant Director, Manuscript Services: Frances M. Perveiler
Production Coordinator: Nancy Baker
Proofroom Supervisor: Barbara M. Kelly

Copyright 1990 by Mosby-Year Book, Inc.
A Year Book Medical Publishers imprint of Mosby-Year Book, Inc.

Mosby-Year Book, Inc.
11830 Westline Industrial Drive
St. Louis, MO 63146

All rights reserved. No part of this publication may be reproduced, stored in a retrieval system, or transmitted, in any form or by any means, electronic, mechanical, photocopying, recording, or otherwise, without prior written permission from the publisher. Printed in the United States of America.

Permission to photocopy or reproduce solely for internal or personal use is permitted for libraries or other users registered with the Copyright Clearance Center, provided that the base fee of $4.00 per chapter plus $.10 per page is paid directly to the Copyright Clearance Center, 21 Congress Street, Salem, MA 01970. This consent does not extend to other kinds of copying, such as copying for general distribution, for advertising or promotional purposes, for creating new collected works, or for resale.

1 2 3 4 5 6 7 8 9 0 Y R 94 93 92 91 90

Library of Congress Cataloging-in-Publication Data

Keats, Theodore E. (Theodore Eliot), 1924-
 Atlas of roentgenographic measurement / Theodore E. Keats. --6th
ed.   p.   cm.
 Includes bibliographical references.
 Includes index.
 ISBN 0-8151-5657-X
 1. Radiography, Medical--Measurement--Tables. 2. Radiography,
Medical--Atlases. I. Title.
 [DNLM: 1. Radiography--atlases. 2. Reference Values--atlases.
3. Tomography, X-Ray Computed--atlases.   WN 17 K25ab]
RC78.K315   1990
616.07'572--dc20
DNLM/DLC
for Library of Congress   90-12741
                                                   CIP

TO
HOWARD L. STEINBACH

FOREWORD TO THE FIRST EDITION

Since the conception of radiology as a medical science, the growth of this field has been truly remarkable. The early pioneers in the field had little or no knowledge of the normal anatomy or physiology of the living human and, of necessity, relied on morbid anatomy and existing texts. The early radiologic literature was based on empiric observation. These observations, when correlated with what was considered normal in the cadaver, led to erroneous concepts of normal anatomy and physiology.

It soon became apparent that a thorough knowledge of the normal roentgenologic anatomy was necessary before the physician could reliably detect the pathologic state. As a result of intensive studies of normal subjects, a great body of statistics has been accumulated representing the wide range in size and form of normal structures. However, the great number and relative inaccessibility of these observations has precluded their routine use by the busy practitioner of radiology.

This book should be of value to the physician because it provides him, in one volume, the most useful roentgenographic measurements in the medical literature. It should point the way to further studies of a statistical nature in those fields in which there is a lack of information or a conflict of observations.

The selection of the most pertinent information to be included in a book such as this is a difficult task. The authors have done their job well; and it is hoped that they will continue to collect new data, as they become available, for future editions.

HOWARD L. STEINBACH

PREFACE TO THE FIRST EDITION

With the discovery of roentgen rays it was possible, for the first time, to make accurate measurements of internal anatomic structures in living subjects. The value of such measurement had been firmly established by the anatomists. It is, therefore, not surprising that the accumulation of roentgen-image measurements was begun and that in a relatively short period of time a great wealth of material was collected.

Because of the large volume of measurement information, it is difficult for the busy practitioner of medicine to find specific data and to recognize that which is valid. Also, it is difficult for him to have at hand the reference material which is necessary in his daily work. These are acute problems for the physician whose practice is not confined to a single location and who does not have a conveniently accessible medical library. This atlas has been compiled to help fill these needs. But, needless to say, the limitation of such an atlas should be recognized by the reader, for it is not possible to present all of the measurements which have been reported. We have included the data that are, in our opinion, most reliable and practical. In some cases the data have a questionable statistical value because of the small sample. In these cases, however, the type of measurement selected was thought to be important and to be the best available.

There are several serious limitations to roentgenographic measurements: first, the roentgenologic image is not sharp; second, the anatomic points for the measurements are not always clearly defined, and they are subject to individual interpretation; and third, in many cases the wide range of normal anatomic variation has not been defined.

The interpretation of a roentgenogram remains an art—an art which depends, in part, upon the gestalt which the physician has developed from his study of many similar roentgenograms. To this interpretation the objective evidence of the roentgenographic measurement can make an important contribution.

There are several areas of roentgenographic measurement which need further investigation. This is particularly true in pediatrics. Undoubtedly, more measurement data will be forthcoming as the result of the brisk activity in pediatric roentgenology.

We wish to thank Dr. Howard L. Steinbach for directing our attention to the need for such an atlas and for his critical review of the manuscript, and we are indebted to Dr. John F. Holt for his suggestions concerning improvement of this presentation and to the University of Missouri Research Council for financial assistance which helped to make the project possible.

Mr. William E. Loechel, of the National Institute of Health, prepared many of the drawings.

We are grateful to the many authors who have allowed us to reproduce their original work in the *Atlas* and to their publishers for kind permission to reproduce the data.

Especially, we thank our secretaries, Lecho Otts, Lillian Worden, Josephyne Corsi and Helena Vatter, for their excellent help in preparing the manuscript.

LEE B. LUSTED, M.D.
THEODORE E. KEATS, M.D.

PREFACE TO THE SIXTH EDITION

This edition of the *Atlas of Roentgenographic Measurement* will mark the first time since 1959 that Lee Lusted's name does not appear with mine as co-author. Lee provided the initial impetus for the compilation of the atlas and has lent wise counsel and guidance in the subsequent editions. His bent for statistics and decision analysis has been an important contribution to the work. He has decided to devote his energies to other vocations, particularly to the area of medical decision making, a subject of great interest for many years. His guidance and help will be sorely missed.

The current edition reflects the many changes in technology and practice patterns in Diagnostic Radiology. These changes have led me to eliminate a variety of measurements that no longer reflect current practice, such as those derived from pneumoencephalography and polytomography. The reader will find new measurements in conventional radiology, nuclear medicine, computed tomography, magnetic resonance imaging, and ultrasound. The large increase in numbers of ultrasound measurements in the literature reflects the ease of obtaining such measurements directly, without problems of distortion by magnification. One gains the impression that virtually everything that can be demonstrated by sonography is being measured. It was imperative to select the most reliable and practical measurements for this large volume.

I have enlisted the help of members of my faculty, who are subspecialists, to advise me in the selection process, and I am indebted to Drs. Patricia L. Abbitt, Wayne S. Cail, Barbara Y. Croft, C. David Teates, and Brian R. J. Williamson for this advice. I must also express my appreciation to Mrs. Carol Chowdhry, my editorial assistant, and to Ms. Patricia West, my secretary, for their diligent assistance in manuscript preparation.

Thanks are also due to the many authors and publishers for permission to reproduce illustrations and data from the original publication, and to our many readers for their continued interest in and support of this work.

THEODORE E. KEATS, M.D.

CONTENTS

CHAPTER 1

Geometric Distortion of the Roentgen Image and Its Correction

The roentgen image of an object is larger than the object. This image distortion is caused by the divergence of the roentgen rays, and the amount of distortion is a function of three factors (Fig 1–1): the object dimension (O), the target-film distance (D), and the object-film distance (d).

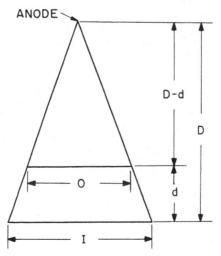

FIG 1–1.
(From Brown GH Jr: *AJR* 1957; 78:1063. Used by permission.)

GEOMETRIC DISTORTION OF THE ROENTGEN IMAGE AND ITS CORRECTION

To find the true object dimension, the image dimension is multiplied by a number less than 1 (correction factor, CF). This correction factor is obtained by means of the following equation, in which

O = Object dimension (cm)
I = Image dimension on the film (cm)
D = Target-film distance (cm)
d = Object-film distance (cm)

It is important to have all dimensions in the same units. Then, by similar triangles,

$$\frac{O}{I} = \frac{D - d}{D} \quad \text{and} \quad O = \frac{(D - d)}{(D)} I$$

Therefore,

$$CF = \frac{D - d}{D}$$

GEOMETRIC DISTORTION OF THE ROENTGEN IMAGE AND ITS CORRECTION*

A number of devices have been constructed that give a fully compensated value of a given object dimension. These devices have usually been made for use in pelvicephalometry.

A nomogram (Fig 1–2) and a base chart (Fig 1–3) may be used for finding corrected dimensions and for converting a given target-film distance to another target-film distance.

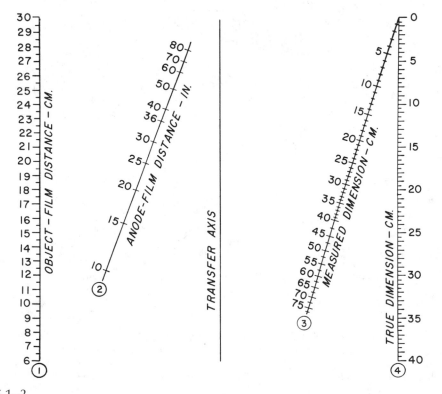

FIG 1–2.

Nomogram (designed by Holmquist) for securing corrected dimensions. (1) Draw a straight line from the object-film distance *(1)* through the anode-film distance *(2)* to the transfer axis. (2) Draw a second line from this point on the transfer axis through the measured dimension *(3)* to the true dimension *(4)*.

*Ref: Ball RP, Golden R: *AJR* 1943; 49:731.

GEOMETRIC DISTORTION OF THE ROENTGEN IMAGE AND ITS CORRECTION*

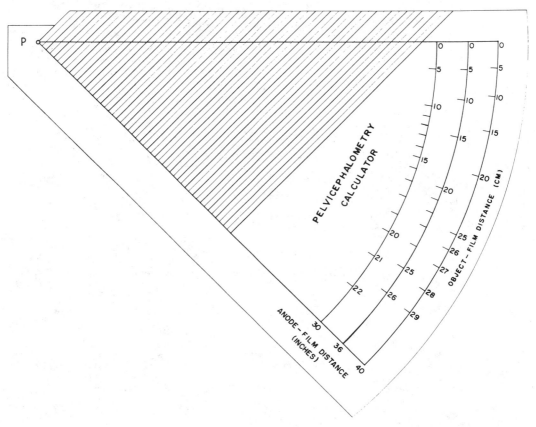

FIG 1–3.
Base chart for constructing a roentgen-image distortion calculator (approx × 1/2). To use the calculator, a centimeter scale, pivoted at P, is set for the correct object-film distance value, which is located on the appropriate target-film scale. The image dimension is measured on the centimeter scale at the top of the calculator. From the scale point so obtained, the corresponding oblique guide line is followed down to the pivoted centimeter scale. The compensated dimension is read from the centimeter scale at the intersection of the guide line and the pivoted scale. (From Brown GH Jr: *AJR* 1957; 78:1063. Used by permission.)

*Ref: Brown GH Jr: *AJR* 1957; 78:1063.

GEOMETRIC DISTORTION OF THE ROENTGEN IMAGE AND ITS CORRECTION

Table 1–1 can be used for converting centimeters to inches, and inches to centimeters.

The amount of shift used to obtain stereo radiographs may be calculated as follows:

TABLE 1–1.

CM	IN	IN	CM
1	0.39	1	2.54
2	0.78	2	5.08
3	1.18	3	7.62
4	1.57	4	10.16
5	1.96	5	12.70
6	2.36	6	15.24
7	2.75	7	17.78
8	3.15	8	20.32
9	3.54	9	22.86
10	3.94	10	25.40
15	5.90	11	27.94
20	7.87	12	30.48
25	9.84	13	33.02
30	11.81	14	35.56
35	13.78	15	38.10
40	15.75	16	40.64
45	17.71	17	43.18
50	19.68	18	45.72
55	21.65	19	48.26
60	23.62	20	50.80
65	25.59	21	53.34
70	27.55	22	55.88
75	29.52	23	58.42
80	31.49	24	60.96
85	33.46	25	63.50
90	35.43	26	66.04
95	37.40	27	68.58
100	39.37	28	71.12
		29	73.66
		30	76.20
		32	81.3
		34	86.4
		36	91.4
		38	96.5
		40	101.6
		48	121.9
		60	152.4
		72	182.9

GEOMETRIC DISTORTION OF THE ROENTGEN IMAGE AND ITS CORRECTION

$$\frac{\text{Target-film distance}}{\left(\dfrac{\text{Film viewing distance}}{\text{Interpupillary distance}}\right)} = \begin{array}{l}\text{Total tube shift} \\ \text{(Half of shift to each side of midline)}\end{array}$$

Examples:

1. Target-film distance = 40 inches
   Film viewing distance = 20 inches
   Interpupillary distance = 2.5 inches
   $$\frac{40}{20/2.5} = 5 \text{ inches}$$
   (2.5-inch shift to each side of midline)

2. Target-film distance = 72 inches
   Other quantities as above
   $$\frac{72}{20/2.5} = 9 \text{ inches}$$
   (4.5-inch shift to each side of midline)

CHAPTER 2

The Central Nervous System

MEASUREMENT OF CEREBRAL VENTRICULAR
SIZE IN INFANTS BY ULTRASOUND*

Technique

Studies performed through the anterior fontanelle with a 5.0 MHz transducer using an ATL portable real time unit.

Measurements

Measurements made with the echo analyzer of the instrument calibrated at five field settings using the electronic calipers in both the coronal and sagittal planes (Figs 2–1 and 2–2).

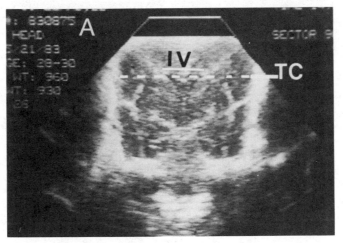

FIG 2–1.
Measurements in the coronal plane. **A,** measurements at the level of the head of the caudate nucleus are obtained by measuring the intraventricular distance *(IV)* and the transcalvarial distance *(TC)*. (From Poland RL, Slovis TL, Shankaran S: *Pediatr Radiol* 1985; 15:12–14. Used by permission.)

*Ref: Poland RL, Slovis TL, Shankaran S: *Pediatr Radiol* 1985; 15:12–14.

MEASUREMENT OF CEREBRAL VENTRICULAR SIZE IN INFANTS BY ULTRASOUND

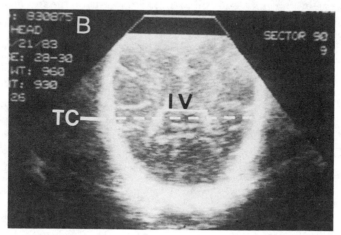

FIG 2–1,B.
Measurements at the level of the midglomus of the choroid plexus in the atria of the lateral ventricle are obtained by measuring the intraventricular distance *(IV)* and the transcalvarial distance *(TC)*. (From Poland RL, Slovis TL, Shankaran S: *Pediatr Radiol* 1985; 15:12–14. Used by permission.)

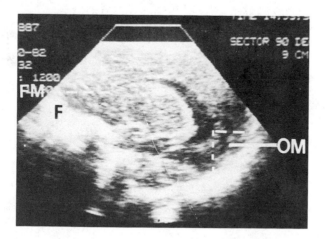

FIG 2–2.
Measurements in the sagittal plane. Evaluation of the frontal cortical mantle thickness *(FM)* is obtained by measuring the distance from the anterior aspect of the frontal horn of the lateral ventricle to the frontal bone *(F)*. Estimation of the occipital cortical mantle thickness *(OM)* is obtained by measuring the greatest distance within a 90° sector shown above. This sector is drawn from the most posterior portion of the occipital horn. (From Poland RL, Slovis TL, Shankaran S: *Pediatr Radiol* 1985; 15:12–14. Used by permission.)

MEASUREMENT OF CEREBRAL VENTRICULAR SIZE IN INFANTS BY ULTRASOUND

The sonographic intracranial measurements and the mean values and 95% confidence limits for ratios are shown in Tables 2−1 and 2−2.

TABLE 2−1.

Sonographic Intracranial Measurements*

	n	Mean (mm)	SD
Frontal mantle thickness	71	26.5	4.9
Occipital mantle thickness	8	20.6	5.1
Ventricular diameter at caudate	72	25.0	5.6
Ventricular diameter at atria	70	37.9	6.0
Brain diameter at caudate	73	77.0	12.4
Brain diameter at atria	72	75.4	10.0

*From Poland RL, Slovis TL, Shankaran S: *Pediatr Radiol* 1985; 15:12−14. Used by permission.

TABLE 2−2.

Mean Values and 95% Confidence Limits for Ratios*

Ratio	n	Mean	95% Confidence Limits
Occipital/frontal mantle	8	0.78	0.49−1.07
Ventricles/brain at caudate	73	0.32	0.23−0.42
Ventricles/brain at atria	73	0.51	0.40−0.60

*From Poland RL, Slovis TL, Shankaran S: *Pediatr Radiol* 1985; 15:12−14. Used by permission.

Source of Material

Data based on 73 sonographic scans on 67 infants between 28 and 48 weeks postconception who had no evidence of intracranial disease.

MEASUREMENT OF THE CEREBRAL VENTRICLES
(Figs 2–3 and 2–4)

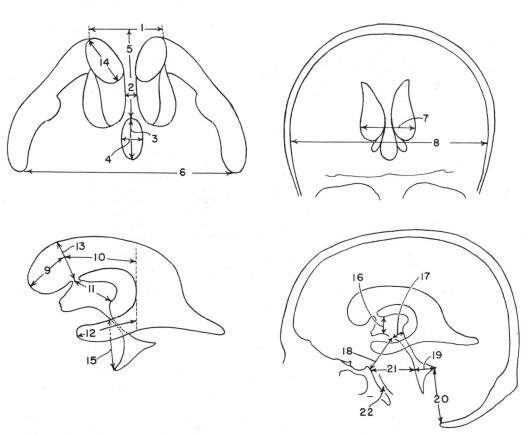

FIG 2–3.
Cerebral ventricles. *Top,* anteroposterior projection. *Bottom,* lateral projection. (Adapted from Orley A: *Neuroradiology.* Springfield, Ill, Charles C Thomas, Publisher, 1949, pp 267–268.)

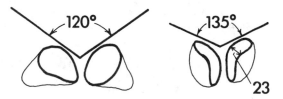

FIG 2–4.
Corpus callosal angle.* *Left,* erect. *Right,* anteroposterior supine. Measurement 23, septum caudate distance: 10 mm ± 0.18 mm (age 1 year to 15 years).†

*Ref: LeMay M, New PFJ: *Radiology* 1970; 96:347.
†Ref: Lodin H: *Acta Radiol Diagn* 1968; 7:385.

MEASUREMENT OF THE CEREBRAL VENTRICLES
(Table 2−3)

TABLE 2−3.

Dimensions of Cerebral Ventricles: Adults*† (See Fig 2−3)

	Lower Limit	Average	Upper Limit
1.		40.0 mm†	45.0 mm†
2.		2.5 mm†	3.0 mm†
3.		2.0 cm†	
4.	2.0 mm§	7.2 mm (anterior)§	10.0 mm§
	4.0 mm§	8.4 mm (posterior)§	10.0 mm§
5.		5.0 mm†	7.0 mm§
6.		90.0 mm†	100.0 mm†
7.		{ratio of 7 to 8 is 0.16−0.29 : 1}	
8.			
9.		25.0 mm‡	
10.		50.0 mm‡	
11.		26.0 mm†	
12.		50.0 mm†	
13.		25.0 mm†	
14.	16.0 mm‡	18.0 mm‡	20.0 mm‡
15.		40.0 mm‡	
16.	11.0 mm†	14.2 mm†	16.0 mm†
17.	1.0 mm†	1.5 mm†	2.0 mm†
18.	30.0 mm†	34.4 mm†	39.0 mm†
19.	10.0 mm†	14.6 mm†	19.0 mm†
20.	30.0 mm†	32.6 mm†	40.0 mm†
21.	33.3 mm†	36.1 mm†	40.0 mm†
22.	5.0 mm†	8.2 mm†	12.0 mm†

*Ventricular size is reliably assessed by computed tomography (CT). Synek et al. (*Neurology* 1976; 26:231) showed good correlation for Evans' Index (ratio of measurements 7 to 8 in above chart—mean value 0.23 ± 0.04 SD) by CT and pneumoencephalography. Hanson et al. (*Acta Radiol Suppl* 1975; 346:98) reported similar findings for cerebral ventricles measured by CT, encephalography, and echoventriculography.
†Davidoff LM, Dyke CG: *AJR* 1940; 44:3; and Davidoff LM, Dyke CG: *The Normal Pneumoencephalogram.* Philadelphia, Lea & Febiger, 1946.
‡Orley A: *Neuroradiology:* Springfield, Ill, Charles C Thomas, Publisher, 1949, pp 267−268.
§Borgersen A: *Acta Radiol Diagn* 1966; 4:645.
Note: Ratios of ventricle-to-skull size are discussed in Berg KJ, Lonnum A: *Acta Radiol Diagn* 1966; 4:65.

MEASUREMENT OF THE CEREBRAL VENTRICLES
(Figs 2–5 to Fig 2–8)

Dimensions of Cerebral Ventricles: Children* (See Fig 2–3)

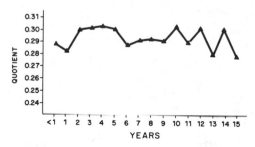

FIG 2–5.
Quotient of the anterior horns in the respective age groups. (From Lodin H: *Acta Radiol Diagn* 1968; 7:385. Used by permission.)

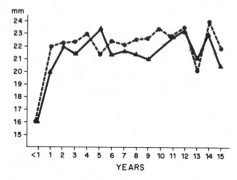

FIG 2–6.
Width of anterior horns in millimeters. Right horn, *solid line;* left horn, *dotted line.* (From Lodin H: *Acta Radiol Diagn* 1968; 7:385. Used by permission.)

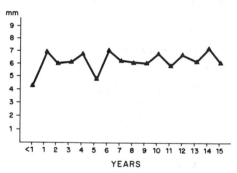

FIG 2–7.
Width of third ventricle. Measurement 4, Fig 2–3. (From Lodin H: *Acta Radiol Diagn* 1968; 7:385. Used by permission.)

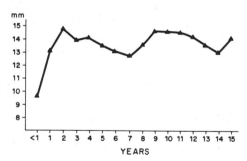

FIG 2–8.
Height of fourth ventricle. Measurement 19, Fig 2–3. (From Lodin H: *Acta Radiol Diagn* 1968; 7:385. Used by permission.)

Technique

1. The anteroposterior projection:

   Central ray: Vertical and enters a point 3 cm in front of the root of the nose.

   Position: Anteroposterior with patient on his back. Position is correct when the line joining the christa galli and the lambda is perpendicular to a line joining two symmetrical points of the right and left petrous bones.

Ref: Lodin H: *Acta Radiol Diagn* 1968; 7:385.

MEASUREMENT OF THE CEREBRAL VENTRICLES

Target-film distance: 29 inches (Davidoff and Dyke)*

70 cm (Orley)†

90 cm (Lodin)‡

2. The lateral projection:

Central ray: Perpendicular to film centered over midportion of skull.

Position: True lateral.

Target-film distance: 29 inches (Davidoff and Dyke)

70 cm (Orley)

90 cm (Lodin)

Measurements (See Fig 2–3)

1 = Distance between the outermost limits of the bodies at the lateral angles.

2 = Width of the shadow of the septum pellucidum.

3 = Vertical diameter of the third ventricle.

4 = Width of the shadow of the third ventricle.

5 = Distance between the tips of the lateral ventricles and the dorsal end of the shadow of the septum pellucidum.

6 = Distance between the two temporal horns.

7 = Transverse diameter of the anterior horns.

8 = Transverse diameter of the skull.

9 = Average length of the anterior horn of the lateral ventricle.

10 = Length of the body of the lateral ventricle.

11 = Diagonal distance between the foramen of Monro and the rostral end of the aqueduct of Sylvius.

12 = Length of the temporal horn of the lateral ventricle.

13 = Distance from the foramen of Monro to the roof of the lateral ventricle.

14 = Diagonal width of the body of the lateral ventricle.

15 = Caudal end of the fourth ventricle to the cephalic end of the aqueduct of Sylvius.

16 = Prepineal ventrodorsal diameter of the third ventricle.

17 = Height of the aqueduct of Sylvius.

18 = Distance from the aqueduct of Sylvius to the dorsum sellae.

19 = Maximum height of the fourth ventricle.

20 = Distance between the superior recess of the fourth ventricle and the floor of the skull.

*Ref: Davidoff LM, Dyke CG: *AJR* 1940; 44:3.

†Ref: Orley A: *Neuroradiology.* Springfield, Ill, Charles C Thomas, Publisher, 1949; pp 267–268.

‡Ref: Lodin H: *Acta Radiol Diagn* 1968; 7:385.

21 = Distance from the dorsum sellae to the floor of the fourth ventricle at the level of the superior recess.

22 = Distance from the dorsum sellae to the anterior margin of the pons varolii.

Source of Material

The dimensions of Davidoff and Dyke were based on 150 encephalograms in which the size of the ventricles appeared to correspond to the accepted size for the normal in standard books on anatomy.

Orley states that the number of encephalograms measured was "fairly substantial."

MEASUREMENT OF NORMAL VENTRICULAR SYSTEM AND HEMISPHERIC SULCI OF 100 ADULTS BY CT

Technique

1. CT studies were performed with EMI scanner using a 160 × 160 matrix and scan time of 4.5 minutes.
2. Patients imaged in supine position with transaxial sections.

Measurements (Table 2–4)

TABLE 2–4.

The Fifth, 50th (Median), and 95th Percentiles of Values of Linear Parameters From the Brains of 100 Normal Adults Measured by Fine Matrix CT, Divided According to Sex in the First Three Columns*†

		Values in Separate Sexes Percentiles			Total Female and Male Values Percentiles		
		5	50	95	5	50	95
LAH	F	13.2	16.5	19.8	13.2	16.5	19.8
	M	14.9	18.2	19.8			
RAH	F	11.6	16.5	19.8	13.2	16.5	19.8
	M	13.2	18.2	18.2			
LSC	F	3.3	8.3	9.9	5.0	8.3	13.2
	M	5.0	8.3	13.2			
RSC	F	5.0	6.6	11.6	5.0	6.6	11.6
	M	5.0	7.5‡	11.6			
CM	F	19.8	28.1‡	33.0	19.8	29.7	36.3
	M	23.1	29.7	36.3			
3V	F	1.7	3.3	6.6	1.7	3.3	6.6
	M	1.7	3.3	8.3			
SU	F	1.7	3.3	5.0	1.7	3.3	5.0
	M	1.7	3.3	5.0			
IS	F	115.5	125.4	135.3	118.8	125.4	135.3
	M	122.1	132.0	135.3			
OS	F	135.3	141.9	151.8	135.3	145.2	155.1
	M	135.3	148.5	155.1			
Left Evans' ratio	F	0.21	0.26	0.32	0.21	0.27	0.32
	M	0.22	0.27	0.32			
Right Evans' ratio	F	0.19	0.26	0.30	0.20	0.26	0.30
	M	0.20	0.27	0.32			
CM index	F	4.2	5.1	6.8	4.2	5.0	6.8
	M	4.2	4.8	6.4			

*From Gyldensted L: *Neuroradiology* 1977; 14:183. Used by permission.
†Values are given in mm, except for last three rows. Abbreviations are defined on page 18.
‡Indicates values obtained by linear interpolation. The 95th percentile is taken as the upper normal limit.

MEASUREMENT OF NORMAL VENTRICULAR SYSTEM AND HEMISPHERIC SULCI OF 100 ADULTS BY CT (Figs 2−9 and 2−10)

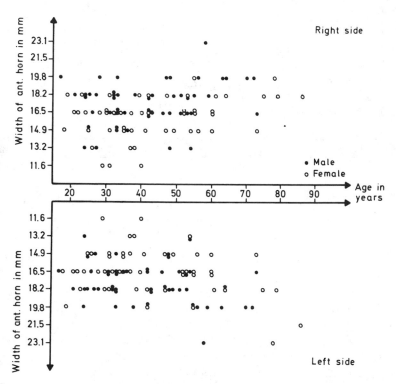

FIG 2−9.

Left and right anterior horn width in 100 normal adults expressed as functions of age. The scatter is considerable both below and above median age, but an increase from the younger to the older group was statistically significant at the 5% level. (From Gyldensted L: *Neuroradiology* 1977; 14:183. Used by permission.)

MEASUREMENT OF NORMAL VENTRICULAR SYSTEM AND HEMISPHERIC SULCI OF 100 ADULTS BY CT (Fig 2–10)

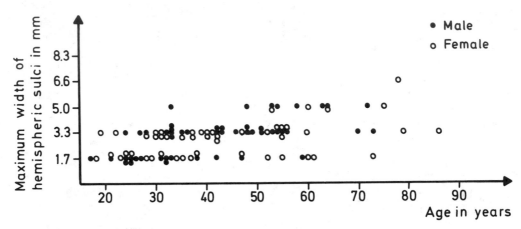

FIG 2–10.
Maximum width of hemispheric sulci in 50 men and 49 women expressed as function of age. A statistically highly significant increase in hemispheric sulci was shown from the younger to the older group by distribution-free analysis. (From Gyldensted L: *Neuroradiology* 1977; 14:183. Used by permission.)

Using Polaroid prints and minification correction, the following distances were measured by dividers:

LAH = Maximum width of left anterior horn
RAH = Maximum width of right anterior horn
LSC† = Maximum left septum-caudate distance
RSC† = Maximum right septum-caudate distance
CM = Minimum width of middle portion of lateral ventricles
3V = Maximum width of third ventricle
SU = Maximum width of hemispheric sulci
IS = Maximum internal width of skull
OS = Maximum external width of skull

†Measured at a 45° angle with the septum pellucidum from the head of the caudate nucleus.

Three ratios were calculated:

$$\text{Left Evan's ratio} \quad \frac{2 \times \text{LAH}}{\text{IS}}$$

$$\text{Right Evan's ratio} \quad \frac{2 \times \text{RAH}}{\text{IS}}$$

$$\text{CM index} \quad \frac{\text{OS}}{\text{CM}}$$

MEASUREMENT OF NORMAL VENTRICULAR SYSTEM AND HEMISPHERIC SULCI OF 100 ADULTS BY CT*

Significant increases were shown with increasing age on all measurements with the exception of skull size. Right and left Evan's ratios also increased, and the CM index decreased with increasing age.

Six parameters were larger in men than in women: LAH, RAH, right Evan's ratio, CM, OS, and IS.

Source of Material

One hundred adults, aged 17 to 86 years. Forty-six were healthy employees from the hospital, and 54 were patients with no evidence of organic brain disease. Half had electroencephalograms performed, which were all normal.

Ref: Gyldensted L: Neuroradiology 1977; 14:183.

POSITION OF THE AQUEDUCT
AND FOURTH VENTRICLE*

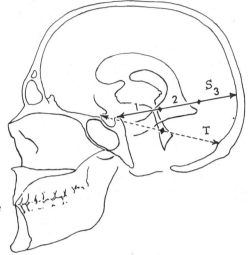

FIG 2–11.
Swedish line† and Twining line.‡ The
Swedish line *(S)* (modified from Sahlstedt) is
drawn from the tip of the dorsum sellae
through the lower part of the aqueduct to the
skull vault. The Twining line *(T)* is drawn
from the tuberculum sellae to the internal
occipital protuberance.

Technique

Central ray: Perpendicular to the film centered 1 inch anterior and 1 inch superior to external auditory meatus.

Position: True lateral of skull (third ventricle and fourth ventricle— views of the pneumoencephalogram or ventriculogram).

Target-film distance: 75 cm used by Sutton, but distance not critical for this study.

Measurements

1. Position of the aqueduct:
   Divide line S (Fig 2–11) into three parts. The aqueduct will lie at about the junction of the first and middle thirds.
2. Position of the fourth ventricle:
   Bisect line T. The midpoint of line T should lie within the fourth ventricle.
   Displacement of the aqueduct or fourth ventricle in the lateral projection is helpful in detecting subtentorial lesions.

Source of Material

Sutton's encephalograms of 100 normal cases were used as a basis. Sutton found no case where the aqueduct was above the junction of the first and mid-

*Ref: Sutton D: Br J Radiol 1950; 23:208.
†Ref: Sahlstedt H: Acta Radiol Suppl 1935; 24.
‡Ref: Twining EW: Br J Radiol 1939; 12:569.

POSITION OF THE AQUEDUCT
AND FOURTH VENTRICLE

dle thirds of the Swedish line. The midpoint of Twining's line lay in the fourth ventricle or posterior to the floor of the fourth ventricle in all 100 cases.

   Note:

$$\text{A ratio} = \frac{\text{Distance of nasion-inion}}{\text{Distance of inion-foramen magnum (posterior lip)}}$$

has been used by Schechter and Zingesser§ in cases of aqueductal stenosis. Normal value of the ratio is 3; for aqueductal stenosis cases the ratio range is 4 to 7.5.¶

§*Ref:* Schechter MM, Zingesser LH: *Radiology* 1967; 88:905.
¶*Ref:* Wolpert SM: *Radiology* 1969; 92:1511.

DISTANCE BETWEEN POSTERIOR MARGIN OF THIRD VENTRICLE AND AMBIENT CISTERN*

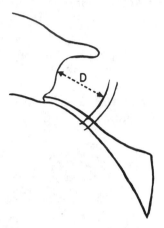

FIG 2–12.
(Adapted from Klaus E: *Acta Radiol* 1958; 50:12.)

Technique

Central ray: Perpendicular to film. Center is 1 inch anterior to and 1 inch superior to external auditory meatus.
Position: True lateral pneumoencephalogram.
Target-film distance: 75 cm.

Measurements

See Figure 2–12. Distance D is the shortest distance between the posterior margin of the third ventricle and the ambient cistern. Normal range, 7–14 mm.

Source of Material

Two hundred normal adult pneumoencephalograms were used as a basis.

*Ref: Klaus E: *Acta Radiol* 1958; 50:12.

MEASUREMENTS FROM CEREBRAL ANGIOGRAMS*

Many meticulous studies of the normal anatomy of intracranial arteries and veins have been made. Some of the more commonly used measurements are provided in this chapter. Other measurements are listed with a reference for each measurement in Table 2–5.

TABLE 2–5.

Studies Used for Measurement of Normal Positions of Vessels on Cerebral Angiograms*

Vessel	View†	Reference
Anterior choroidal artery	Lateral internal carotid arteriogram	Newton TH, Potts DG: *Radiology of the Skull and Brain*. St Louis, CV Mosby Co, 1974, vol 2, p 1634.
Middle cerebral artery	Anteroposterior internal carotid arteriogram	
Measurement A		Taveras JM, Wood EH: *Diagnostic Neuroradiology*, ed 2. Baltimore, Williams & Wilkins Co, 1976, vol 2, p 610.
Measurement B		Chase NE, Taveras JM: Temporal tumors studied by serial angiography: A review of 150 cases, *Acta Radiol Diagn* 1963; 1:225–235.
Measurement C		Taveras and Wood (see above)
Lenticulostriate artery	Anteroposterior internal carotid arteriogram	Leeds NE, Goldberg HI: Lenticulostriate artery abnormalities: Value of direct serial magnification. *Radiology* 1970; 97:377–383.
Middle cerebral artery	Lateral internal carotid arteriogram	Jimenez JP, Goree JA: The normal middle cerebral artery axis. *AJR* 1967; 101:88–93.

*Adapted from Ross P: *Med Radiogr Photogr* 1977; 53:10–11. Used by permission.
†Approximately 10% magnification at center of head.

(Continued.)

*Ref: Ross P: Cerebral angiography: A chart. *Med Radiogr Photogr* 1977; 53:10–11.

MEASUREMENTS FROM CEREBRAL ANGIOGRAMS

TABLE 2−5 (cont.).

Vessel	View†	Reference
Ophthalmic artery	Lateral internal and external carotid arteriogram	Vignaud J, Clay C, Aubin ML: Orbital arteriography. *Radiol Clin North Am* 1972; 10:39−61.
Thalamostriate vein	Anteroposterior internal carotid venogram	Richardson HD, Bednarz WW: The depiction of ventricular size by the striothalamic vein in the anteroposterior phlebogram. *Radiology* 1963; 81:604−609.
Venous angle	Lateral internal carotid venogram	Fischer E: Localisation of the venous angle with consideration paid to the size and shape of the cranial vault. *Acta Radiol Diagn* 1966; 5:173−179.
Choroidal point of posterior inferior cerebellar artery	Lateral vertebrobasilar arteriogram	Huang YP, Wolf BS: Angiographic features of fourth ventricle tumors with special reference to the posterior inferior cerebellar artery. *AJR* 1969; 107:543−564. Belloni G, du Boulay G: The choroidal point and copular point. *Br J Radiol* 1974; 47:261−264.
Precentral cerebellar vein	Lateral vertebrobasilar venogram	Huang YP, Wolf BS: Precentral cerebellar vein in angiography. *Acta Radiol Diagn* 1966; 5:250−262.
Thickness of midbrain	Lateral vertebrobasilar venogram	Huang and Wolf, 1966 (see above)
Inferior vermian vein	Lateral vertebrobasilar venogram	Huang YP, Wolf BS, Okudera T: Angiographic anatomy of the inferior vermian vein of the cerebellum. *Acta Radiol Diagn* 1969; 9:327−344.

MEASUREMENT OF THE SYLVIAN TRIANGLE*†

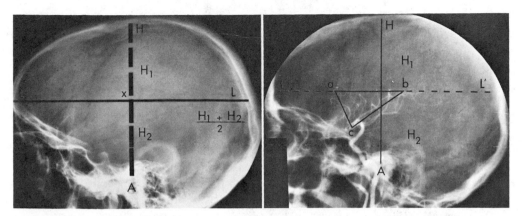

FIG 2–13.
A and **B,** lines of reference to determine displacement of the superior insular line on the vertical plane. (From Gonzalez C, Kricheff II, Lin JP, et al: *Radiology* 1970; 94:535. Used by permission.)

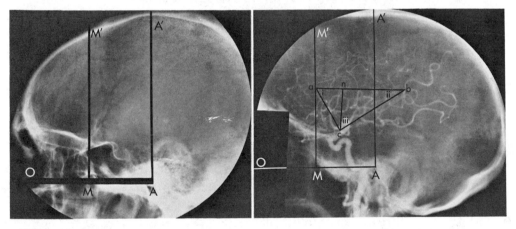

FIG 2–14.
A and **B,** lines of reference to determine displacement of the triangle on the sagittal plane. (From Gonzalez C, Kricheff II, Lin JP, et al: *Radiology* 1970; 94:535. Used by permission.)

Technique

Central ray: To a point 1 inch anterior and 1 inch superior to external auditory meatus.

Position: True lateral carotid arteriogram.

Target-film distance: 44 inches.

*Ref: Fernandez-Serrats AA, Vlahovitch B, Parker SA: *J Neurol Neurosurg Psychiatry* 1968; 31:379.

†Ref: Gonzalez C, Kricheff II, Lin JP, et al: *Radiology* 1970; 94:535.

MEASUREMENT OF THE SYLVIAN TRIANGLE

Measurements

1. Construction of the sylvian triangle (Figs 2–13,B and 2–14,B).

ab = Superior insular line or sylvian line. Line joining the highest points of the first loops of the insular arteries, excepting the first, the fronto-orbital.

bc = Lower border of triangle. A line along the segment of the middle cerebral artery lying within the sylvian fissure. This line joins the origin of the first superior branch of the artery to the highest point of the curve of the middle cerebral trunk.

ac = Anterior border of triangle. A line joining the origin of the first superior branch (the inferior point, *c*) to the most anterosuperior vascular loop.

2. Construction of reference lines (Fig 2–13,A and B).

AH = Hemisphere height. Line from superior border of the external auditory meatus to inner table of the skull. Line is drawn perpendicular to sylvian line, *ab*. *AH* is divided by the sylvian line into two portions, H_1 and H_2, which are used to determine variations of the sylvian triangle in the vertical plane.

See Figure 2–14,A and B.

OA = Anthropometric base line (Frankfurt plane). Line from orbital floor (*O*) to superior border of external auditory meatus (*A*).

AA^1 = Intra-auricular line. Line perpendicular to line *OA* at the level of the external auditory meatus.

MM^1= Line perpendicular to line *OA* halfway between points *O* and *A*.

3. Extremities of the sylvian triangle (Fig 2–14,B).

Gonzalez et al.	*Vlahovitch*
Point *a:* 1.31 mm (SD ± 1.72 mm) posterior to MM^1	0.57 mm (SD ± 2.27 mm) posterior to MM^1
Point *b:* 5 to 25 mm posterior to AA^1	10 to 25 mm posterior to AA^1
Point *c:* Within ± 4.5 mm in any direction from a point at the junction of lower one fourth of AA^1 and posterior one third of *OA*.	

MEASUREMENT OF THE SYLVIAN TRIANGLE

4. Angles of the sylvian triangle (Fig 2–14,B).

	Vlahovitch	Gonzalez et al.
Anterosuperior angle (i) =	65° (P = 95_ ± 11°)	61° (P = 95_ ± 12°)
Posterior angle (ii) =	30° (P = 95_ ± 7.8°)	35° (P = 95_ ± 21°)
Inferior angle (iii) =	85° (P = 95_ ± 10°)	79° (P = 95_ ± 15°)

(From Gonzalez C, Kricheff II, Lin JP, et al: *Radiology* 1970; 94:535. Used by permission.)

5. Height of the sylvian triangle (Fig 2–14,B).
   Height *cn* is one-fourth the hemisphere height, *AH*.
6. Superior border of the sylvian triangle (Fig 2–13,A and B).

The superior insular line (Table 2–6) is at one-half the hemisphere height, *AH*. Standard deviation is 2.5 mm. In 95% of cases the superior insular line will lie within 5 mm of point x.

TABLE 2–6.
Superior Insular Line Relative to Hemisphere Height With Calculation of Standard Deviations*

Height of Hemisphere	Position of Superior Insular Line (SD = 1σ)	Position of Superior Insular Line (SD = 2σ)
11	5.60 ± 0.40	5.60 ± 0.80
12	5.90 ± 0.21	5.90 ± 0.42
12.2	6.10 ± 0.25	6.10 ± 0.52
12.3	6.00 ± 0.11	6.00 ± 0.22
12.5	6.27 ± 0.11	6.27 ± 0.22
12.8	6.30 ± 0.14	6.30 ± 0.28
13.0	6.57 ± 0.28	6.57 ± 0.56
13.4	6.36 ± 0.35	6.36 ± 0.70
13.5	6.77 ± 0.26	6.77 ± 0.52
14.0	6.96 ± 0.23	6.96 ± 0.46
14.5	7.12 ± 0.25	7.12 ± 0.50
Average SD	±0.23	±0.47

*From Gonzalez C, Kricheff II, Lin JP, et al: *Radiology* 1970; 94:535. Used by permission.

Particular attention should be given to displacement of the superior insular line. Concavity in any border of the triangle or deformation of the angles of the triangle is found with space-occupying lesions.

Rotation of the skull changes all the normal relationships and makes the measurements worthless.

Source of Material
Fernandez-Serrats et al. studied 100 normal angiograms. Gonzalez et al. studied 100 normal angiograms.

SIZE OF THE INTERNAL CAROTID, MIDDLE CEREBRAL, AND ANTERIOR CEREBRAL ARTERIES*

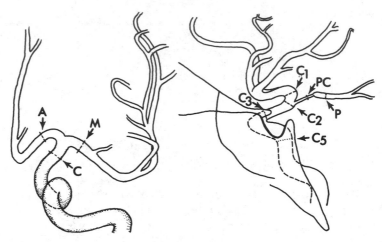

FIG 2–15.
(Adapted from Gabrielsen TO, Greitz T: *Acta Radiol Diagn* 1970; 10:1.)

Technique
    Central ray: Anteroposterior: Directed to superior forehead with the
                    beam angulated 20° cranially.
                Lateral: Perpendicular to the film centered 1 inch anterior
                    and 1 inch superior to the external auditory meatus.
    Position: Anteroposterior and lateral.
    Target-film distance: 85 cm, using a 10-by-12-inch Elema-Schönander
    film changer.

Measurements (Fig 2–15; Tables 2–7 and 2–8)
1. Anteroposterior view:
    C = Diameter of internal carotid artery 5 mm proximal to its bifurca-
        tion into the anterior and middle cerebral arteries.
    A = Diameter of the anterior cerebral artery 5 mm distal to origin.
    M = Diameter of the middle cerebral artery 5 mm distal to origin.
2. Lateral view:
    C_1 = Diameter of the internal carotid artery 5 mm distal to its junction
        with the posterior communicating artery.
    C_2 = Diameter of the internal carotid artery just proximal to the junc-
        tion with the posterior communicating artery.
    C_3 = Diameter of the internal carotid artery at the level of the tubercu-
        lum sellae.
    C_5 = Diameter of the internal carotid artery just proximal to its bend at
        the posterior aspect of the cavernous sinus.

Ref: Gabrielsen TO, Greitz T: *Acta Radiol Diagn* 1970; 10:1.

SIZE OF THE INTERNAL CAROTID, MIDDLE CEREBRAL, AND ANTERIOR CEREBRAL ARTERIES

C_6 = Diameter of the internal carotid artery at the level of the atlas.

PC = Diameter of the posterior communication artery 5 mm distal to its junction with the internal carotid artery.

P = Diameter of the posterior cerebral artery 5 mm distal to its junction with the posterior communicating artery.

TABLE 2–7.

Mean Values for Various Diameters of Normal Cerebral Arteries*†

Measurement	Mean Diameter (mm)	SD (mm)
M	3.82	0.43
A	3.02	0.50
C	4.57	0.46
C_1	3.78	0.43
C_2	4.08	0.47
C_3	5.12	0.63
C_5	5.80	0.76
C_6	5.90	0.73
Siphon length	15.1	2.45

*From Gabrielsen TO, Greitz T: *Acta Radiol Diagn* 1970; 10:1. Used by permission.
†Based on 156 normal carotid angiographies. No correction for sex and skull size.

TABLE 2–8.

Influence of Sex and External Biparietal Diameter (W in cm) on Size of Internal Carotid and Middle Cerebral Arteries (in mm)*

Measurement	Male	Female
M	1.97 + 0.118 W	1.78 + 0.118 W
C	2.99 + 0.100 W	2.81 + 0.100 W
C_5	4.56 + 0.112 W	3.91 + 0.112 W
$M + C + C_5$	9.52 + 0.330 W	8.50 + 0.330 W

*From Gabrielsen TO, Greitz T: *Acta Radiol Diagn* 1970; 10:1. Used by permission.

Source of Material

One hundred fifty-six angiograms from 72 males and 84 females, ranging in age from 13 to 69 years. Mean age was 33 years. Great care was taken to select normal cases. Excluded from the study were cases with even minimal atherosclerosis or cerebral spasm.

DISTANCE FROM LENTICULOSTRIATE ARTERIES TO MIDLINE OF SKULL*

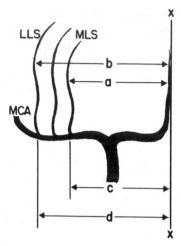

FIG 2–16.
(Adapted from Anderson PE: *Acta Radiol* 1958; 50:84.)

Technique
Central ray: Vertical and enters a point 3 cm in front of the root of the nose.
Position: Anteroposterior.
Target-film distance: 75 cm.

Measurements (Fig 2–16)

X = Midplane of skull.
MLS = Most medial lenticulostriate artery.
LLS = Most lateral lenticulostriate artery.
MCA = Middle cerebral artery.

Distances		Average Normal Values
a	=	26 mm
b	=	38 mm
c	=	17 mm
d	=	30 mm

Source of Material
Studies were made of an unselected series of 300 consecutive adult carotid angiographies.

*Ref: Anderson PE: *Acta Radiol* 1958; 50:84.

QUANTITATION OF CAROTID STENOSES WITH CONTINUOUS-WAVE DOPPLER ULTRASOUND*

Technique

1. Carotid blood velocity was measured with a 5 MHz continuous-wave directional Doppler ultrasound unit (Fig 2–17).
2. The probe is placed against the neck and a Doppler image of the carotid bifurcation (DOPSCAN) including the common carotid and its external and internal branches is obtained. Magnetic tape recordings were made for later spectral analysis.

Measurement

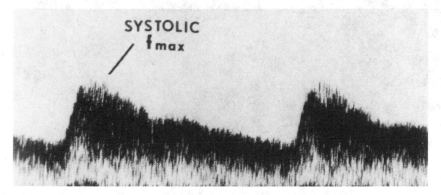

FIG 2–17.
Doppler spectrum of frequencies (velocities) in the normal internal carotid. (From Spencer MP, Reid JM: *Stroke* 1979; 10:326–330. Used by permission.)

*Ref: Spencer MP, Reid JM: *Stroke* 1979; 10:326–330.

QUANTITATION OF CAROTID STENOSES WITH
CONTINUOUS-WAVE DOPPLER ULTRASOUND

To determine the luminal cross section at the angle of the internal carotid artery the frequency ratio between the internal carotid artery signals found at the angle of the jaw $f_{2_{max}}$, downstream to the origin and $f_{1_{max}}$ is determined (Fig 2–18).

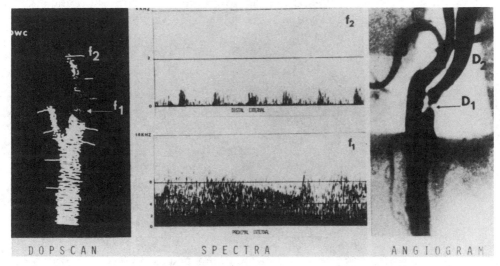

DOPSCAN   SPECTRA   ANGIOGRAM

FIG 2–18.
DOPSCAN image of the carotid bifurcation in a patient with a "tight" stenosis of the internal carotid. Frequencies within the stenosis (f_1) are elevated while downstream frequencies (f_2) are decreased below normal. (From Spencer MP, Reid JM: *Stroke* 1979; 10:326–330. Used by permission.)

QUANTITATION OF CAROTID STENOSES WITH CONTINUOUS-WAVE DOPPLER ULTRASOUND

The relationship between Doppler frequency ratios and x-ray diameters in normal and stenotic carotid arteries is given in Fig 2–19.

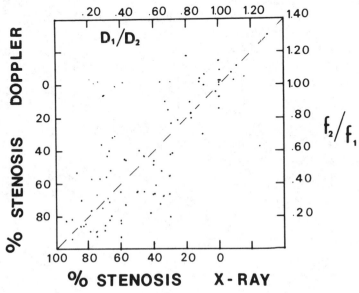

FIG 2–19.
Relationship between Doppler frequency ratios f_2/f_1 and x-ray diameter ratios D_1/D_2 in normal and stenotic internal carotid arteries. The use of f_2/f_1 assuming stenoses are asymmetric without a square root function improves the fit between x-ray and Doppler data. Horizontal bars represent unusual uncertainty in measuring the x-ray diameter. (From Spencer MP, Reid JM: Stroke 1979; 10:326–330. Used by permission.)

Source of Material
Data are based on a study of 95 internal carotid arteries from 64 patients.

MEASUREMENT OF RECORDING OF FLOW VELOCITY IN BASAL CEREBRAL ARTERIES BY DOPPLER ULTRASOUND*

Technique

Range-gated Doppler ultrasound unit with frequency 2MHz; burst repetition rate 6.8 to 18 kHz; burst length 10 μ sec; high pass filter 100 Hz; low pass filter 3.4 to 9 kHz; and emitted ultrasonic power 350 mW. Transducer equipped with a polystyrene acoustic lens with a focal length of 5 cm. Focused beam had a width of 4 mm. The Doppler frequency spectrum was displayed on an Angioscan frequency analyzer. The location of the probe is shown in Figure 2–20.

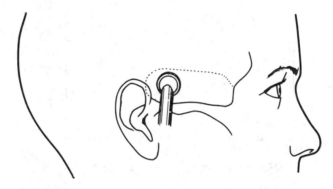

FIG 2–20.
Diagram of the area *(dotted line)* where Doppler signals from intracranial arteries were obtained. The zygomatic arch is indicated. The most likely location to obtain signals is shown by the position of the probe. (From Aaslid R, Markwelder T-M, Nornes H: *J Neurosurg* 1982; 57:769–774. Used by permission.)

*Ref: Aaslid R, Markwalder T-M, Nornes H: *J Neurosurg* 1982; 57:769–774.

MEASUREMENT OF RECORDING OF FLOW VELOCITY IN BASAL CEREBRAL ARTERIES BY DOPPLER ULTRASOUND

Measurement

Figure 2–21 illustrates a spectrum analysis of the Doppler signal from the middle cerebral artery in a healthy 38-year-old man.

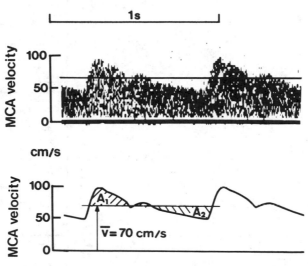

FIG 2–21.

Top, spectral display of the Doppler signal from the middle cerebral artery *(MCA)*. The *horizontal line* through the spectra represents a cursor that can be controlled up or down on the display. **Bottom,** the outline of the spectra shown above. The cursor was placed so that the areas A_1 and A_2 were judged equal. The velocity $\bar{V}$ corresponding to this cursor position was calculated using the Doppler equation. (From Aaslid R, Markwelder T-M, Nornes H: *J Neurosurg* 1982; 57:769–774. Used by permission.)

MEASUREMENT OF RECORDING OF FLOW VELOCITY IN BASAL CEREBRAL ARTERIES BY DOPPLER ULTRASOUND

The velocities in the middle cerebral arteries in 10 normal individuals are shown in Figure 2–22.

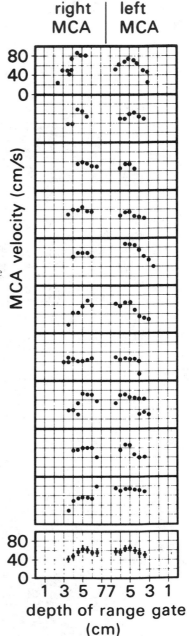

FIG 2–22.
Diagram of the velocities in the middle cerebral artery *(MCA)* in 10 normal subjects *(10 upper panels)*. The abscissae are the depth settings at which the velocity determinations were made. Notice that the depths of the left and right sides run toward the midline from each side. If more than one velocity is given at a certain depth, it indicates that determinations in two branches were made. The *lower panel* represents the means of the MCA velocities in 10 subjects. The standard deviations are indicated by *vertical bars*. (From Aaslid R, Markwelder T-M, Nornes H: *J Neurosurg* 1982; 57:769–774. Used by permission.)

MEASUREMENT OF RECORDING OF FLOW VELOCITY IN BASAL CEREBRAL ARTERIES BY DOPPLER ULTRASOUND

Source of Material

Data are based on a study of 50 healthy subjects with no history of cerebral vascular disease. Their ages ranged from 20 to 65 years with a mean of 36 years.

MEASUREMENT OF THE POSTERIOR
CHOROIDAL ARTERIES (Tables 2–9 and 2—10)*

TABLE 2–9.

Results of Measurements in Normal Patients and Pathological Material

	Measurement A*	Measurement B*	Measurement C*
Normal patients (no.)			
All patients (68)	36.8–56.2%	43.8–63.5%	5.2–9.5%
	Mean 46.1% ± 0.56	Mean 53.4% ± 0.58	Mean 7.3% ± 0.11
	SD 4.6	SD 4.8	SD 0.93
Adults (54)	36.8–52.1%	43.8–58.6%	5.2–8.7%
	Mean 44.6% ± 0.53	Mean 51.9% ± 0.55	Mean 7.2% ± 0.13
	SD 3.8	SD 4.8	SD 0.95
Children (14)	47.9–56.2%	55.2–63.5%	6.2–9.5%
	Mean 51.5% ± 0.70	Mean 50.2% ± 0.64	Mean 7.6% ± 0.23
	SD 2.61	SD 2.4	SD 0.85
Hydrocephalus (10 patients)	30.0–46.5%	30.8–52.1%	1.6–5.6%
Brainstem tumors (5 patients)	45.5–54.3%	48.2–59.6%	2.7–5.3%
Tumors of the pineal region (19 patients)	19.0–55.3%	43.9–70.8%	0.0–41.8%

*See Table 2–10.

TABLE 2–10.

Results of Measurements in Normal Patients and Pathological Material*

Measurement A = distance between the dorsum sellae and the medial choroidal artery

DA, expressed as a percentage of the base line DT: $\dfrac{DA}{DT} \times 100$

Measurement B = distance between the dorsum sellae and the lateral choroidal artery

DB, expressed as a percentage of the base line DT: $\dfrac{DB}{DT} \times 100$

Measurement C = interchoroidal distance AB, expressed as a percentage of the base

line DT: $\dfrac{AB}{DT} \times 100$

*From Pachtman H, et al: *Radiology* 1974; 112:343. Used by permission.

*Ref: Pachtman H, et al: *Radiology* 1974; 112:343.

MEASUREMENT OF THE POSTERIOR CHOROIDAL ARTERIES

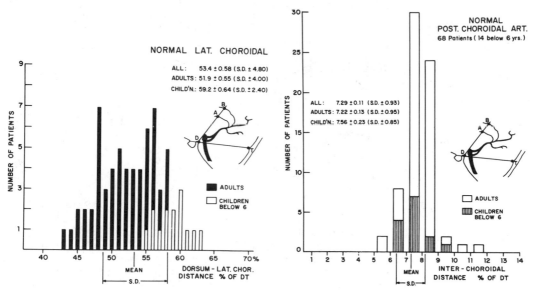

FIG 2–23.
A, normal variation of measurement B in 68 patients. Measurement B is the distance DB between the lateral choroidal artery and the dorsum sellae, expressed as a percentage of the reference line DT. The difference in the range of measurements between adults and children is illustrated well. **B,** normal variation of measurement C, the interchoroidal distance AB expressed as a percentage of reference line DT. Note the values for adults and children are quite similar. (From Pachtman H, et al: *Radiology* 1974; 112:343. Used by permission.)

Technique
Central ray: Perpendicular to plane of film.
Position: Lateral.
Target-film distance: Immaterial.

Measurements (Tables 2–9 and 2–10; Fig 2–23)
Twining's line (DT) is drawn between the tuberculum sellae and the internal occipital protuberance, and the point of intersection with the posterior cortex of the dorsum sellae is noted. A second line is then extended posterosuperiorly from this point at a 60° angle to intersect the posterior choroidal arteries. The distance (DT) between the dorsum sellae (D) and the torcular Herophili (T) was taken as the reference length, and all other measurements were expressed as percentages of it.

Source of Material
Based on a total of 102 patients, 68 of whom were found to be normal; 14 were 5 years of age or younger.

MEASUREMENT OF THE VENOUS ANGLE OF THE BRAIN*

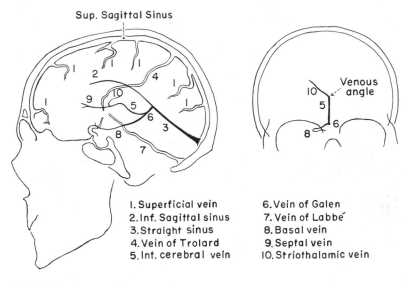

Sup. Sagittal Sinus

Venous angle

1. Superficial vein
2. Inf. Sagittal sinus
3. Straight sinus
4. Vein of Trolard
5. Int. cerebral vein
6. Vein of Galen
7. Vein of Labbé
8. Basal vein
9. Septal vein
10. Striothalamic vein

FIG 2–24.
Deep venous circulation of brain.

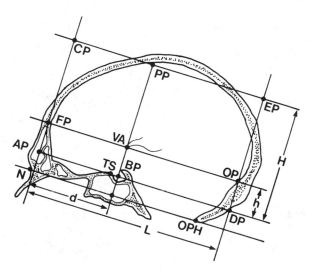

FIG 2–25.
(Adapted from Probst FP: *Acta Radiol Diagn* 1970; 10:271.)

*Ref: Probst FP: *Acta Radiol Diagn* 1970; 10:271.

MEASUREMENT OF THE VENOUS ANGLE OF
THE BRAIN

Technique
  Central ray: To a point 1 inch anterior and 1 inch superior to the external auditory meatus.
  Position: True lateral.
  Target-film distance: 100 cm.

Measurements (Figs 2–24 and 2–25)
1. Construction of reference lines:

Line N-OPH = A line from nasion to opisthion.
Line AP-TS = Base line drawn parallel to line N-OPH through the tuberculum sellae *(TS)*.
Line FP-VA = Venous angle horizontal line is drawn parallel to line N-OPH through the venous angle *(VA)*. VA is the point at which the striothalamic vein joins the internal cerebral vein. The anterior convexity point is usually directed anteriorly, but it may point anteroinferiorly. If the angle takes the form of a large arc, one should choose the anteroinferior convexity point of the arc for the orientation study.
Line CP-PP = Parietal line drawn parallel to line N-OPH through a point on the inner table of the parietal bone *(PP)*.
Line AP-CP = Frontal line drawn perpendicular to line N-OPH through a point on the inner table of the frontal bone *(FP)*.
Line BP-PP = Venous angle vertical line drawn perpendicular to line N-OPH through point *VA*.
Line DP-EP = Occipital line drawn perpendicular to line N-OPH through a point on the inner table at the occipital bone *(OP)*.

2. Measure the following lengths in millimeters:

Frontal distance *(d)* = FP-VA
Total length *(L)*   = FP-OP
Basal distance *(h)*   = BP-VA
Total height *(H)*   = BP-PP

  Plot the distances on the two charts in Figure 2–26.
  The two charts are integrated in Figure 2–27.
  The regression line in each chart in Figure 2–26 is identical with the *y* and *x* axes, respectively, in Figure 2–27.

MEASUREMENT OF THE VENOUS ANGLE OF
THE BRAIN

The range of variation is indicated by the ellipses in Figure 2–27: 99% of normals ($P = 0.01$) will fall inside the larger ellipse and 95% of normals ($P = 0.05$) will fall inside the smaller ellipse.

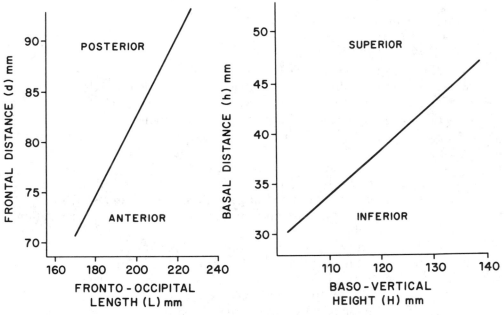

FIG 2–26.
(Adapted from Probst FP: *Acta Radiol Diagn* 1970; 10:271.)

MEASUREMENT OF THE VENOUS ANGLE OF THE BRAIN

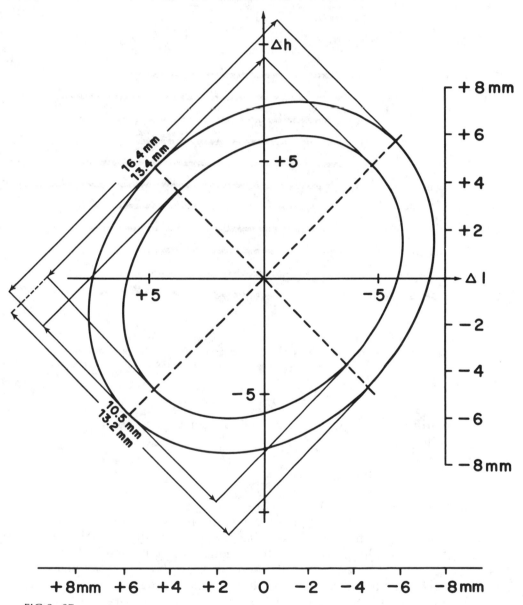

FIG 2–27.
(Adapted from Probst FP: *Acta Radiol Diagn* 1970; 10:271.)

Source of Material
Two hundred sixteen carotid angiograms from adults judged to be normal.

CIRCULATION TIME IN VESSELS OF THE BRAIN*

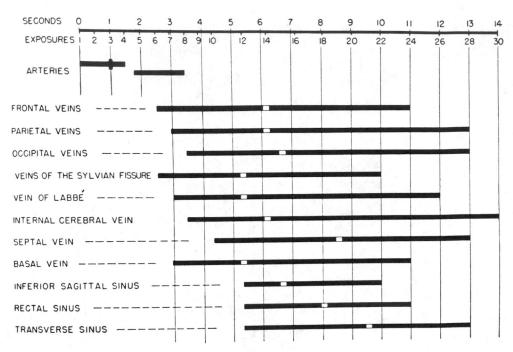

FIG 2–28.
Sequence of contrast filling of different veins in the normal case. The lines are broken at the point of maximum filling, i.e., the transition between filling and emptying phases. This point determined for parietal veins roughly coincides with the average for cerebral veins. (From Greitz T: *Acta Radiol* 1956; 46:285. Used by permission.)

Technique
Central ray: To a point 1 inch anterior and 1 inch superior to external auditory meatus.
Position: Lateral.
Target-film distance: Immaterial.

Measurements (Fig 2–28)
The head of the column of contrast medium is taken as the point of reference for the measurement of the arterial filling phase, the arterial emptying phase, the venous filling phase, and the venous emptying phase. It is not possible to determine with accuracy the termination of the emptying phase, because the contrast filling seems to decrease asymptotically.

For this study, Greitz used a cut-film changer with a program technique: 2 films/sec for the first 5 seconds and then 1 film/sec for 10 seconds.

Source of Material
Cerebral arteriograms from 120 cases were studied.

*Ref: Greitz T: *Acta Radiol* 1956; 46:285.

MEASUREMENT OF NORMAL PITUITARY GLAND BY CT*

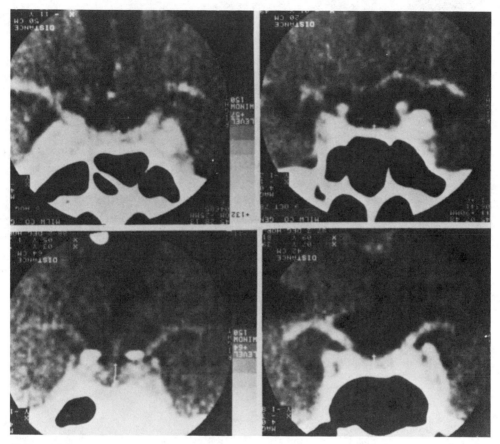

FIG 2–29.

The pituitary gland on coronal CT images. Measurement of gland height is illustrated with cursor in four patients. (From Syvertsen A, et al: *Radiology* 1979; 133:385. Used by permission.)

Technique

1. GE 8800 CT/T scanner with 5-mm thick sections in the coronal plane.
2. Localization with lateral scout image, with the head hyperextended in the auxiliary head holder. Coronal sections set perpendicular to the sellar floor.
3. One hundred fifty milliliters of 30% iodinated contrast were infused in 3 to 4 minutes. The infusion was then slowed during coronal imaging.

*Ref: Syvertsen A, et al: *Radiology* 1979; 133:385.

MEASUREMENT OF NORMAL PITUITARY GLAND
BY CT

4. Axial images with and without enhancement were compared, but not measured.

Measurement (Fig 2–29)

The pituitary was homogeneously isodense or slightly hyperdense with respect to brain tissue. The top of the gland was outlined with cerebrospinal fluid and was flat or concave.

The lateral margin of the gland was difficult to distinguish from the cavernous sinus on routine and enhanced views.

Height of the pituitary gland:

Females: 4.8 + 1.3 mm* (range 2.7–6.7 mm)

Males: 3.5 + 1.5 mm* (range 1.4–5.9 mm)

*Plus 1 SD.

The infundibulum could be identified between the top of the gland and the infundibular recess of the third ventricle, often slightly off midline.

Source of Material

Twenty patients (14 females and 6 males) between the ages of 6 and 74 years. These subjects had no clinical suspicion of pituitary adenoma.

MEASUREMENT OF THE NORMAL PITUITARY STALK BY CT IN CHILDREN*

Technique

1. Scans were obtained on a GE 8800 scanner. 10 mm slice thickness was used.
2. Scans were begun during a bolus injection of 2 ml/kg of Hypaque meglumine 60%.

Measurement (Fig 2–30)

The ideal stalk diameter is made through the midstalk in the suprasellar cisterns. Measurement of the basilar artery is made on the same slice.

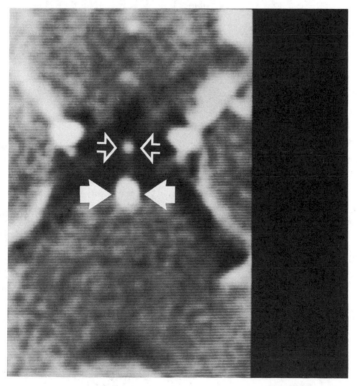

FIG 2–30.
Normal pituitary stalk with pituitary stalk/basilar artery ratio less than 1.0. Pituitary stalk diameter *(open arrows)*; basilar artery diameter *(closed arrows)*. (From Seidel FG, Towbin R, Kaufman RA: *AJR* 1985; 145:1297–1302. Used by permission.)

Ref: Seidel FG, et al: *AJR* 1985; 145:1297–1302.

MEASUREMENT OF THE NORMAL PITUITARY STALK BY CT IN CHILDREN

The absolute pituitary stalk and basilar artery diameters are shown in Tables 2–11 and 2–12.

TABLE 2–11.

Pituitary Measurements in "Pure" Population of Normal Boys Aged 0–19 Years*

Age (Months)	Minimum No. (n = 659)	Mean Diameter in mm (SD)		Mean Stalk/Basilar Ratio (SD)
		Pituitary Stalk	Basilar Artery	
0–6	11	1.9 (0.34)	2.7 (0.74)	0.73 (0.20)
7–12	12	1.9 (0.35)	3.4 (0.54)	0.57 (0.10)
13–24	37	2.0 (0.31)	3.6 (0.43)	0.55 (0.10)
25–36	22	1.9 (0.37)	3.9 (0.57)	0.50 (0.11)
37–48	23	2.1 (0.47)	3.8 (0.40)	0.57 (0.12)
49–60	23	2.1 (0.36)	3.9 (0.53)	0.52 (0.09)
61–72	23	2.1 (0.36)	3.9 (0.46)	0.56 (0.12)
73–84	29	2.2 (0.31)	3.7 (0.46)	0.60 (0.12)
85–96	27	2.1 (0.31)	3.8 (0.46)	0.56 (0.11)
97–108	35	2.2 (0.37)	3.9 (0.56)	0.57 (0.12)
109–120	25	2.4 (0.42)	3.9 (0.40)	0.62 (0.11)
121–132	22	2.4 (0.47)	3.9 (0.51)	0.62 (0.16)
133–144	14	2.6 (0.46)	4.1 (0.56)	0.64 (0.15)
145–156	20	2.3 (0.38)	3.7 (0.65)	0.62 (0.12)
157–168	9	2.4 (0.55)	3.8 (0.54)	0.62 (0.10)
169–180	11	2.4 (0.34)	3.5 (0.51)	0.68 (0.10)
181–192	4	2.8 (0.74)	3.8 (0.46)	0.72 (0.20)
193–204	5	2.3 (0.49)	3.8 (0.46)	0.61 (0.13)
205–216	3	2.3 (0.50)	3.6 (0.05)	0.64 (0.13)
217–228	1	1.8	3.2 (0.23)	0.54

*From Seidel FG, Towbin R, Kaufman RA: *AJR* 1985; 145:1297–1302. Used by permission.

MEASUREMENT OF THE NORMAL PITUITARY STALK BY CT IN CHILDREN

TABLE 2–12.

Pituitary Measurements in "Pure" Population of Normal Girls Aged 0–19 Years*

Age (Months)	Minimum No. (n = 659)	Mean Diameter in mm (SD)		Mean Stalk/Basilar Ratio (SD)
		Pituitary Stalk	Basilar Artery	
0–6	8	1.9 (0.41)	2.5 (0.47)	0.74 (0.09)
7–12	9	1.8 (0.34)	3.3 (0.47)	0.57 (0.13)
13–24	37	2.1 (0.42)	3.5 (0.56)	0.59 (0.11)
25–36	30	2.0 (0.31)	3.6 (0.66)	0.57 (0.15)
37–48	28	2.0 (0.40)	3.5 (0.44)	0.58 (0.11)
49–60	17	2.0 (0.31)	3.6 (0.63)	0.60 (0.16)
61–72	22	2.2 (0.48)	3.7 (0.47)	0.60 (0.18)
73–84	24	2.2 (0.33)	3.5 (0.52)	0.62 (0.09)
85–96	19	2.2 (0.52)	3.7 (0.51)	0.61 (0.10)
97–108	20	2.2 (0.45)	3.9 (0.53)	0.57 (0.15)
109–120	9	2.4 (0.57)	3.5 (0.53)	0.69 (0.13)
121–132	11	2.2 (0.28)	3.6 (0.50)	0.60 (0.09)
133–144	15	2.5 (0.39)	3.7 (0.51)	0.68 (0.08)
145–156	13	2.8 (0.50)	3.5 (0.30)	0.80 (0.17)
157–168	10	2.6 (0.49)	3.7 (0.49)	0.70 (0.10)
169–180	5	2.5 (0.63)	3.2 (0.69)	0.73 (0.10)
181–192	10	2.7 (0.68)	3.6 (0.71)	0.74 (0.21)
193–204	1	2.7	3.4 (0.54)	0.64
205–216	4	3.0 (0.82)	3.8 (0.59)	0.79 (0.21)
217–228	3	2.4 (0.32)	3.1 (0.47)	0.79 (0.18)

*From Seidel FG, Towbin R, Kaufman RA: AJR 1985; 145:1297–1302. Used by permission.

The pituitary stalk to basilar artery ratio is easily estimated visually. Ratios greater than or equal to 1 are unusual in normal children. A ratio greater than or equal to 1 should prompt direct measurement of the stalk and comparison with age-matched normal values. A stalk measurement greater than 2 SD above the age-matched mean is presumably abnormal.

Source of Material

Data are based on a study of 1,005 normal CT scans in 990 patients aged newborn to 18 years. Fifty-three percent were boys and 47% were girls.

MEASUREMENT OF THE NORMAL PITUITARY STALK BY CT IN ADULTS*

Technique

1. Scans were performed on a GE 8800 immediately after drip infusion of 150 cc Conray 60.
2. Scan plane was parallel to the orbitomeatal line. Five or 10 mm slices were obtained.

Measurement (Fig 2–31)

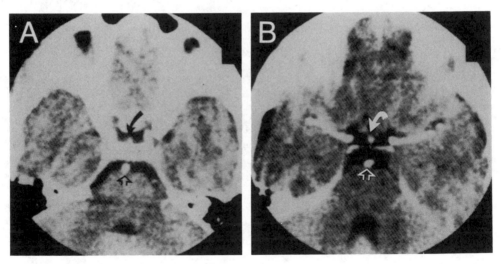

FIG 2–31.
Two contiguous axial CT sections. Normal pituitary stalk *(solid arrow)* and basilar artery *(open arrow)*. **A,** stalk is seen at level of dorsum. **B,** stalk is slightly above level of dorsum and just posterior to optic chiasm. (From Peyster RG, Hoover ED, Adler LP: *AJNR* 1984; 5:45–47. Used by permission.)

Measurements were taken to the nearest half millimeter of the smallest diameter of the stalk and basilar artery when both were visualized at the level of the dorsum sellae and at the suprasellar levels.

*Ref: Peyster RG, et al: *AJNR* 1984; 5:45–47.

MEASUREMENT OF THE NORMAL PITUITARY STALK BY CT IN ADULTS

Table 2–13 shows the normal measurements of normal pituitary stalk and basilar artery.

TABLE 2–13.

Statistical Measurements of Normal Pituitary Stalk and Basilar Artery on High-Resolution Axial CT With Contrast Enhancement*†

Structure and Level	No. Visualized	Dimensions (mm)		Confidence Intervals (mm)	
		Mean±SD	Range	95%	99%
Pituitary stalk					
At dorsum sellae	137	2.1±0.7	0.5–4.0	0.5–3.5	0.0–4.0
Above dorsum sellae	32	2.8±0.6	1.5–4.0	1.5–4.0	1.0–4.5
Basilar artery					
At dorsum sellae	152	3.2±0.8	1.5–7.5	1.5–4.5	1.5–5.5
Above dorsum sellae	29	3.6±0.9	2.5–6.0	2.0–5.5	1.0–6.0

*From Peyster RG, Hoover ED, Adler LP: *AJNR* 1984; 5:45–47. Used by permission.
†Subjects were 184 normal patients.

The upper size limit of the normal pituitary stalk is 4 mm at the level of the dorsum sellae and 4.5 mm above the dorsum. Stalks longer than this should be viewed with suspicion. Comparison with the size of the basilar artery is a quick and reliable visual check of stalk size with a 1:1 ratio.

Source of Material

Data are based on a CT study of 98 male and 86 female subjects 9 to 84 years of age.

MEASUREMENT OF NORMAL BRAIN STEM IN ADULTS AND CHILDREN BY CT CISTERNOGRAPHY*

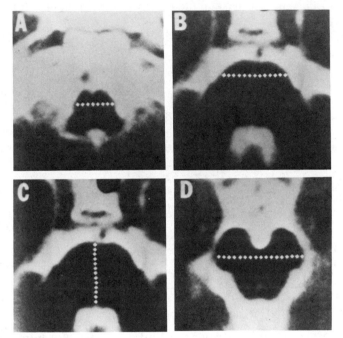

FIG 2–32.
Locations at which transverse medullary (A), transverse pontine (B), pons–fourth ventricle (C), and transverse peduncular (D) dimensions were obtained. (From Steele JR, Hoffman JC: *AJR* 1981; 136:287. Used by permission.)

Technique
1. GE 8800 CT/T scanner with 10-mm slices (occasional 5 mm).
2. Patient lies supine with transverse slices, parallel to the canthomeatal line. Coronal scanning is used in some, depending on individual circumstances.
3. Six milliliters of metrizamide (190 mg iodine/ml) are injected in the lumbar subarachnoid space (proportionately smaller volume in younger patients). The prone patient is tilted into a 45° angle Trendelenburg position with head flexed for 2 minutes to fill the intracranial cisterns. The patient remains in the prone hanging-head position during transport to the CT suite.

Ref: Steele JR, Hoffman JC: *AJR* 1981; 136:287.

MEASUREMENT OF NORMAL BRAIN STEM IN ADULTS AND CHILDREN BY CT CISTERNOGRAPHY

Measurement (Fig 2−32 and Table 2−14)

Measurements were done on hard copy images, corrected for minification.

Transverse measurements of the medulla, pons, and cerebral peduncles were made when possible. These are easily made, except at the level of the brachium pontis, where lateral margins are not readily defined; at that level, the transverse measurement is 5 mm posterior to the anterior pontine margin.

Distance from the anterior pons to the floor of the fourth ventricle is sometimes not possible because of incomplete mixing of contrast with cerebrospinal fluid in the fourth ventricle.

Measurements on young and elderly patients tend to be in the lower end of the normal range.

Minor asymmetry was noted in about 10% of normal patients, particularly in the cerebral peduncles. Causes include positioning and ectatic arteries.

TABLE 2−14.

Normal Brain Stem Measurements*

Location	No. of Cases	Mean (mm)	SD (σ)	Range ($\pm 2\sigma$) (mm)
Transverse peduncular	41	25.4	3.1	19.5−31.5
Transverse pontine	43	24.8	2.2	20.4−29.2
Transverse medullary	29	13.8	1.9	10.0−17.6
Pons−fourth ventricle	39	22.8	2.3	18.1−27.4

*From Steele JR, Hoffman JC: *AJR* 1981; 136:287. Used by permission.

Sources of Material

Seventy-eight CT cisternograms were reviewed. About half had satisfactory images of the basal cisterns. All such patients examined for reasons unrelated to brain stem or posterior fossa were considered "normal."

CHAPTER 3

The Neck

MEASUREMENT OF THE SOFT TISSUES OF THE NECK: RATIO METHOD*

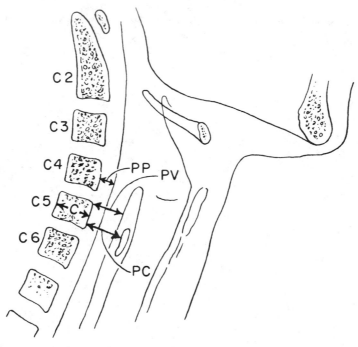

FIG 3–1.
(From Hay PD: in *Annals of Roentgenology*. New York, Paul B Hoeber, Inc, 1939, vol 9. Used by permission.)

TABLE 3–1.

Upper Normal Limits of the Soft Tissue Spaces of the Neck

Age	Postpharyngeal Soft Tissue		Postventricular Soft Tissue	
0–1	1.5C5		2.0C5	
1–2	0.5C5		1.5C5	
2–3	0.5C5		1.2C5	
3–6	0.4C5		1.2C5	
6–14	0.3C5		1.2C5	
			Postcricoid	
	Male	Female	Male	Female
Adult	0.3C5	0.3C5	0.7C5	0.6C5

*Ref: Hay PD: In *Annals of Roentgenology*. New York, Paul B Hoeber, Inc, 1939, vol 9.

MEASUREMENT OF THE SOFT TISSUES OF THE NECK: RATIO METHOD

Technique

Central ray: On coronal plane at the level of the thyroid cartilage.
Position: Lateral at rest.
Target-film distance: Immaterial.

Measurements (Fig 3 1 and Table 3–1)

PV = Postventricular soft tissue for use in children where the cricoid cartilage is not visible. The distance is measured between the posterior commissure of the larynx and the nearest portion of the cervical spine.

PP = Postpharyngeal soft tissue, measured at a point where the soft tissues run parallel to the vertebrae.

PC = Postcricoid soft tissue, measured between the posterior surface of the cricoid cartilage and the anterior surface of the adjacent cervical vertebra.

C = Anteroposterior dimension of C5 vertebral body at its middle.

All measurements are given as multiples of the AP width of the C5 body. The adult anteroposterior diameter of the trachea at the point of greatest construction equals 1.2C5. The retrocricoid space equals 0.6C5.

Adran and Kemp[†] state that in children the thickness of the soft tissue between the pharyngeal lumen and the vertebrae should be about three-fourths the diameter of the adjacent vertebra.

Direct measurement of the retropharyngeal soft tissues as a sign of cervical trauma is of limited usefulness due to large overlap in measurement of normal and abnormal patients. It has been stated[‡] that in films made in the lateral projection using a 40-inch focus film distance, values between 7 and 10 mm at C2, C3, or C4 should suggest possible abnormality. Values of 10 mm or more definitely indicate the need for additional investigation.

Source of Material

Fifty normal adults and 25 normal infants were studied.

Adran and Kemp's data are based on a study of 100 infants aged 6 months to 5 years.

[†]*Ref:* Adran GM, Kemp FH: *Med Radiogr Photogr* 1968; 44:26.
[‡]*Ref:* Templeton PA, et al: *Skeletal Radiol* 1987; 16:98–104.

MEASUREMENT OF THE PREVERTEBRAL SOFT TISSUES IN ADULTS: DIRECT MEASUREMENT (PENNING)*

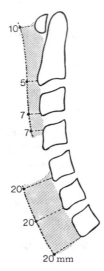

FIG 3–2.

Normal prevertebral space measurements show upper limits of normal width. (From Penning: *AJR* 1981; 136:553. Used by permission.)

TABLE 3–2.

Normal Prevertebral Soft Tissue Width*

| Level | Average Width (Range in mm) | | |
	Flexion	Midposition	Extension
C1	5.6 (2–11)	4.6 (1–10)	3.6 (1–8)
C2	4.1 (2–6)	3.2 (1–5)	3.8 (2–6)
C3	4.2 (3–7)	3.4 (2–7)	4.1 (3–6)
C4	5.8 (4–7)	5.1 (2–7)	6.1 (4–8)
C5	17.1 (11–22)	14.9 (8–20)	15.2 (10–20)
C6	16.3 (12–20)	15.1 (11–20)	13.9 (7–19)
C7	14.7 (9–20)	13.9 (9–20)	11.9 (7–21)

*From Penning L: *AJR* 1981; 136:553. Used by permission.

Technique

Central ray: Perpendicular to plane of film centered over midneck.

Position: Lateral (shoulder against cassette holder).

Target-film distance: 120 cm; magnification factor 1.3.

*Ref: Penning L: *AJR* 1981; 136:553.

MEASUREMENT OF THE PREVERTEBRAL SOFT TISSUES IN ADULTS: DIRECT MEASUREMENT (PENNING)

Measurement (Fig 3−2 and Table 3−2)

Measurement made a line describing the shortest distance between (1) the anterior arch of the atlas and the anterosuperior or anteroinferior edges of the vertebral bodies C2 to C7 and (2) the air shadows of the pharynx and trachea.

Table 3−2 shows the values for normal individuals. These data may be useful in detecting occult fractures of the cervical vertebrae.

Source of Material

Fifty noninjured adults ranging in age from 15 to 78 years. Flexion and extension films were made on 20 adults aged 16 to 67 years.

MEASUREMENT OF THE SOFT TISSUES OF THE NECK*

Technique
   Central ray: perpendicular to midpoint of the neck
   Position: Lateral supine
   Target film distance: 40 inches, midline of spine to film 9 inches

Measurements
See Fig 3–3. Measurements are in millimeters.

NORMAL ADULT CERVICO-CRANIAL
SOFT TISSUE MEASUREMENTS (mm)*
N=66

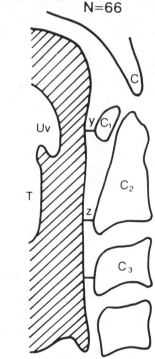

Y 5.26 ± 0.17 SD 1.41 SE 0.17

Z 4.67 ± 0.13 SD 1.04 SE 0.13

C_3 4.95 ± 0.14 SD 1.13 SE 0.14

* SUPINE; TFD=40"; MID-LINE SPINE TO FILM=9"

C=CLIVUS; Uv=UVULA; T=TONGUE

Source of Material
Data derived from radiographs of 66 normal individuals.

Ref: Harris, J: Personal communication.

MEASUREMENT OF SIZE OF CERVICAL AND RETROPHARYNGEAL LYMPH NODES BY CT*

Technique

1. Studies performed on a Siemens Somatom II and a Phillips 300 CT scanner.
2. Position: supine.
3. Section thickness varied between 4 and 8 mm. All studies were contrast enhanced.

Measurement

Nodes were measured using cursors. The largest cross-sectional diameter of the node was recorded. Nodes smaller than 3 mm were assigned a measurement of 3 mm. The size range of nodes in the various anatomic sites is shown in Table 3–3.

TABLE 3–3.

Size and Frequency of Visualization of Normal Cervical and Retropharyngeal Nodes*

Group	No. of Patients in Which It Was Seen	Size Range (mm)	No. of Patients With Nodes at Upper Limit of Range
Occipital	0/30	—	—
Mastoid	0/30	—	—
Facial	0/30	—	—
Lingual	0/30	—	—
Parotid	7/30	3–5	1/7
Retropharyngeal			
Median	0/30	—	—
Lateral	20/30	3–7	2/20
Submental-submandibular	28/30	3–10	3/28
Internal jugular			
Superior	30/30	3–10	6/30
Middle	30/30	3–10	2/30
Inferior	30/30	3–5	5/30
Anterior jugular:			
juxtavisceral-scalene	0/30	—	—
Spinal accessory	28/30	3–5	5/28

*From Mancuso AA, et al: *Radiology* 1983; 148:709–714. Used by permission.

Source of Material

Data derived from CT study of 30 patients.

*Ref: Mancuso AA, et al: *Radiology* 1983; 148:709–714.

MEASUREMENT OF THE POSITION OF THE HYOID BONE AS A SIGN OF TRACHEAL TRANSECTION*

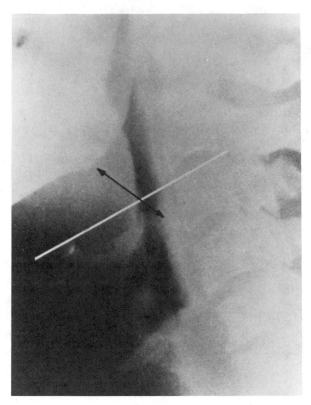

FIG 3–4.

Normal anatomy: lines for measurement of the position of the hyoid bone. (From Polansky A, et al: *Radiology* 1984; 150:117. Used by permission.

Technique

Central ray: Perpendicular to plane of the film over midneck.
Position: True lateral, upright with neck in neutral position.
Target-film distance: 40 inches.

Measurements (Fig 3–4)

Normally, the hyoid bone lies below the level of the third cervical vertebral body *(white line)*. The distance between the cornua and the angle of the mandible *(black line)* should not be less than 2 cm. In the normal group, the distance ranged from 1.9 to 5 cm with an average of 2.95 cm + 0.76 cm (standard deviation).

Source of Material

Data derived from 30 normal patients.

*Ref: Polansky A, et al: *Radiology* 1984; 150:117.

PRETRACHEAL MEASUREMENTS FOR DETECTION OF ECTOPIC THYROID*

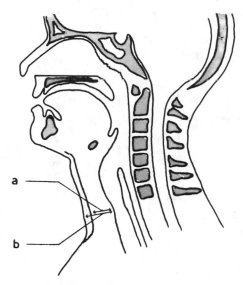

FIG 3–5.
Measurement of pretracheal ratio (a/b × 100). (From Mahboubi S, et al: *AJR* 1981; 137:717. Used by permission.)

Technique
    Central ray: Perpendicular to plane of film directed over midneck.
    Position: True lateral with hyperextended neck.
    Target-film distance: Immaterial.

Measurements (Figs 3–5 and 3–6)
A ratio (a/b × 100) is determined for the distance between the anterior wall of the trachea and both the outer margins of the skin (b) and the interface of the subcutaneous fat and the pretracheal fascia (a) at the level of the calcified cricoid cartilage, or its equivalent area, demonstrated by the constriction of the airway immediately below the larynx.

*Ref: Mahboubi S, et al: *AJR* 1981; 137:717.

PRETRACHEAL MEASUREMENTS FOR DETECTION
OF ECTOPIC THYROID

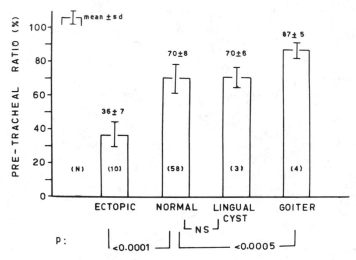

FIG 3–6.

Mean and range of 1 standard deviation of mean for pretracheal ratios in normal ectopic thyroid and goiter patients. Numbers in parentheses are numbers of patients. *NS* = not significant. (From Mahboubi S, et al: *AJR* 1981; 137:717. Used by permission.)

Source of Material

Normal measurements based on a study of 58 normal euthyroid subjects, aged newborn to 16 years.

MEASUREMENT OF THE LATERAL
THORACIC INLET*

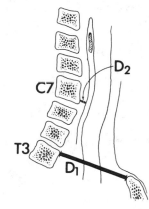

FIG 3–7.
(From Kendall BE, Ashcroft K, Whiteside CG: *Br J Radiol* 1962; 35:769. Used by permission.)

Technique
   Central ray: Perpendicular to plane of the film directed to the level of the seventh cervical and first thoracic vertebrae.
   Position: True lateral.
   Target-film distance: 72 inches.

Measurements (Fig 3–7)

   D_1 = Minimum distance between posterior cortex of manubrium and spine.
   D_2 = Minimum distance between trachea and spine.

   Sagittal inlet (D_1): average = 6.2 cm; range = 5.0 to 8.7 cm.
   Distance from spine to trachea (D_2): average = 1.3 cm; range = 0.5 to 2.5 cm.

Source of Material
   Sixty-seven patients who had routine barium swallows.
   Note: A narrow thoracic inlet may cause compression of the esophagus by the trachea. This compression is seen as a smooth, crescent-shaped defect on the barium-filled esophagus at the C7 to T3 level. The defect usually is on the right side of the esophagus in the PA projection.

Ref: Kendall BE, Ashcroft K, Whiteside CG: *Br J Radiol* 1962; 35:769.

SCINTILLATION SCAN MEASUREMENTS OF THE THYROID GLAND*

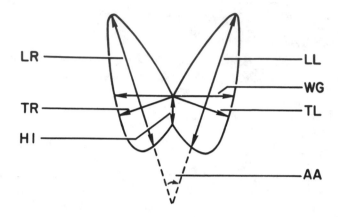

FIG 3–8.

Diagram to illustrate 6 parameters and 1 angle to be measured in each thyroid scan. *LR* = longitudinal length of the right lobe; *LL* = longitudinal length of the left lobe; *TR* = width of the right lobe; *TL* = width of the left lobe; *WG* = width of the whole gland; *HI* = height of the isthmus; *AA* = axial angle. (From Tong EC, Rubenfeld S: *AJR* 1972; 115:706. Used by permission.)

TABLE 3–4.

Mean Measurements of the Normal and Enlarged Glands in Different Parameters*

Measurement	Normal Glands†	Enlarged Glands†
Longitudinal length		
Right lobe	4.8 ± 0.9 cm	6.6 ± 1.3 cm
Left lobe	4.7 ± 1.0 cm	6.4 ±1.4 cm
Width of the whole gland	5.2 ± 0.7 cm	6.5 ± 1.7 cm
Width of lobes		
Right Lobe	2.3 ± 0.5 cm	3.2 ± 0.9 cm
Left Lobe	2.3 ± 0.6 cm	3.0 ± 0.7 cm
Height of isthmus	1.7 ± 0.8 cm	2.6 ± 1.2 cm
Axial angle	25.5 ± 12.8°	25.5 ± 12.8°

*From Tong EC, Rubenfeld S: *AJR* 1972; 115:706. Used by permission.
†Mean ± 1 SD.

Technique

1. Collimator centered on anterior neck over thyroid gland. The focal plane of the collimator passes through the thyroid gland.
2. Position: Supine, anteroposterior.
3. Equipment used by authors included a Nuclear Chicago scanner with a 61-hole collimator and a Picker Magna scanner with a 3-inch fine

Ref: Tong EG, Rubenfeld S: *AJR* 1972; 115:706.

SCINTILLATION SCAN MEASUREMENTS OF THE THYROID GLAND

collimator. Scans done on a thyroid phantom containing 30 μc of I^{131} showed the size of the image in the scan precisely matched the size of the thyroid phantom.

Measurements (Fig 3—8 and Table 3—4)

The longitudinal length of the lobes and the width of the whole gland were found to be essential parameters. When either dimension measures 6.5 cm or more, the thyroid gland should be considered to be enlarged.

Source of Material

Two hundred fifty-six patients from the thyroid clinic. The thyroid gland was normal by palpation in 159 patients; 97 patients had diffuse goiter or a palpably enlarged thyroid mass.

CHAPTER 4

The Skeletal System

The Skull

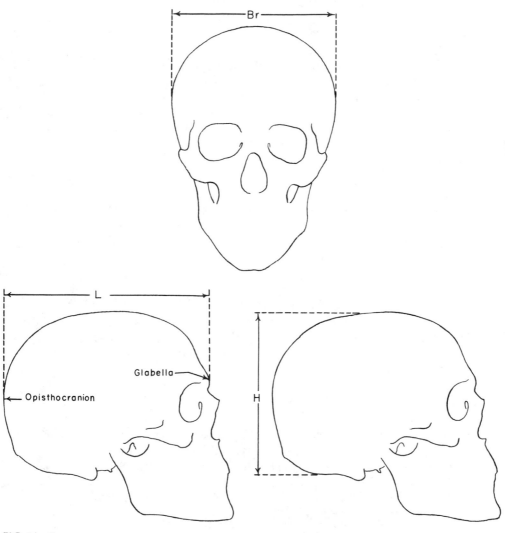

FIG 4A–1.

MEASUREMENT OF THE NORMAL SKULL*

Technique
    Central ray: Posteroanterior: to glabella; Lateral: to a point 1 inch anterior and 1 inch superior to external auditory meatus.
    Positions: Posteroanterior; lateral.
    Target-table distance: 91.4 cm (36 inches).
    Table-film distance: 5.6 cm (enlargement factor of 16%).
    Target-film distance: 97.0 cm (38 inches).

Measurements (Fig 4A−1)

Br = Greatest transverse diameter of skull in posteroanterior position.
L = Greatest length of skull, which equals distance from the glabella to the opisthocranion.
H = Height of skull, which equals total height from the basion to the vertex.

Note:

1. In roentgenograms the breadth averages from 4 to 8 mm less on the anteroposterior view than on the posteroanterior view.
2. Haas believes that it is best to measure breadth at the upper margin of the squamous suture, or slightly above it at the level of the stephanion, when the skull is wider there.

The modulus $M = \dfrac{L + H + Br}{3}$ is a better indicator of skull size than a single diameter. The computed modulus values conform to anthropologic data.
    The cephalic index, $CI = Br_L \times 100$, is characteristic of skull shape.

    Mesocephalic skull, $CI = 75-84$.
    Brachycephalic skull, $CI = 84$ or greater.
    Dolichocephalic skull, $CI = 75$ or less.

    Skull size and measurements have diagnostic value. Deformity itself does not necessarily mean clinical pathology, but deviations in size call for detailed clinical and roentgenologic studies.
    In Tables 4A−1 to 4A−5 which follow:

$$\text{Modulus } (M) = \frac{L + H + Br}{3} \qquad \text{Cephalic index } (CI) = \frac{Br}{L} \times 100$$

*Ref: Haas LL: AJR 1952; 67:197.

MEASUREMENT OF THE NORMAL SKULL

TABLE 4A–1.

Breadth (cm) of Skull on Roentgenograms (Distortion: 16%)*†

	Male			Female			Total		
Age	n	V_{min}–V_{max}	M	n	V_{min}–V_{max}	M	n	V_{min}–V_{max}	m
−4 wk	2	11.1–11.6	11.3	3	10.0–12.0	10.8	5	10.0–12.0	11.0
2–6 mo	8	11.0–14.1	12.2	7	10.1–12.8	11.6	15	10.1–12.8	11.9
7–12 mo	14	12.7–15.6	13.9	12	12.0–15.0	13.2	26	12.0–15.6	13.6
13–18 mo	12	12.8–15.8	14.1	17	12.4–15.6	13.9	29	12.4–15.8	14.0
19–30 mo	22	14.0–16.7	15.1	9	13.2–16.0	14.4	31	13.2–16.7	14.9
3–5 yr	38	14.1–17.0	15.3	30	13.1–16.4	14.9	68	13.1–17.0	15.1
6–8 yr	32	14.1–17.2	15.9	27	13.6–16.6	15.3	59	13.6–17.2	15.6
9–11 yr	29	14.9–17.6	16.0	23	14.3–17.2	15.5	52	14.3–17.6	15.8
12–14 yr	29	15.2–17.3	16.2	23	14.7–17.0	15.7	52	14.7–17.3	16.0
15–17 yr	32	15.0–17.8	16.5	18	14.7–17.1	15.7	50	14.7–17.8	16.2
18–20 yr	31	14.7–18.9	16.5	24	15.5–17.2	16.1	55	14.7–18.9	16.3
21–	369	14.9–19.0	16.8	356	14.2–17.9	16.2	725	14.2–19.0	16.5

$$\sigma = -0.79 + 0.65 \qquad\qquad \sigma = -0.43 + 0.65$$
$$M \pm \sigma = 16.0\text{--}17.4 = 70.9\% \qquad M \pm \sigma = 15.4\text{--}16.8 = 65.7\%$$
$$M \pm 2\sigma = 15.2\text{--}18.1 = 95.4\% \qquad M \pm 2\sigma = 14.7\text{--}17.4 = 96.3\%$$

| Total | 618 | | | 549 | | | 1167 | | |

*From Haas LL: *AJR* 1952; 67:197. Used by permission.
†m = mean value; n = number of individuals; M = modulus.

V_{min} − V_{max} = variation range from minimum to maximum. Values outside this range are definitely abnormal.

Adults: $M \pm \sigma$ = range of variation for mesocephalic skull; σ (standard deviation) not computed for children.

Values of M outside of $M \pm 2\sigma$ indicate hyperdolichocephaly, and in adults suggest previous pathology in childhood.

n = Number of individuals; m = mean value

Source of Material

Studies were made of 1,300 racially mixed patients of various age groups and both sexes.

MEASUREMENT OF THE NORMAL SKULL

TABLE 4A–2.

Length Diameter (cm) of Racially Mixed Skulls on Roentgenograms (Distortion: 16%) of Various Age Groups of Both Sexes*†

Age	Male			Female			Total		
	n	$V_{min}-V_{max}$	M	n	$V_{min}-V_{max}$	M	n	$V_{min}-V_{max}$	m
−4 wk	2	13.7−14.2	13.9	3	12.6−14.0	13.2	5	12.6−14.2	13.5
2−6 mo	8	13.5−16.2	14.7	7	13.4−14.8	14.3	15	13.4−15.0	14.5
7−12 mo	14	14.0−17.8	16.4	12	14.5−16.9	15.8	26	14.0−17.6	16.1
13−18 mo	12	15.8−18.2	17.1	17	15.8−18.1	17.1	29	15.8−18.2	17.1
19−30 mo	22	16.1−19.8	18.1	12	15.7−19.5	17.7	34	15.7−19.8	17.9
3−5 yr	40	16.4−20.4	18.9	30	16.2−20.4	18.8	70	16.2−20.4	18.8
6−8 yr	33	17.1−20.8	19.4	29	16.0−20.7	19.0	62	16.0−20.8	19.2
9−11 yr	34	17.9−21.1	19.6	26	16.6−21.3	19.3	60	16.6−21.3	19.5
12−14 yr	32	18.3−21.8	20.3	26	17.9−21.0	19.7	58	17.9−21.8	20.0
15−17 yr	34	19.0−22.2	20.6	20	18.7−21.8	20.1	54	18.7−22.2	20.4
18−20 yr	33	19.6−22.6	20.8	29	19.2−21.0	20.1	62	19.2−22.6	20.5
21−	395	18.9−23.2	21.2	363	18.0−22.3	20.1	758	18.0−23.2	20.7

$$\sigma = -8.0 + 7.9 \qquad\qquad \sigma = -7.5 + 7.4$$
$$M \pm \sigma = 20.4-22.0 = 69.8\% \qquad M \pm \sigma = 19.4-20.9 = 74.5\%$$
$$M \pm 2\sigma = 19.6-22.8 = 96.7\% \qquad M \pm 2\sigma = 18.7-21.6 = 95.5\%$$

Total	659		574		1233

*From Haas LL: *AJR* 1952; 67:197. Used by permission.
†m = mean value; n = number of individuals; M = modulus.

MEASUREMENT OF THE NORMAL SKULL

TABLE 4A–3.

Height (cm) of Skull on Roentgenograms (Roentgenological Enlargement: 16%)*†

Age	Male			Female			Total		
	n	V_{min}–V_{max}	M	n	V_{min}–V_{max}	M	n	V_{min}–V_{max}	m
−4 wk	2	10.2−11.2	10.7	3	9.8−13.0	11.1	5	9.8−13.0	11.0
2 6 mo	8	10.5−13.7	11.7	7	10.8−13.5	11.8	15	10.5−13.7	11.7
7−12 mo	10	12.1−14.3	13.3	12	11.4−13.6	12.4	22	11.4−14.3	12.8
13−18 mo	9	12.6−15.0	14.0	17	12.1−15.5	13.6	26	12.1−15.5	13.8
19−30 mo	22	13.6−15.7	14.7	9	13.2−15.3	14.2	31	13.2−15.7	14.5
3−5 yr	40	13.5−16.3	14.9	26	13.5−16.0	14.6	66	13.5−16.3	14.7
6−8 yr	33	14.2−16.7	15.2	27	13.2−16.3	14.8	60	13.2−16.7	15.1
9−11 yr	34	14.0−17.0	15.3	25	13.8−15.8	14.8	59	13.8−17.0	15.1
12−14 yr	32	14.4−17.0	15.6	24	13.8−16.3	15.1	56	13.8−17.0	15.4
15−17 yr	32	14.5−17.1	15.7	19	13.8−15.7	15.0	51	13.8−17.1	15.4
18−20 yr	29	14.0−17.4	15.6	26	13.0−16.3	15.1	55	13.0−17.4	15.4
21−	379	13.4−17.7	15.6	353	13.4−17.1	15.1	732	13.4−17.7	15.3

$$\sigma = -0.72 + 0.68 \qquad\qquad \sigma = -0.64 + 0.64$$
$$M \pm \sigma = 14.9-16.3 = 75.7\% \qquad M \pm \sigma = 14.5-15.8 = 70.0\%$$
$$M \pm 2\sigma = 14.1-16.9 = 95.0\% \qquad M \pm 2\sigma = 13.8-16.4 = 95.3\%$$

Total	630			548			1178		

*From Haas LL: *AJR* 1952; 67:197. Used by permission.
†m = mean value; n = number of individuals; M = modulus.

MEASUREMENT OF THE NORMAL SKULL

TABLE 4A–4.

Modulus (cm) of Skull on Roentgenograms*†

Age	Male			Female			Total		
	n	$V_{min}-V_{max}$	M	n	$V_{min}-V_{max}$	M	n	$V_{min}-V_{max}$	m
−4 wk	2	11.6−12.3	12.0	3	10.8−12.8	11.6	5	10.8−12.3	11.8
2−6 mo	8	11.9−14.6	12.9	7	12.1−14.1	12.7	15	11.9−14.6	12.8
7−12 mo	11	13.0−15.3	14.9	12	12.9−15.0	13.8	23	12.9−15.3	14.2
13−18 mo	9	14.3−16.1	15.3	17	13.5−16.0	14.8	26	13.5−16.1	15.0
19−30 mo	23	14.5−16.8	15.9	12	13.6−16.6	15.1	35	13.6−16.8	15.7
3−5 yr	33	14.8−17.4	16.3	26	14.2−17.4	16.0	59	14.2−17.4	16.2
6−8 yr	29	15.5−17.7	16.8	27	14.3−17.5	16.3	56	14.3−17.7	16.6
9−11 yr	30	15.7−18.1	16.9	23	15.2−17.6	16.5	53	15.2−18.1	16.7
12−14 yr	30	16.4−18.5	17.4	23	16.0−17.6	16.7	53	16.0−18.5	17.1
15−17 yr	32	16.6−18.8	17.6	18	15.9−17.7	16.9	50	15.9−18.8	17.3
18−20 yr	30	16.3−19.2	17.7	22	16.3−17.8	17.1	52	16.3−19.2	17.5
21−	360	16.3−19.5	17.8	355	15.7−18.5	17.1	715	15.7−19.5	17.5

$$\sigma = -\ 0.52 + 0.51 \qquad\qquad \sigma = -0.54 + 0.39$$
$$M \pm \sigma = 17.3-18.4 = 72.1\% \qquad M \pm \sigma = 16.4-17.6 = 70.2\%$$
$$M \pm 2\sigma = 16.8-18.9 = 94.2\% \qquad M \pm 2\sigma = 16.0-18.1 = 95.7\%$$

Total	597			545			1142		

*From Haas LL: *AJR* 1952; 67:197. Used by permission.
†m = mean value; n = number of individuals; M = modulus.

MEASUREMENT OF THE NORMAL SKULL

TABLE 4A–5.

Cephalic Index on Roentgenograms*†

Age	Male			Female			Total		
	n	$V_{min}–V_{max}$	M	n	$V_{min}–V_{max}$	M	n	$V_{min}–V_{max}$	m
–4 wk	2	81.0–81.7	81.3	3	79.4–85.7	81.6	5	79.4–85.7	81.5
2–6 mo	11	73.5–88.1	81.7	12	72.7–87.7	80.8	23	72.7–87.7	81.4
7–12 mo	12	73.8–89.5	81.8	12	75.9–90.4	82.5	24	73.8–90.4	82.1
13–18 mo	11	78.3–90.3	82.3	11	73.7–87.9	81.5	22	73.7–90.3	81.8
19–30 mo	21	71.7–90.4	81.2	10	77.4–88.4	81.4	31	74.3–90.4	81.3
3–5 yr	35	72.4–90.0	81.2	26	72.7–91.1	81.0	61	72.4–91.1	81.1
6–8 yr	30	71.8–88.6	81.4	24	73.0–88.3	81.5	54	71.8–88.6	81.4
9–11 yr	30	72.0–89.8	81.1	22	74.9–88.5	80.3	52	72.0–89.8	80.8
12–14 yr	30	73.1–88.3	80.5	23	73.9–89.4	80.2	53	73.1–89.4	80.3
15–17 yr	35	72.8–87.7	80.6	17	72.0–83.4	79.6	52	72.8–87.7	80.0
18–20 yr	31	72.8–85.7	79.3	24	73.8–89.6	80.0	55	72.8–89.6	79.6
21–	351	71.3–89.4	79.5	354	71.0–90.4	80.0	705	71.0–90.4	79.8

$$\sigma = -3.66 + 3.87$$
$$M \pm \sigma = 75.9–83.4 = 65.7\%$$
$$M \pm 2\sigma = 72.2–87.3 = 96.5\%$$

$$\sigma = -3.87 + 3.33$$
$$M \pm \sigma = 76.1–84.2 = 66.2\%$$
$$M \pm 2\sigma = 72.3–88.3 = 94.0\%$$

Total 599   538   1137

*From Haas LL: *AJR* 1952; 67:197. Used by permission.
†m = mean value; n = number of individuals; M = modulus.

MEASUREMENT OF NORMAL
CRANIAL GROWTH*

Technique

1. GE 8800 CT scanner with JC software package. Scan time 9.6 seconds.
2. *Position:* Supine with 5° to 10° tilt from the canthomeatal line.

Measurement (Fig 4A–2)
The midventricular slice that shows the most prominent frontal horns was selected for estimation of cranial area.

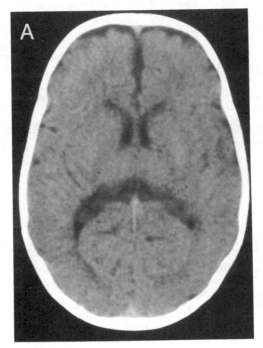

FIG 4A–2,A.
Midventricular slice of head CT scan showing prominent frontal horns of lateral ventricles selected for measurement of cranial area and linear dimensions. (From Hahn FJ, Chu W-K, Cheung JY: *AJR* 1984; 142:1253–1255. Used by permission.)

*Ref: Hahn FJ, et al: *AJR* 1984; 142:1253.

MEASUREMENT OF NORMAL CRANIAL GROWTH

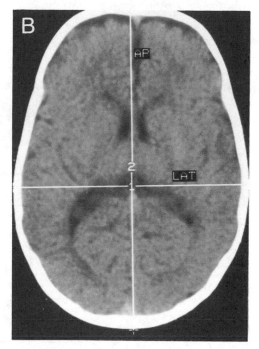

FIG 4A–2,B.
Measurements of maximum anteroposterior *(AP)* and lateral *(LAT)* dimensions of outer margin of cranium. (From Hahn FJ, Chu W-K, Cheung JY: *AJR* 1984; 142:1253–1255. Used by permission.)

Using a built-in cursor, the outer edge of the cranial vault was traced and the enclosed cranial area automatically calibrated by the computer. Maximum anteroposterior *(AP)* dimension and maximum width of the cranium were also measured. The regression formula for cranial area as a function of age for ages less than or equal to 24 months is:

$$\text{Area (cm}^2\text{)} = 75.55 + 26.5 \times \log_n \text{(age in months)}$$

For this equation, r = 0.96.

MEASUREMENT OF NORMAL
CRANIAL GROWTH

The regression formula for ages more than 2 years is:

$$\text{Area (cm}^2) = 140.11 + 21.44 \times \log_n \text{(age in years)}$$

For this equation, $r = 0.86$.

The mean cranial areas and their normal ranges are given in Table 4A–6.

TABLE 4A–6.

Mean Head Areas and Their Normal Ranges
as Measured by CT*

Age	No. of Subjects	Mean Area* in cm² (Range†)
Subject ≤2 years old (months)		
1	17	75.5 (63.0–88.0)
2	6	93.9 (81.4–106.4)
3	4	104.7 (92.2–117.2)
4	6	112.3 (99.8–124.8)
5	8	118.2 (105.7–130.7)
6	6	123.0 (110.5–135.5)
7	3	127.1 (114.6–139.6)
8	7	130.7 (118.2–143.2)
9	7	133.8 (121.3–146.3)
10	1	136.6 (124.1–149.1)
11	3	139.1 (126.6–151.6)
12	9	141.4 (128.9–153.9)
13	1	143.5 (131.0–156.0)
14	1	145.5 (133.0–158.0)
15	1	147.3 (134.8–159.8)
16	3	149.0 (136.5–161.5)
17	3	150.6 (138.1–163.1)
18	3	152.1 (139.6–164.6)
19	1	153.6 (141.1–166.1)
20	1	154.9 (142.4 167.4)
21	2	156.2 (143.7–168.7)
22	1	157.5 (145.0–170.0)
23	2	158.7 (146.2–171.2)
24	14	159.8 (147.3–172.3)

MEASUREMENT OF NORMAL CRANIAL GROWTH

TABLE 4A−6 (cont.).

Age	No. of Subjects	Mean Area* in cm^2 (Range†)
Subjects ≥3 years old (years)		
3	13	163.0 (146.4−179.4)
4	14	169.4 (152.9−185.9)
5	5	174.4 (157.9−190.9)
6	8	178.6 (162.1−195.1)
7	7	182.0 (165.5−198.5)
8	8	185.0 (168.5−201.6)
9	6	187.7 (171.2−204.2)
10	8	190.1 (173.6−206.6)
11	7	192.2 (195.7−208.7)
12	1	194.2 (177.7−210.7)
13	11	196.0 (179.6−212.6)
14	5	197.7 (180.7−213.7)
15	6	199.2 (182.7−215.7)
16	6	200.7 (184.2−217.2)
17	7	202.1 (185.6−218.6)
18	3	204.4 (187.9−220.9)

*Mean area is derived from the regression formula provided in the text.
†Range reflects the 90% of the population closest to the mean.

Source of Material

Data based on CT study of 215 subjects, 125 boys and 90 girls with ages ranging from birth to 18 years.

MEASUREMENT OF CRANIAL CAPACITY
IN CHILDREN*

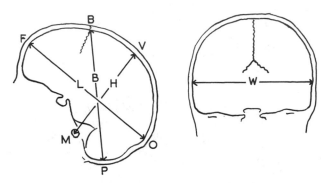

FIG 4A–3.
Dimensions to be measured from the anteroposterior and lateral radiographs. (From Gordon IRS: *Br J Radiol* 1966; 39:377. Used by permission.)

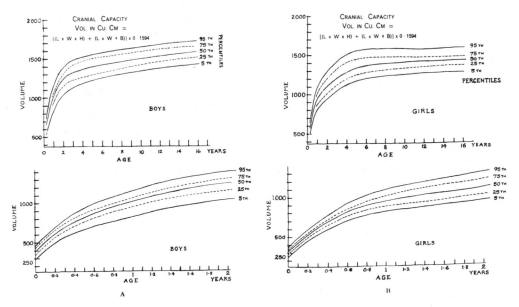

FIG 4A–4.
Percentile curves for cranial capacity (also expressed in cubic centimeters). (From Gordon IRS: *Br J Radiol* 1966; 39:377. Used by permission.)

*Ref: Gordon IRS: *Br J Radiol* 1966; 39:377.

MEASUREMENT OF CRANIAL CAPACITY
IN CHILDREN

Technique
  Central ray: Perpendicular to plane of film directed to midplane of skull.
  Position: Posteroanterior and lateral.
  Target-film distance: 100 cm.

Measurements (Figs 4A–3 and 4A–4)

L = The greatest longitudinal diameter from the frontal pole *(F)* to the occipital pole *(O)*.

B = The vertical height from the bregma *(B)* to the deepest point of the posterior fossa *(P)*.

A = The vertical height from the external auditory meatus *(M)* to the most distant point in the vertex *(V)*.

W = The greatest width from the posteroanterior view.

The cranial volume is calculated by the formula:

$$V = [(L \times W \times B) + (L \times W \times H) \times 0.1594]$$

Source of Material
  Two hundred thirteen children, 104 boys and 109 girls, ranging in age from birth to 15 years.

NORMAL WIDTH OF CRANIAL SUTURES*

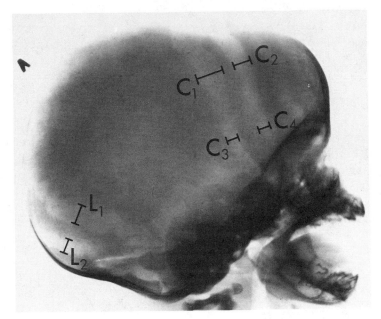

FIG 4A–5.
Sites of measurement indicated on the lateral film of a child with increased intracranial pressure. The projected course of the coronal suture is divided in three approximately equal parts and the lambdoid suture in two. (From Erasmie O, Ringertz H: *Acta Radiol* 1976; 17:565. Used by permission.)

*Ref: Erasmie O, Ringertz H: *Acta Radiol* 1976; 17:565.

NORMAL WIDTH OF CRANIAL SUTURES

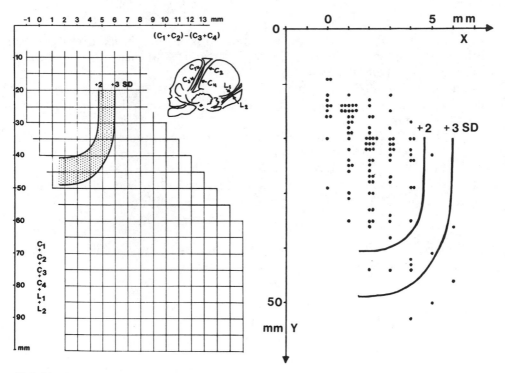

FIG 4A–6.

A, upper normal limits for the measurements of V-shape along horizontal axis and sum of suture width along the vertical axis. The *dotted area* represents values between +2 and +3 SD. **B,** the left upper part of the diagram in A with the distribution of the 107 normal cases. (From Erasmie O, Ringertz H: *Acta Radiol* 1976; 17:565. Used by permission.)

Technique

Central ray: Perpendicular to the plane of the film centered over the midskull.

Position: Lateral.

Target-film distance: 90 cm.

Measurements (Figs 4A–5 and 4A–6)

Both coronal sutures are assessed at levels located at approximately one third (C1 and C2) and two thirds (C3 and C4) of their course between the crown and the skull base. In the same manner, the lambdoid sutures are estimated halfway between the calvarium and the base of the skull (L1 and L2). The sum of these 6 measurements (4) is used as one of the parameters expressing suture width.

NORMAL WIDTH OF CRANIAL SUTURES

When the coronal suture is V-shaped, this feature is expressed as the difference between the sums of the top-near and basal measurements (C1 + C2) − (C3 + C4) and denoted X.

In Figure 4A−6,A the values of Y and X are presented. In Figure 4A−6,B the Y and X values are plotted in a diagram demonstrating the average and the ± 1 SD range.

In normal neonates, between 0 and 45 days of age, the mean and SD of X is 2.1 ± 1.3 mm. The corresponding figures for Y are 23.8 ± 8.3 mm. The application of the charts should be reserved for skulls with a length of the cranium below 149 mm and a height below 110 mm. With marked molding deformity of the vault, the method should be applied with caution.

Source of Material
Data based on a study of 64 girls and 86 boys in the age interval 0 to 60 days after birth. All but 13 were considered mature at delivery.

MEASUREMENT OF THE THICKNESS OF THE SKULL*†

Technique
  Central ray: To a point 1 inch anterior and 1 inch superior to external auditory meatus.
  Position: Lateral.
  Target-film distance: 70 cm (Orley*); 7 feet (Hansman†).

Measurements

Outer table: Average thickness, 1.5 mm.*
Inner table: Average thickness, 0.5 mm.*
Cranial wall: Frontal region, average thickness, 5.0 mm.* Parietal region (measured on anteroposterior skull film) also has an average thickness of 5.0 mm except in the region of parietal thinning.*
Floor of skull: Average thickness, 2.0 to 3.0 mm.*
Occipital (lambda†): See Figures 4A–7 and 4A–8.

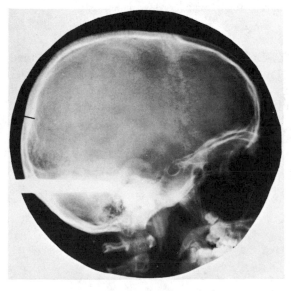

FIG 4A–7.
Straight line at lambda indicates site of measurement of skull thickness. (From Hansman CF: *Radiology* 1966; 86:87. Used by permission.)

*Ref: Orley A: *Neuroradiology*. Springfield, Ill, Charles C Thomas, Publisher, 1949, p 3.
†Ref: Hansman CF: *Radiology* 1966; 86:87.

MEASUREMENT OF THE THICKNESS OF
THE SKULL

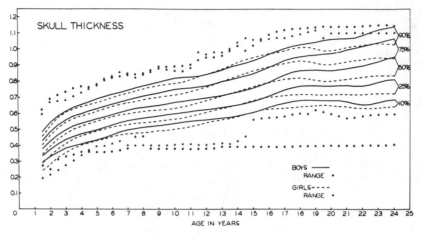

FIG 4A–8.

Percentile standards for measurements of skull thickness for both sexes. The ranges for the two dimensions are indicated. (From Hansman CF: *Radiology* 1966; 86:87. Used by permission.)

Source of Material

These dimensions are from Dr. Orley's extensive experience in skull measurement. No statistics were available.

Hansman used several hundred normal individuals who have been studied by the Child Research Council of the University of Colorado.

LOCALIZATION OF THE PINEAL GLAND:
LATERAL PROJECTION

Vastine-Kinney Method*

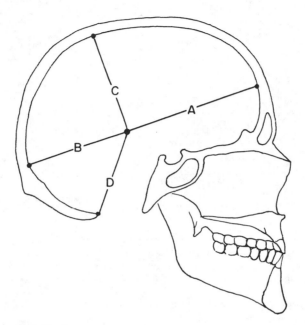

FIG 4A–9.
Vastine-Kinney chart for pineal position measurements.

*Ref: Vastine JH, Kinney KK: AJR 1927; 17:320.

LOCALIZATION OF THE PINEAL GLAND:
LATERAL PROJECTION

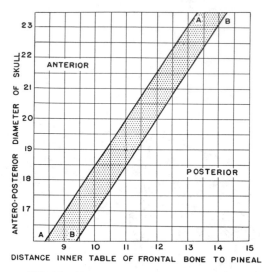

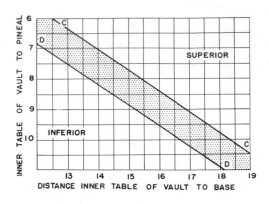

FIG 4A–10.

Dyke modification of Vastine-Kinney chart for pineal position measurements.† **A,** normal anteroposterior variation. The measurement of A is plotted against the sum of A + B. This sum is approximately equal to the greatest anteroposterior diameter of the skull. The pineal glands of normal skulls lie between A-A and B-B. **B,** normal vertical variation. The measurement of C is plotted against the sum of C + D. This sum is approximately equal to the vertical diameter of the skull. The pineal glands of normal skulls lie between C-C and D-D. *Note:* Dyke advocates moving forward 4 mm the normal zone of Vastine and Kinney. (From Dyke CG, *AJR* 1930; 23:598. Used by permission.)

Vastine-Kinney Method

Technique
Central ray: Perpendicular to film centered over midportion of skull.
Position: True lateral.
Target-film distance: Immaterial.

Measurements (Figs 4A–9 and 4A–10)

A = The greatest distance from the pineal body to the inner table of the frontal bone.

B = The greatest distance from the pineal body to the inner table of the occiput.

C = The greatest distance from the pineal body to the inner table of the vault.

D = The greatest distance from the pineal body to the occipital bone in the vertical direction.

†*Ref:* Dyke CG: *AJR* 1930; 23:598.

LOCALIZATION OF THE PINEAL GLAND:
LATERAL PROJECTION

Source of Material

This material is based on the roentgen examination of 200 skull films that were essentially negative for intracranial lesions.

Pawl-Walter Method*

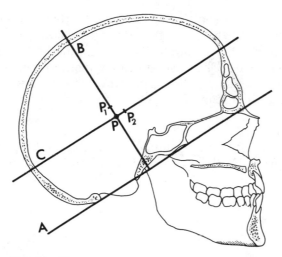

FIG 4A–11.
(Adapted from Pawl RP, Walter AK: *AJR* 1969; 105:287.)

Technique

Central ray: Perpendicular to film centered over midportion of skull.
Position: True lateral.
Target-film distance: Immaterial.

Measurements (Fig 4A–11)

Line *A* is drawn from nasion to lowest point of basiocciput just posterior to the opisthion.

Line *B* is drawn perpendicular to line *A* and passes through the center of the calcified pineal body *(P)*.

Ref: Pawl RP, Walter AK: *AJR* 1969; 105:287.

LOCALIZATION OF THE PINEAL GLAND: LATERAL PROJECTION

Pawl-Walter Method

Point P_1 is one-half the distance from the baseline A to the inner table of the cranial vault.

Line C is drawn through the pineal body (P) perpendicular to line B.

Point P_2 is one-half the distance from the inner table of the frontal bone to the outer table of the occipital bone.

The pineal body (P) should lie 1 cm below point P_1 and 1 cm posterior to point P_2.

The range of normal is 5 mm superior, inferior, anterior, or posterior to this calculated point.

The accuracy in Pawl and Walter's series was 100% in the superoinferior dimension and 98.5% in the anteroposterior dimension.

Note: Pawl and Walter reviewed the various methods for localization of the calcified pineal body. The Vastine-Kinney method has been included because it is familiar to many radiologists. However, the Pawl-Walter method, which does not require use of overlays and tables, has much to recommend it.

Source of Material

One hundred twenty skull examinations at Tripler Army Medical Center.

Note: A calcified pineal may normally be shifted 2 to 3 mm from the midline on a good PA skull. This is considered a normal variation.

MEASUREMENT OF THE BASE OF THE SKULL
FOR BASILAR INVAGINATION

Chamberlain's Line* (Fig 4A–12)

The odontoid process should not project above this (Chamberlain's) line in the normal case (SD ± 3.3 mm).† In any individual case an odontoid process 6.6 mm (2 SD) or more above this line should be considered strongly indicative of basilar impression.

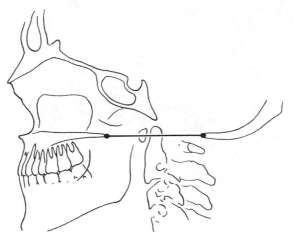

FIG 4A–12.

*Ref: Chamberlain WE: *Yale J Biol Med* 1939; 11:487.
†Ref: Poppel MH, et al: *Radiology* 1953; 61:639.

MEASUREMENT OF THE BASE OF THE SKULL
FOR BASILAR INVAGINATION

McRae's Line*

If the line of the occipital squama is convex upward or if it lies above the line of the foramen magnum (Fig 4A–13), basilar impression is present. In addition, a perpendicular drawn from the apex of the odontoid to the reference line should intersect it in its ventral quarter.

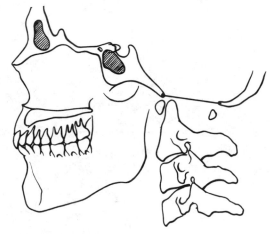

FIG 4A–13.
(From Hinck V, et al: *Radiology* 1961; 76:572. Used by permission.)

*Ref: McRae DL, Barnum AS: *AJR* 1953; 70:23.

MEASUREMENT OF THE BASE OF THE SKULL FOR BASILAR INVAGINATION

Method of Bull*

If angle B in Figure 4A–14 is more than 13°, the position of the odontoid process is abnormal.

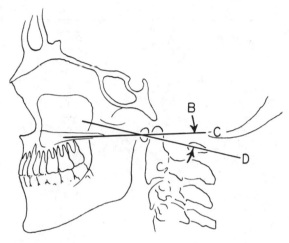

FIG 4A–14.

McGregor's Line† (Fig 4A–15; Tables 4A–7 and 4A–8)

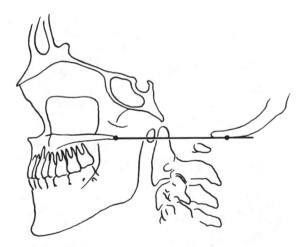

FIG 4A–15.

*Ref: Bull JW, et al: Brain 1955; 78:229.
†Ref: Hinck VC, Hopkins CE: AJR 1960; 84:945.

MEASUREMENT OF THE BASE OF THE SKULL
FOR BASILAR INVAGINATION

TABLE 4A–7.

Children: Both Sexes (mm)*

Age (Yrs)	Mean Base Line	90% Tolerance Range
3	1.94	−0.8 + 4.7
4	2.07	−0.7 + 4.8
5	2.17	−0.6 + 4.9
6	2.24	−0.5 + 5.0
7	2.29	−0.4 + 5.1
8	2.31	−0.4 + 5.1
9	2.30	−0.4 + 5.1
10	2.27	−0.5 + 5.0
11	2.21	−0.5 + 5.0
12	2.13	−0.6 + 4.9
13	2.01	−0.7 + 4.8
14	1.88	−0.9 + 4.6
15	1.71	−1.0 + 4.5
16	1.52	−1.2 + 4.3
17	1.31	−1.4 + 4.1
18	1.07	−1.7 + 3.8

TABLE 4A–8.

Adults (mm)*

	Mean	SD	90% Tolerance Range for Normals
Male subjects	0.33	3.81	−7.4 to + 8.0 mm
Female subjects	3.67	1.69	−2.4 to + 9.7 mm
Male-female average difference	−3.06	. . . .	. . . .

MEASUREMENT OF THE BASE OF THE SKULL FOR BASILAR INVAGINATION

Digastric Line (Fig 4A−16; Tables 4A−9 and 4A−10)

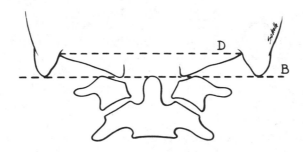

FIG 4A−16.
D = digastric line; B = bimastoid line. (From Hinck VC, Hopkins CE: *AJR* 1960; 84:945. Used by permission.)

TABLE 4A−9.

Adults: Measured on Laminagrams
to Atlanto-occipital Joint (mm)*

	Mean	SD	90% Tolerance Range for Normals
Either sex	11.66	4.04	3.8−19.5 mm

TABLE 4A−10.

Adults: Measured on Laminagrams to Apex
of Dens (mm)*

	Mean	SD	90% Tolerance Range for Normals
Either sex	10.70	5.06	1.0−20.4 mm

Technique
1. McGregor's, McRae's, and Chamberlain's lines:
     Central ray: Perpendicular to lateral skull.
     McGregor's: centered to C2.
     McRae's and Chamberlain's: over midportion of skull.
     Position: McGregor's: true lateral of cervical spine and skull. Patient sitting with head in neutral position.
     McRae's and Chamberlain's: true lateral of skull. Include upper portion of cervical spine.
     Target-film distance: 72 inches for McGregor's measurements.
                                         36 inches for Chamberlain's measurements.

*Ref: Hinck VC, Hopkins CE: AJR 1960; 84:945.

MEASUREMENT OF THE BASE OF THE SKULL
FOR BASILAR INVAGINATION

2. Method of Bull:
    As above, except that the roentgenograms must be made with the patient in the prone position and the chin in neutral position, neither flexed nor extended. Criteria do not apply in the erect position.
3. Digastric line:
    Central ray: To line connecting outer canthus of eye and external auditory meatus.
    Position: Patient supine and skull so positioned that line connecting outer canthus of eye and external auditory meatus is perpendicular to the table top. Anteroposterior tomograms used.
    Target-film distance: 40 inches.

Measurements

Chamberlain's line (Fig 4A–12): Line from the posterior margin of the hard palate to the posterior margin of the foramen magnum.

McRae's line (Fig 4A–13): Foramen magnum line. Line from the anterior margin of the foramen magnum (basion) to the posterior border (opisthion).

Method of Bull (Fig 4A–14):

C = Line drawn along plane of hard palate.
D = Line drawn along plane of atlas.

McGregor's line (Fig 4A–15): Line from the posterosuperior margin of the hard palate to the lowermost point on the midline occipital curve.

Digastric line (Fig 4A–16): Line between the two digastric grooves that lie just medial to the bases of the mastoid processes.

Source of Material

The measurements of the normal position of the odontoid process in relationship to Chamberlain's line were based on a series of roentgenograms of 102 normal skulls (Poppel).

McRae's measurements were based on roentgenograms of 26 skulls.

Bull's measurements were based on roentgenograms of 120 normal skulls.

Hinck's measurements of McGregor's line were based on roentgenograms of 66 normal adult skulls and a series of 258 films taken at yearly intervals on 43 normal children, aged 3 to 18 years.

Hinck's measurements of the digastric line were based on skull laminagrams of 68 normal adults.

Note: Studies by Hinck show that, of the various diagnostic systems to determine basilar invagination, McRae's line and the digastric line appear to be the best. McGregor's line seems to be the best measurement for use on the lateral skull film.

MEASUREMENT OF THE BASE OF THE SKULL
FOR PLATYBASIA

The Basal Angle*

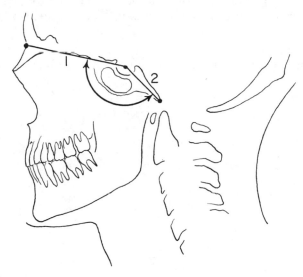

FIG 4A–17.

TABLE 4A–11.

Normal Range of the Basal Angle

Maximum	152°
Minimum	123°
Mean	137°

Technique
  Central ray: Perpendicular to film centered over midportion of skull.
  Position: True lateral. Midline tomogram may be used.
  Target-film distance: Immaterial.

Measurements (Fig 4A–17 and Table 4A–11)

1 = Line drawn from the nasion to the center of the sella turcica.
2 = Line drawn from the center of the sella turcica to the anterior margin
    of the foramen magnum.

Ref: Poppel MH, et al: *Radiology* 1953; 61:639.

MEASUREMENT OF THE BASE OF THE SKULL
FOR PLATYBASIA

The basal angle is not a measurement of degree of impression of the base but is an index of the position of one part of the base relative to another. The base may be impressed with or without disturbance of this relationship.

Source of Material

These measurements were based on roentgen examination in 102 normal cases.

MEASUREMENT OF THE HARD PALATE IN THE NEWBORN*

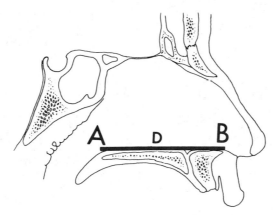

FIG 4A–18.
(Adapted from Austin JHM, et al: *Radiology* 1969; 92:775.)

Technique

Central ray: Perpendicular to plane of film centered over the midportion of the skull.

Position: Lateral.

Target-film distance: 40 inches.

Measurements (Fig 4A–18)

Length of hard palate (*AB*) extends from the anterior maxillary process to posterior termination.

$D = 31$ mm $\pm$ 3 mm.

Note: In a newborn term infant, roentgenographic hard-palate length of 26 mm or less is a sign of mongolism. Hard-palate length of 27 mm or 28 mm is indeterminate, and 29 mm or more is within normal limits.

Source of Material

One hundred eighty-two newborn full-term infants considered to be normal at birth.

Ref: Austin JHM, et al: *Radiology* 1969; 92:775.

MEASUREMENT OF ADENOIDAL SIZE IN CHILDREN*

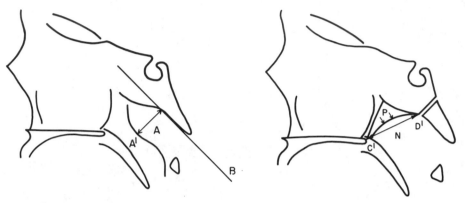

FIG 4A–19.

A, adenoidal measurement. **B,** nasopharyngeal measurement. (From Fujioka M, et al: *AJR* 1979; 133:401. Used by permission.)

Technique

Central ray: Perpendicular to plane of film centered over midskull.

Position: True lateral erect.

Target-film distance: Immaterial.

Measurements (Fig 4A–19)

See Figure 4A–19,A, adenoidal measurement: A represents the distance from A^1, point of maximal convexity, along inferior margin of adenoid shadow to line B, drawn along straight part of anterior margin of the basiocciput. A is measured along a line perpendicular from point A^1 to its intersection with B.

See Figure 4A–19,B, nasopharyngeal measurement: N is the distance between C^1, posterior superior edge of hard palate, and D^1 anteroinferior edge of sphenobasiocccipital synchondrosis. When synchondrosis is not clearly visualized, point D^1 can be determined as 5.6 of the crossing of the posteroinferior margin of the lateral pterygoid plates P and the floor of the bony nasopharynx. The AN ratio is obtained by dividing the measurement for A by the value for N (Table 4A–12).

*Ref: Fujioka M, et al: *AJR* 1979; 133:401.

MEASUREMENT OF ADENOIDAL SIZE IN CHILDREN

TABLE 4A–12.

Adenoidal-Nasopharyngeal Ratios (AN Ratio) in Infants and Children*

Median Ages (yrs, mos)	No. of Children (n = 1,398)	Mean	SD
0, 1.5	33	0.329	0.1154
0, 4.5	51	.457	.1242
0, 9	74	.508	.1087
1, 3	56	.548	.1023
1, 9	45	.538	.0940
2, 6	78	.555	.0991
3, 6	82	.567	.1021
4, 6	85	.588	.1129
5, 6	79	.586	.1046
6, 6	98	.575	.1182
7, 6	85	.555	.1174
8, 6	73	.568	.1108
9, 6	74	.536	.1372
10, 6	79	.511	.1515
11, 6	93	.532	.1401
12, 6	81	.518	.1542
13, 6	84	.458	.1521
14, 6	85	.435	.1436
15, 6	63	.380	.1533

*From Fujioka M, et al: *AJR* 1979; 133:401. Used by permission.

Source of Material

Data taken from 1,398 children, 812 boys and 586 girls. Patients with sinus or lung abnormality were excluded.

NORMAL LATERAL MEASUREMENTS OF THE ADULT NASOPHARYNX*

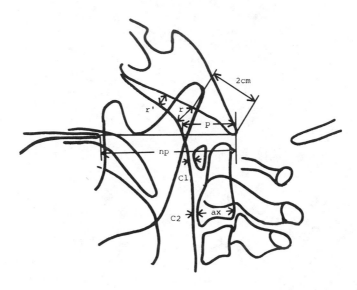

FIG 4A–20.
Measured section of the nasopharynx on the lateral view. r' = middle third roof thickness; r = roof thickness; p = posterior wall thickness; $C1 = c_1$ − postpharyngeal distance; $C2 = c_2$ − postpharyngeal distance; ax = thickness of axis (c_1 vertebral body); np = depth of nasopharynx. (From Okimura T, et al: *Nippon Acta Radiol* 1977; 37:429. Used by permission.)

Technique
    Central ray: To nasopharynx at level of the posterior angle of the mandible.
    Position: True lateral of the nasopharynx.
    Target-film distance: 100 cm.

Measurements (Fig 4A–20; Tables 4A–13 and 4A–14)

Ref: Okimura T, et al: *Nippon Acta Radiol* 1977; 37:429.

NORMAL LATERAL MEASUREMENTS OF THE ADULT NASOPHARYNX

TABLE 4A–13.

Measurement of Thickness of Nasopharyngeal Soft Tissue*

Diameter of the Nasopharynx	Male (Mean ± SD mm)	Female (Mean ± SD mm)
Middle third roof thickness (r′)	5.2 ± 1.6	4.8 ± 1.4
Roof thickness (r)	8.4 ± 2.4	7.0 ± 1.9
Posterior wall thickness (p)	19.2 ± 2.9	17.6 ± 2.9
C1-postpharyngeal space (C1)	4.5 ± 1.7	4.2 ± 1.3
C2-postpharyngeal space (C2)	2.9 ± 0.8	3.1 ± 0.8
Thickness of axis (ax)	19.2 ± 1.6	17.8 ± 1.2
Depth of nasopharynx (np)	50.0 ± 4.8	47.5 ± 3.5

*From Okimura T, et al: *Nippon Acta Radiol* 1977; 37:429. Used by permission.

NORMAL LATERAL MEASUREMENTS OF THE
ADULT NASOPHARYNX*†

TABLE 4A–14.

Comparison of the Thickness of
Nasopharyngeal Tissue Measured by Three
Investigators*†

	Thickness of Pharynx (mm)		
	Khoo	Eller	Okimura
MALE			
r′	8.4 ± 3.6 (7.5)	. . .	5.2 ± 1.6
r	. . .	11.5 ± 4.4	8.4 ± 2.4
p	17.2 ± 2.7 (16.9)	21.0 ± 3.8	19.2 ± 2.9
C1	3.9 ± 1.9 (3.8)	. . .	4.5 ± 1.7
C2	3.1 ± 0.9 (3.1)	. . .	2.9 ± 0.8
FEMALE			
r′	6.7 ± 3.0 (5.8)	. . .	4.8 ± 1.4
r	. . .	8.9 ± 3.6	7.0 ± 1.9
p	16.1 ± 2.3 (15.9)	19.0 ± 3.6	17.6 ± 2.9
C1	3.8 ± 1.6 (3.7)	. . .	4.2 ± 1.3
C2	2.8 ± 0.7 (2.8)	. . .	3.1 ± 0.8

*From Okimura T, et al: *Nippon Acta Radiol* 1977;
37:429. Used by permission.
†Brackets show the mean for adults excluding minors in
Khoo's measurements.

Source of Material

Two hundred one normal Japanese adults (92 males and 109 females)
from age 20 to 70+ years.

*Ref: Khoo FY, et al: *Br J Radiol* 1974; 47:763. Source of material: 640 Chinese patients
(355 males and 285 females) from age 10 to 70+ years.

†Ref: Eller JL, et al: *AJR* 1971; 112:537. Source of material: 300 United States patients with
an equal number of males and females from age 16 to 80 years. (Eller identified the patients as
4% black, 12% Spanish-American, and 84% white.) Eller used a target-film distance of 36
inches.

MEASUREMENT OF NASOPHARYNGEAL SOFT TISSUES FOR THE DIAGNOSIS OF FRACTURES OF THE BASE OF THE SKULL*

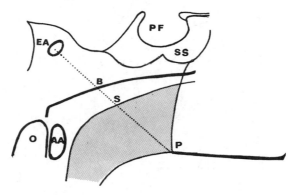

FIG 4A–21.
Measurements of nasopharyngeal soft tissues. (From Andrew WK: *Clin Radiol* 1978; 29:443.

Technique
Central ray: Perpendicular to film centered over midportion of skull.
Position: True lateral, brow up.
Target-film distance: 115 cm.

Measurements (Fig 4A–21)
EA is external auditory meatus, from which a line is drawn to *P,* the posterior end of the hard palate. The distance measured *BS* is from *B,* the skull base to *S,* the anterior margin of the soft tissue. *PF* is the pituitary fossa, *SS* the sphenoid sinus, *O* the odontoid process, and *AA* the anterior arch of the atlas. The shaded area is the posterior nasopharyngeal air space.

The average measurement of *BS* (in millimeters) of adolescents was 10.68, ranging from 5 to 16. The average in adults was 10.03, ranging from 5 to 15. The measurement in patients with fractured bases of the skull was nearly twice normal.

Source of Material
Data are based on a study of 60 normal adults and 20 normal adolescents and compared with 45 patients with fractures.

*Ref: Andrew WK: *Clin Radiol* 1978; 29:443.

NORMAL LATERAL MEASUREMENTS
OF THE SELLA TURCICA

Children*

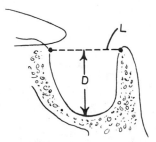

FIG 4A–22.

TABLE 4A–15.

Mean Area of Pituitary Fossa for Given Combinations of Length and Depth (Boys)*

Length in mm	Depth in mm (D)							
	3	4	5	6	7	8	9	10
5	14.5	15.0	13.0	. . .	. . .	. . .	. . .	. . .
6	14.1	18	19.0	. . .	. . .	. . .	. . .	. . .
7	17.8	20.2	25.5	35.7	36	61	. . .	. . .
8	17.2	22.3	30.0	36.8	47.4	55.9	61.0	. . .
9	13.0	27.3	34.2	42.0	51.4	60.2	69.9	. . .
10	. . .	31.7	38.1	46.7	55.8	65.0	74.8	87.5
11	. . .	29.0	41.9	51.7	60.9	69.9	81.9	85.3
12	. . .	45.0	47.0	57.6	64.3	72.9	81.3	92.3
13	. . .	. . .	43.9	55.2	69.7	78.1	87.3	95.0
14	. . .	. . .	61.0	66.8	73.6	81.0	87.6	97.0
15	. . .	. . .	. . .	58.0	71.3	90.6	103.3	97.0
16	. . .	. . .	. . .	. . .	84.0	90.0	96.7	. . .

*Adapted from Silverman F: AJR 1957; 78:451.

*Ref: Silverman F: AJR 1957; 78:451.

NORMAL LATERAL MEASUREMENTS OF THE SELLA TURCICA

TABLE 4A–16.

Mean Area of Pituitary Fossa for Given Combination of Length and Depth (Girls)*

Length in mm	Depth in mm (D)							
	3	4	5	6	7	8	9	10
5	14.4	16.0	22.7	42.0	43.2	39.0	. . .	. . .
6	17.4	22.0	28.2	39.1	41.9	51.1	55.0	. . .
7	19.8	24.7	30.5	40.4	46.8	56.6	81.7	89.0
8	21.0	28.0	35.6	43.1	52.5	61.0	74.8	. . .
9	. . .	32.0	41.0	47.9	55.2	66.7	75.7	84.9
10	. . .	37.5	42.7	55.9	59.1	69.4	80.6	86.2
11	. . .	. . .	49.2	60.3	68.3	78.6	85.7	92.7
12	. . .	. . .	52.0	65.8	73.2	81.4	88.4	96.2
13	. . .	. . .	. . .	65.4	78.6	85.4	93.8	. . .
14	. . .	. . .	. . .	. . .	. . .	. . .	. . .	. . .
15	. . .	. . .	. . .	. . .	. . .	. . .	. . .	. . .
16	. . .	. . .	. . .	. . .	. . .	. . .	. . .	. . .

*Adapted from Silverman F: *AJR* 1957; 78:451.

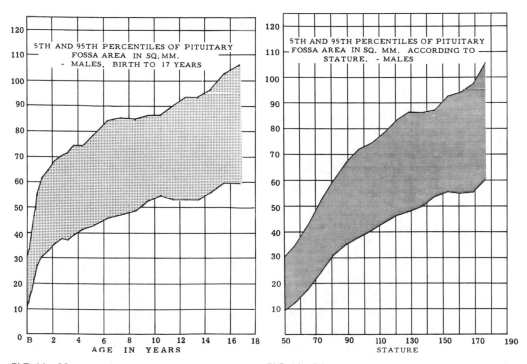

FIG 4A–23.
(From Silverman F: *AJR* 1957; 78:451. Used by permission.)

FIG 4A–24.
(From Silverman F: *AJR* 1957; 78:451. Used by permission.)

NORMAL LATERAL MEASUREMENTS
OF THE SELLA TURCICA*

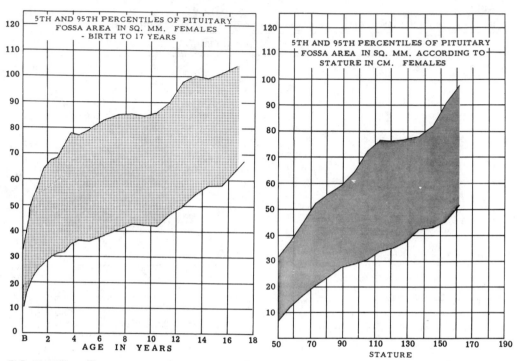

FIG 4A–25.
(From Silverman F: *AJR* 1957; 78:451. Used by permission.)

FIG 4A–26.
(From Silverman F: *AJR* 1957; 78:451. Used by permission.)

Technique
 Central ray: Perpendicular to plane of film centered over midportion of skull.
 Position: Lateral.
 Target-film distance: 5 feet.

Measurements
 The area of the pituitary fossa is measured with a compensating polar planimeter. Conversion to the metric system (square millimeters) is made by multiplying by the factor 6.45. The area is measured by tracing the contour from the tip of the dorsum sellae clockwise to the tuberculum sellae and then following a straight line from the tuberculum sellae back to the point of origin. In cases where the tip of the dorsum sellae could be visualized through the clinoid processes, the line of reference is drawn to the visual boundaries

Ref: Silverman F: *AJR* 1957; 78:451.

NORMAL LATERAL MEASUREMENTS
OF THE SELLA TURCICA*

of the dorsum sellae, disregarding the superimposition of the clinoid processes.

The length (L, Fig 4A−22) is the distance from the dorsum sellae to the tuberculum sellae corresponding to the position of the diaphragmatic sellae. The depth is a perpendicular line dropped to the deepest point (D, Fig 4A−22). In the absence of a compensating polar planimeter, the measurements of the pituitary fossa are obtained as outlined. The tables for boys and girls (Tables 4A−15 and 4A−16) show the mean areas. The mean figure is located on graphs where the area is plotted against age (Figs 4A−23 and 4A−25), or on graphs where the area is plotted against height (Figs 4A−24 and 4A−26). The height of the subject is probably a better standard for evaluation of pituitary fossa area than age. These graphs indicate the position of the pituitary fossa with respect to pituitary fossae from a group of normal children of the same age and the same height. A value for the area obtained from Table 4A−15 or 4A−16 that lies outside the 5th and 95th percentiles would have real significance with respect to indicating a deviation from the normal.

Note: The significance of the small sella turcica is open to question in the light of Di Chiro's work on the small sella turcica. See "Measurement of the Hard Palate in the Newborn" in this chapter.

Source of Material

These data have been based on measurements of the pituitary fossa seen in lateral roentgenograms of the skull on 2,137 films from 168 boys, and on 1,899 films from 152 girls, between the ages of 1 month and 18 years. The children were participants in the longitudinal growth study of the Fels Research Institute.

NORMAL LATERAL MEASUREMENTS
OF THE SELLA TURCICA*

Adults*

Line of Diaphragma Sellae

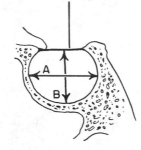

FIG 4A–27.

Technique

Central ray: 2.5 cm in front and 1.9 cm above the external auditory meatus.

Position: True lateral. Essential that sagittal plane of the head be parallel with the film and perpendicular to the central ray.

Target-film distance: 36 inches.

Measurements (Fig 4A–27 and Table 4A–17)

A = Greatest anteroposterior diameter.
B = Greatest depth.

Source of Material

These measurements were based on a study of 500 roentgenograms that had been reported as roentgenologically negative. The dimensions coincide with those obtained by direct measurement of anatomic specimens by Camp.*

TABLE 4A–17.

Normal Range of Measurements

	Max	Min	Av
A (anteroposterior diameter, in mm)	16	5	10.6
B (depth, in mm)	12	4	8.1

*Ref: Camp JD: *Radiology* 1923; 1:65.

NORMAL VOLUME MEASUREMENTS
OF THE SELLA TURCICA

Children*

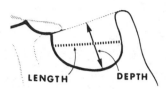

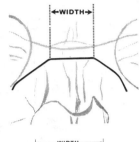

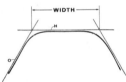

FIG 4A–28.
Diagrams illustrating method for measurement of sellar dimensions. The lowest figure indicates method of width measurement for the "rounded edge" sellar floor. (From Underwood E, et al: *Radiology* 1976; 119:651.)

Technique
Central ray: Perpendicular to plane of film, centered over midportion of the skull.
Positions: Posteroanterior; lateral.
Target-film distance: 60 inches.

Measurements (Fig 4A–28)
The skull films were taken at a 60-inch (152.4 cm) source-to-film distance rather than the usual 34-inch (86.4 cm) to 40-inch (101.6 cm) distance used in clinical radiology. If the sella is about 3 inches (7.6 cm) from the film, a 60-inch source-to-film distance produces magnification of 5.2%. The volume will be magnified 16.6% and correspondingly 31.7% for a 34-inch distance and 26.3% for a 40-inch distance. Therefore, to obtain the "actual" sellar volume (see Tables 4A–18 and 4A–19), measured volumes have been multiplied by the factor 1/1.17 or 0.86. To convert the volumes given in the tables and figures to observed sellar volume on a 34-inch film, multiply the values by the factor 1.32; for a 40-inch source-to-film distance, multiply by 1.26.

Source of Material
Measurements were made on 960 sets of skull films of 427 children aged 6 to 16 years with no known neurologic, endocrine, or skeletal disease.

*Ref: Underwood LE, et al: *Radiology* 1976; 119:651.

NORMAL VOLUME MEASUREMENTS OF THE SELLA TURCICA*

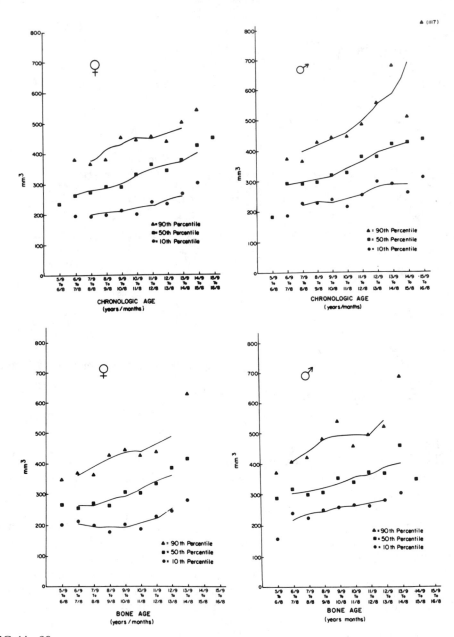

FIG 4A–29.
Volume of sella turcica corrected for magnification for boys and girls by chronologic age and bone age. Lines represent 10th, 50th, and 90th percentiles, calculated by a method of moving averages. (From Chilton LA, et al: *AJR* 1983; 140:797. Used by permission.)

*Ref: Chilton LA, et al: *AJR* 1983; 140:797.

NORMAL VOLUME MEASUREMENTS
OF THE SELLA TURCICA

Children and Adults

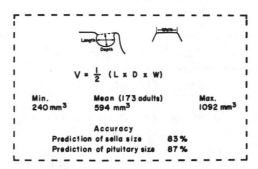

FIG 4A–30.
The volume of the sella turcica. (From Di Chiro
G, Nelsen KB: *AJR* 1962; 87:989. Used by
permission.)

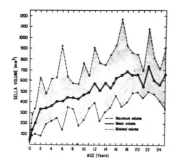

FIG 4A–31.
Sellar volumes of 347 "normal"
controls. (From Fisher RL, Di Chiro G:
AJR 1964; 91:996. Used by
permission.)

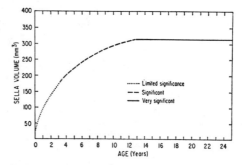

FIG 4A–32.
Minimal expected normal sellar volumes. (From
Fisher RL, Di Chiro G: *AJR* 1964; 91:996. Used
by permission.)

Technique
  Central ray: Posteroanterior: to glabella; lateral: to a point 1 inch ante-
  rior and 1 inch superior to external auditory meatus.
  Positions: Posteroanterior; lateral.
  Target-film distance: 36 inches.

NORMAL VOLUME MEASUREMENTS
OF THE SELLA TURCICA

Measurements (Figs 4A–30, Fig 4A–31, and Fig 4A–32)

Source of Material

These measurements were based on 60 cases* in a series that was later extended to 80 cases.† The sellar volume was calculated from posteroanterior and lateral roentgenograms and was compared with the volume determined by filling the sella turcica with dentist's wax. The method was then tested on 347 "normals."†

Di Chiro has pointed out that the sellar size cannot be reliably estimated from the lateral roentgenogram alone. If the three linear dimensions of the sella are known, it is possible to state pituitary gland size and sellar size so that 90% of the cases will be accurate within approximately 30%. The "best estimate" of pituitary gland volume from pituitary fossa measurements requires the use of regression analysis.‡

*Ref: Di Chiro G, Nelsen KB: *AJR* 1962; 87:989.

†Ref: Fisher RL, Di Chiro G: *AJR* 1964; 91:996.

‡Ref: McLachlan MSF, Williams ED, Fortt RW, et al: *Br J Radiol* 1968; 41:323.

MEASUREMENT OF INTRASELLAR CONTENTS IN NORMAL WOMEN OF CHILDBEARING AGE BY HIGH-RESOLUTION CT*†

Technique

1. GE 8800 CT/T scanner with 1.5-mm thick sections in the coronal plane.
2. Scan localization with lateral scout image. Most patients were scanned in prone position.
3. Bolus injection of 100 ml Reno-M-60 (Squibb) and a continuous drip of Reno-M-DIP during scanning.

Measurement (Tables 4A−18 and 4A−19)

TABLE 4A−18.

The Normal Intrasellar Contents: Childbearing Age Females*

	Mean	SD
Height (mm)	7.1	1.1
Width (mm)	12.8	1.6

*From Swartz JD, et al: *Radiographics* 1983; 3:228. Used by permission.

TABLE 4A−19.

Intrasellar Contents: Statistical Analysis*

Measurement	No.	Mean	SD	Range	Median
Height (mm)	49	7.1	1.1	5.4−9.7	6.9
Width (mm)	38	12.9	1.6	9.5−16.7	13.1
Height × width	38	9.3	0.9	6.3−14.2	8.9

*From Swartz JD, et al: *Radiology* 1983; 147:115. Used by permission.

Height and width measurements were performed with electronic calipers.

The intrasellar contents usually enhanced less than the surrounding cavernous sinus and could be distinguished from it.

Scans were also evaluated for homogeneity of the contents and upward convexity or concavity.

*Ref: Swartz JD, et al: *Radiographics* 1983; 3:228.
†Ref: Swartz JD, et al: *Radiology* 1983; 147:115.

MEASUREMENT OF INTRASELLAR CONTENTS IN NORMAL WOMEN OF CHILDBEARING AGE BY HIGH-RESOLUTION CT

Source of Material

Fifty normal female volunteers were studied who were between the ages of 18 and 35, had normal menstrual periods, and were not currently taking birth control medication. Blood was drawn to measure prolactin and thyroxin levels and thyroid stimulating hormone on all subjects with intrasellar height greater than 7 mm. Four subjects had elevated prolactin and one had hyperthyroidism, but their data were included because all were asymptomatic and none had intrasellar height greater than 7 mm.

THE SELLAR-CRANIAL INDEX*

Technique
Same as used for lateral measurements of the sella turcica.

Measurements

$$\text{Index} = \frac{\text{Greatest anteroposterior diameter of sella}}{\text{Maximum length between inner table of frontal bone and inner table of occipital bone}} \times 100$$

Index in 200 normal subjects: 26% had index of 5, 53% had index of 6, 21% had index of 7.

Source of Material
Two hundred normal subjects.

*Ref: Martinez-Farinas, LO: *Radiology* 1967; 88:264.

MEASUREMENT OF THE OPTIC FORAMINA*

Right   Left

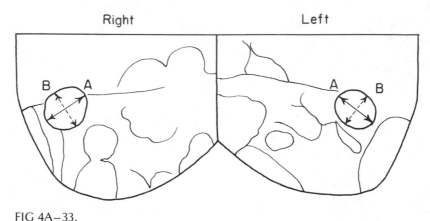

FIG 4A–33.

TABLE 4A–20.

Measurements Corrected for Roentgenographic Distortion*†

	A (in mm)			B (in mm)		
	Max	Min	Av	Max	Min	Av
Right side	5.3	3.5	4.26	5.6	3.0	4.33
Left side	5.6	3.5	4.49	5.5	3.5	4.30

*Data from Goalwin HA: *AJR* 1925; 13:480; and Young BR: *The Skull, Sinuses, Mastoids: A Handbook of Roentgen Diagnosis.* Chicago, Year Book Medical Publishers, 1948.
†Newborn: average maximum diameter is 4 mm. Age 6 months: average maximum diameter is 5 mm. Optic foramina reach adult size at about 5 years.

Technique

Central ray: Perpendicular to film passing through center of orbit being examined. Pfeiffer method†: 37° to sagittal plane and 30° to canthomeatal plane.

Position: Rotate the head 53° from the true frontal position toward the orbit under study, so that the supraorbital ridge and zygomatic arch rest firmly on the plate. Pfeiffer method†: requires V-shaped cassette tunnel to support patient's head.

Target-film distance: Pfeiffer method†: 25 inches. Immaterial for adult measurements.

*Ref: Goalwin HA: *AJR* 1925; 13:480; and Young BR: *The Skull, Sinuses, Mastoids: A Handbook of Roentgen Diagnosis.* Chicago, Year Book Medical Publishers, Inc, 1948.

†Ref: Evans RA, et al: *Radiol Clin North Am* 1963; 1:459. Contains description of Pfeiffer method.

MEASUREMENT OF THE OPTIC FORAMINA

Measurements (Fig 4A–33 and Table 4A–20)

A = Line from the superomesial margin of the canal to the inferolateral
extremity at an angle of 45°.

B = Line from the superolateral edge to the inferomesial border at a right
angle to A.

Source of Material

These measurements were based on a radiographic study of 80 normal
skulls and have been corrected for radiographic distortion.

MEASUREMENT OF THE OPTIC CANALS
IN CHILDREN BY POLYTOMOGRAPHY*

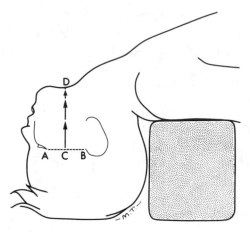

FIG 4A–34.
The position of the head and the landmarks needed for axial tomography of the optic canals. (From Harwood-Nash DC: *Radiol Clin North Am* 1972; 10:83. Used by permission.)

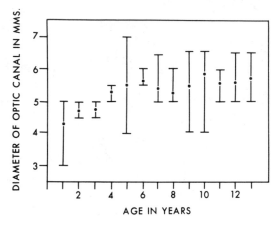

FIG 4A–35.
The age and diameter of normal optic canals (From Harwood-Nash DC: *Radiol Clin North Am* 1972; 10:83. Used by permission.)

Technique

Central ray: Perpendicular: aligned to Point D (Fig 4A–34), marked on the child's neck at the junction of the sagittal plane, and a line extrapolated upward from the midpoint (C) between A-B.

Position: The child is placed in a supine position on a padded box, 6 inches high, with the neck hyperextended over the edge. The vertex

*Ref: Harwood-Nash DC: *Radiol Clin North Am* 1972; 10:83.

MEASUREMENT OF THE OPTIC CANALS
IN CHILDREN BY POLYTOMOGRAPHY

touches the table top. The line *A-B* joins the outer canthus of the eye *(A)* and the upper junction of the ear at the scalp *(B)*. *A-B* is a parallel to the table top. Three exposures are obtained, the middle exposure at the level of *A-B* and the other two 0.5 cm above and below this line respectively. The optimum tomographic level is measured from the vertex on the table top. Six exposures, 1 mm apart, are performed on one film around this optimum level.

Target-film distance: 56 inches (Phillips Polytome).

Measurements (Fig 4A–35)

The true anatomical measurement is used. With the Phillips Polytome the true anatomical measurement is obtained by multiplication of the measurements made on the roentgenogram by a factor of 0.77.

MEASUREMENT OF THE OPTIC CANALS IN
CHILDREN BY POLYTOMOGRAPHY

The diameters, measured to the nearest 0.5 mm at their midpoint, were equal in 41 children, differed by 0.5 mm in 17 children and differed by 1 mm in one child. The average diameter in infants under 1 year of age was 4.5 mm, increasing to 5.5 mm in children of 4 years of age and older. This average size does not increase thereafter.

A difference of diameter of more than 1 mm between one canal and the other is abnormal, as is a diameter of more than 7 mm.

Source of Material

These measurements are based on examination of 59 children of varying ages in whom no pathology of the eyes, optic nerves or intracranial structures was present or suspected.

DEVELOPMENT OF THE PARANASAL SINUSES*

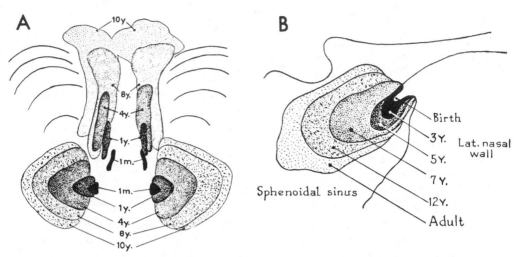

FIG 4A–36.
A, composite drawing showing the changes in size and shape of the maxillary and frontal sinuses in one individual during infancy and childhood (*m* = month; *y* = year). **B,** diagram illustrating the postnatal growth of the sphenoid sinus from birth to maturity. (From Caffey J: *Pediatric X-ray Diagnosis,* ed 8. Chicago, Year Book Medical Publishers, 1956, p 97. Used by permission.)

Frontal and Maxillary Sinuses

Technique
    Central ray: Perpendicular to table top.
    Position: Posteroanterior. Head on 23° board.
    Target-film distance: 28 inches.

Measurements
None

Source of Material
Figure 4A–36 was made from tracings of roentgenograms of 100 children who were examined periodically from birth to maturity.

Sphenoid Sinus

Technique
    Central ray: Perpendicular to table top.
    Position: True lateral.
    Target-film distance: Irrelevant.

*Ref: Caffey J: *Pediatric X-ray Diagnosis,* ed 8. Chicago, Year Book Medical Publishers, Inc, 1956, pp 97–98.

DEVELOPMENT OF THE PARANASAL SINUSES

Measurements
None

Source of Material
Maresh studied the frontal, ethmoid, and maxillary sinuses on routine anteroposterior roentgenograms of 100 children who were being examined from birth to maturity by the Child Research Council.

For studies on the sphenoid sinus, see the work of Schaeffer (*Pa Med J* 1936; 39:395). Schaeffer measured 3,000 sphenoid sinus specimens.

MEASUREMENT OF THE MAXILLARY, FRONTAL, AND SPHENOID SINUSES*

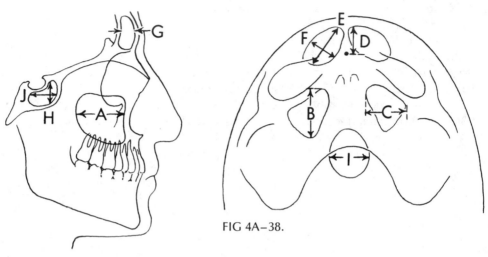

FIG 4A–38.

FIG 4A–37.

TABLE 4A–21.

Maxillary Sinuses (in mm)

Age	A	B	C
Newborn	7.0–8.0	4.0–6.0	3.0–4.0
9 mo	11.0–14.0	5.0–5.0	5.0–5.0
1 yr	14.0–16.0	6.0–6.5	5.0–6.0
2 yr	21.0–22.0	10.0–11.0	8.0–9.0
3 yr	22.0–23.0	11.0–12.0	9.0–10.0
6 yr	27.0–28.0	16.0–17.0	16.0–17.0
10 yr	30.0–31.0	17.5–18.0	19.0–20.0
15 yr	31.0–32.0	18.0–20.0	19.0–20.0
18 yr	31.0–33.0	20.0–21.0	19.0–21.0

*Ref: Schaeffer JP: *Pa Med J* 1936; 39:395.

MEASUREMENT OF THE MAXILLARY, FRONTAL, AND SPHENOID SINUSES

TABLE 4A–22.

Frontal Sinuses (in mm)

Age	D	E	F	G
6–12 mo	2.0	2.0	2.0	3.5
1–2 yr	1.8	5.0	2.5	4.5
3–4 yr	2.5	7.0	4.0	5.5
7–8 yr	9.5	13.0	10.0	8.5
10–11 yr	12.5	16.0	10.0	9.0
13–14 yr	12.0	16.0	9.5	10.0
17–18 yr	15.0	18.0	20.0	16.0
19–20 yr	28.0	26.0	26.0	17.0

TABLE 4A–23.

Sphenoid Sinuses (in mm)

Age	Side	H	I	J
1 yr	R	2.5	2.5	1.5
	L	2.5	2.5	1.5
2 yr	R	4.0	3.5	2.2
	L	4.0	3.5	2.2
5 yr	R	7.0	6.5	4.5
	L	6.5	6.8	4.7
9 yr	R	15.0	12.0	10.0
	L	14.5	11.5	11.0
14 yr	R	14.0	9.0	12.0
	L	15.0	14.0	7.0

Technique

The charted measurements are actual anatomical dimensions.

Measurements (Figs 4A–37 and 4A–38; Tables 4A–21, 4A–22, and 4A–23)

A = Anteroposterior dimension of maxillary sinus.
B = Vertical height of maxillary sinus.
C = Width of maxillary sinus.
D = Distance of cupola of frontal sinus above nasion.
E = Height of frontal sinus.
F = Width of frontal sinus.
G = Length of frontal sinus.

MEASUREMENT OF THE MAXILLARY, FRONTAL, AND SPHENOID SINUSES

H = Height of sphenoid sinus.
I = Width of sphenoid sinus.
J = Length of sphenoid sinus.

Source of Material
These measurements represent actual anatomic measurements based on a study of more than 3,000 specimens.

MEASUREMENT OF PARANASAL SINUS MUCOUS MEMBRANE THICKNESS*

Technique

Central ray: Caldwell: To nasion.

Waters: To anterior nasal spine.

Anteroposterior basal: Perpendicular to base of skull and to midpoint of inferior orbitomeatal line on median plane.

Position: Caldwell projection.

Waters projection.

Anteroposterior basal.

Target-film distance: The measurements given below are anatomic thicknesses. Therefore, if sinus films are taken at a target-film distance of 36 inches, a correction should be made to a 72-inch target-film distance.

Measurements

Frontal sinus: Caldwell projection. 0.06−0.5 mm

Ethmoid sinus: Caldwell projection. 0.08−0.45 mm

Sphenoid sinus: Anteroposterior basal projection. 0.07−0.6 mm

Maxillary sinus: Waters projection. Medial wall, 0.2−1.2 mm. Lateral wall, 0.1−0.5 mm

Average thickness in health varies from 0.6 mm for the medial wall of the maxillary sinus to 0.1 mm for the ethmoid, sphenoid, and frontal sinuses. Thicknesses varying from 2.0 to 6.0 mm are found in pathologic states.

Source of Material

Measurements were made of 3,000 sinus specimens. The measurements given above are anatomic thicknesses.

*Ref: Schaeffer JP: Pa Med J 1936; 39:395.

MEASUREMENT OF INTERORBITAL DISTANCE*

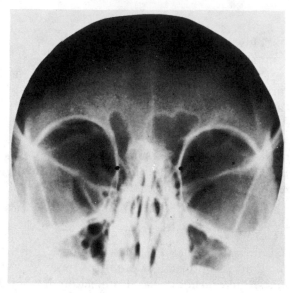

FIG 4A–39.

Black dots indicate the points at which the interorbital distance is measured. (From Hansman CF: *Radiology* 1966; 86:87. Used by permission.)

Technique

Central ray: To anterior nasal spine.

Position: Sinus film, using an angle board with nose and forehead touching the cassette and the tube in a vertical position.

Target-film distance: 28 inches.

*Ref: Hansman CF: *Radiology* 1966; 86:87.

MEASUREMENT OF INTERORBITAL DISTANCE

Measurements (Figs 4A−39 and 4A−40)

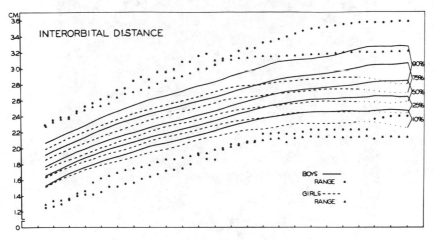

FIG 4A−40.
Percentile standards for measurement of interorbital distance for both sexes. Distance (cm) on the left and percentile scale on the right. (From Hansman CF: *Radiology* 1966; 86:87. Used by permission.)

Source of Material

Hansman used several hundred normal individuals who have been studied by the Child Research Council, University of Colorado.

MEASUREMENT OF THE HEIGHT OF THE ORBIT*

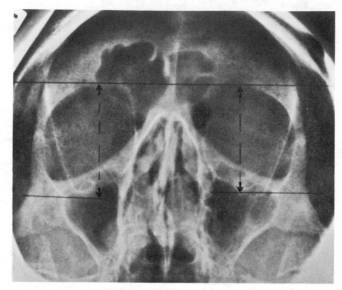

FIG 4A–41.
Method of orbital measurement from plain film. (From Lloyd GAS: *Radiology of the Orbit.* Philadelphia, WB Saunders, 1975, pp 8–11. Used by permission.)

Technique
Central ray: Perpendicular to plane of film centered over the midportion of the skull.
Position: Posteroanterior with the head in nose-chin position.
Target-film distance: Immaterial.

Measurements (Fig 4A–41)
The measurement is taken from the highest point of the orbit to the lowest part of the floor, ignoring the intraorbital margin or supraorbital ridge. A difference of 2 mm in height of the orbits is likely to be of significance in a patient with unilateral exophthalmos. Dysthyroid patients do not show any variation from normal. Over 25% of proved intraorbital space-occupying lesions show a significant increase in vertical diameter of the affected orbit.

Source of Material
Measurements were made on a control series of 200 consecutive nonproptosed patients, 61 patients with unilateral proptosis caused by dysthyroid disease, and 78 patients with proved intraorbital space-occupying lesions of the orbit.

*Ref: Lloyd GAS: *Radiology of the Orbit.* Philadelphia, WB Saunders Co, 1975, pp 8–11.

NORMAL MEASUREMENTS OF THE SUPERIOR ORBITAL FISSURE*

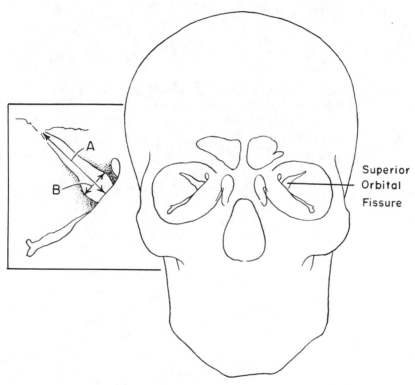

Superior
Orbital
Fissure

FIG 4A–42.

TABLE 4A–24.

Measurements of Anatomic Specimens

A (length)	15 mm (av.)
B (maximal width)	5 mm (av.)

Technique

Central ray: Directed toward external occipital protuberance and angulated 15° toward the feet.

Position: Posteroanterior. Head placed with forehead and nose touching table top.

Target-film distance: 40 inches.

*Ref: Kornblum K, Kennedy GR: *AJR* 1942; 47:845.

NORMAL MEASUREMENTS OF THE SUPERIOR ORBITAL FISSURE

Measurements (Fig 4A–42 and Table 4A–24)

A = Greatest length.
B = Maximum width.

Normal sphenoid fissures showed asymmetric development, compared with the opposite side, in 9% of cases measured.

Source of Material
These measurements were based on a study of 157 anatomic specimens.

MEASUREMENT OF THE INTERNAL AUDITORY CANAL*

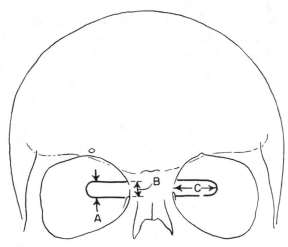

FIG 4A–43.

Technique
   Central ray: To glabella.
   Position: Anteroposterior, with the head placed at such an angle that the shadow of the petrous pyramids is cast through the orbits.
   Target-film distance: 84 inches.

Measurements (Fig 4A–43)

A = Canal diameter = Greatest diameter of canal. Average, 5.2 mm; maximum, 11 mm; minimum, 2.5 mm.
B = Open or medial end of canal. Average width, 6.2 mm.
C = Length of canal from the superior part of the area cribosa to the most mesial point on the concave margin of the posterior wall of the canal. Average, 7.9 mm; maximum, 16 mm; minimum, 3 mm.

From the study of 100 bones, Camp and Cilley* found that in approximately 30% of the bones the right and left canals differed by less than 1 mm in depth and 0.5 mm in diameter.

The thin posterior wall of the internal meatus is usually destroyed to some extent by a tumor mass, which causes dilatation of the porus acusticus with consequent shortening of the canal.

Ref: Camp JD, Cilley EIL: *AJR* 1939; 41:713.

MEASUREMENT OF THE INTERNAL
AUDITORY CANAL

Source of Material

The measurements were based on the examination of 509 individual bones. The bones were normal specimens obtained at necropsy, and in no instance was there evidence of erosion or other abnormality.

MEASUREMENT OF THE FORAMEN MAGNUM
IN CHILDREN AND ADULTS*

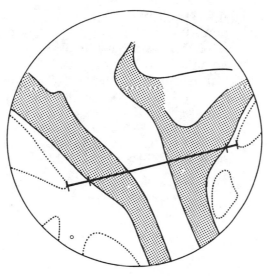

FIG 4A–44.
Landmarks used for measurement of the bony canal and subarachnoidal canal at the level of the foramen magnum. (From Schmeltzer A, et al: *Neuroradiology* 1971; 2:162. Used by permission.)

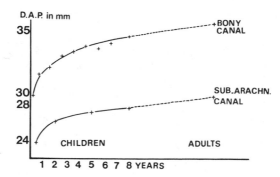

FIG 4A–45.
Normal measurements of the anteroposterior diameter of the bony canal and subarachnoidal canal at the foramen magnum. (From Schmeltzer A, et al: *Neuroradiology* 1971; 2:162. Used by permission.)

Technique
  Central ray: Horizontal: directed at posterior fossa.
  Position: Lateral upright midsagittal pneumotomograms.
  Target-film distance: Immaterial.

Ref: Schmeltzer A, et al: *Neuroradiology* 1971; 2:162.

MEASUREMENT OF THE FORAMEN MAGNUM IN CHILDREN AND ADULTS

Measurements (Figs 4A–44 and 4A–45)

Measurements made on a line drawn between the lower margin of the occipital bone and the basion. The measurements of the width of the subrachnoidal canal were made as indicated in Figure 4–43. Normal measurements given here have been corrected for magnification. The average length of the foramen in adults is 35 mm, and the average length of the subarachnoidal canal is 28 mm. Children reach adult size at 3 to 4 years of age.

Source of Material

Based on measurements obtained on 200 children of all ages and 100 adults.

MEASUREMENT OF FORAMINA
IN THE SKULL BASE*

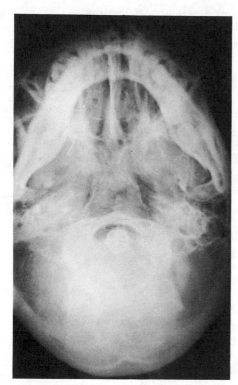

FIG 4A–46.

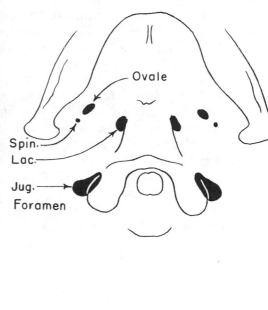

FIG 4A–47.

Technique
Central ray: Perpendicular to inferior orbitomeatal line at angle of mandible.
Position: Basal (anteroposterior).
Target-film distance: 70 cm.

Measurements (Figs 4A–46 and 4A–47)
Foramen spinosum: Contains middle meningeal vessels. Average length of short diameter, 2 mm. Minimum length, 1 mm; maximum length, 3.5 mm. The shape of the canal on radiographic projection is oval. The round artery fills the foramen from side to side in the short diameter. In 97% of the cases the right and left foramen are almost equal in size.

*Ref: Orley A: Neuroradiology. Springfield, Ill, Charles C Thomas, Publisher, 1949, p 45.

MEASUREMENT OF FORAMINA
IN THE SKULL BASE

Foramen ovale: Contains mandibular nerve and accessory meningeal artery. Length, 5 to 11 mm; width, 3–7 mm.

Foramen lacerum (carotid canal): Contains internal carotid artery. Average diameter, 6.4 mm. Minimum diameter, 5.5 mm; maximum diameter, 7.0 mm. Measurements are taken in the lateral portion of the canal corresponding to its narrowest point.

Jugular foramen: Consists of three portions: (1) lateral portion: corresponds to jugular vein. Right side average, 12.9 × 8.6 mm. Left side average, 11.6 × 7.6 mm. Minimum, 6 × 7 mm; maximum, 12 × 16 mm. (2) medial portion: Minimum, 2 × 4 mm; maximum, 3 × 5 mm. (3) intermediate portion: contains 9th, 10th, and 11th cranial nerves. Minimum, 3 × 5 mm; maximum, 4 × 6 mm.

Source of Material
These measurements are from Orley's extensive experience in skull measurement. No statistics were available.

DEVELOPMENT OF THE TEETH* (FIG 4A–48 AND TABLE 4A–25)

TABLE 4A–25.

Approximate Periods of Eruption*

Deciduous Teeth	Eruption Occurs	Shedding Begins
Medial incisors	6–8 mo	7th yr
Lateral incisors	7–12 mo	8th yr
First molars	14–15 mo	10th yr
Canines	18–19 mo	10th yr
Second molars	20–24 mo	11th–12th yr

	Year Eruption Occurs	
Permanent Teeth	Girls	Boys
First molars	6.0	6.5
Medial incisors	6.5	7.0
Lateral incisors	8.0	8.5
First premolars	9.0	10.0
Second premolars	10.0	11.0
Canines	11.0	11.5
Second molars	11.5	12.0
Third molars	17–25	17–25

*From Pendergrass EP, Schaeffer JP, Hodes P: *The Head and Neck in Roentgen Diagnosis.* Springfield, Ill, Charles C Thomas, Publisher, 1956, vol 1, p. 442. Used by permission.

*Ref: Schour I, Poncher H: Publication copyright 1940 and 1945 by Mead Johnson & Company.

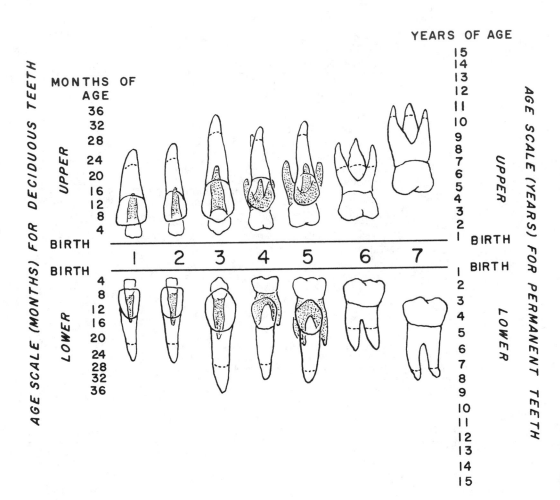

FIG 4A–48.
Schematic representation of the velocity of calcification and eruption of the teeth. The position of the biting edge of the crowns in the age scale indicates the age at which calcification of each tooth begins. Dotted lines on the roots signify the age at which each tooth erupts and its approximate size at that time. The position of the ends of the roots on the age scale measures the age at which calcification of each tooth is completed. The third permanent molar is not shown because of its great normal developmental variation. It usually begins to calcify between ages 7 and 10, erupts between ages 17 and 21, and completes calcification between ages 18 and 25. Deciduous teeth are *shaded;* permanent teeth are *unshaded.* (Adapted from Schour I, Poncher H: Publication copyright 1940 and 1945 by Mead Johnson & Company.)

MEASUREMENTS OF THE AUDITORY OSSICLES AND TYMPANIC CAVITY*

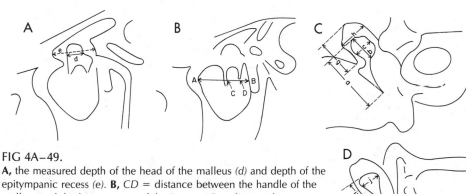

FIG 4A–49.
A, the measured depth of the head of the malleus *(d)* and depth of the epitympanic recess *(e)*. **B,** *CD* = distance between the handle of the malleus and the long process of the incus; *AC* = distance between the anterior wall of the tympanic cavity and the handle of the malleus; and *AB* = depth of the tympanic cavity. **C,** *a* = height of the malleus; *b* = height of the head of the malleus; *c* = width of the head of the malleus; *g* = height of the epitympanic recess; and *h* = width of the epitympanic recess. **D,** *i* = height of the body of the incus; *j* = width of the body of the incus; *k* = height of the tympanic cavity; and *l* = width of the tympanic cavity. (From Lin S-R et al: *Invest Radiol* 1972; 7:539. Used by permission.)

Ref: Lin S-R, et al: *Invest Radiol* 1972; 7:539.

MEASUREMENTS OF THE AUDITORY OSSICLES AND TYMPANIC CAVITY

TABLE 4A–26.

Result of Measurements*†

Measurements		Total Number for Measurements	Maximum (mm)	Minimum (mm)	Mean (mm)	Standard Deviation
Distance between the handle of the malleus and the long process of the incus		100	3.6	2.3	2.9	0.3
Distance between the anterior wall of the tympanic cavity and the handle of the malleus		100	5.9	3.1	4.5	0.5
Size of the head of the malleus	H	92	4.1	2.3	3.2	0.4
	W	92	3.8	2.2	3.1	0.4
	D	77	3.3	2.1	2.8	0.3
Size of the body of the incus	H	87	5.0	3.0	4.1	0.4
	W	87	5.3	3.3	4.3	0.4
Height of the malleus		78	11.6	7.0	9.2	1.0
Size of the epitympanic recess	H	100	11	4.4	8.3	1.2
	W	100	12	5.0	8.0	1.2
	D	70	10	6.0	8.2	0.9
Size of the tympanic cavity	H	100	17	9.6	12.8	1.7
	W	100	10	4.0	7.0	1.2
	D	100	12.5	7.4	10.0	1.2

*From Lin S-R, et al: *Invest Radiol* 1972; 7:539. Used by permission.
†H = height; W = width; D = depth.

Technique

Polytomography with 48° swing.

Central ray: Frontal; directed 1 to 2 cm medial to the lateral canthus; *lateral*; directed toward the root of the tragus.

Position: Frontal; supine with a line that joins the external canthus of the eye and the tragus in perpendicular to the plane of the film; *lateral*; prone with the head rotated so that a line through both external auditory canals lies perpendicular to the film.

Target-film distance: 110 cm with a magnification factor of 1.3.

MEASUREMENTS OF THE AUDITORY OSSICLES AND TYMPANIC CAVITY

Measurements (Fig 4A–49 and Table 4A–26)
Measurements given are not corrected for magnification.

Source of Material
Based on 81 normal examinations of 43 women and 38 men.

Skeletal Maturation

SKELETAL MATURATION: METHOD OF SONTAG, SNELL, AND ANDERSON*

TABLE 4B–1.

List of Centers (Total, 67)

Shoulder	Femur
Coracoid process	Proximal epiphysis
Humerus	Greater trochanter
Proximal medial epiphysis	Distal epiphysis
Proximal lateral epiphysis	Knee
Capitellum	Patella
Medial epicondyle	Tibia
Radius	Proximal epiphysis
Proximal epiphysis	Distal epiphysis
Distal epiphysis	Fibula
Hand	Proximal epiphysis
Capitatum	Distal epiphysis
Hamatum	Foot
Triquetrum	Cuboid
Lunate	First cuneiform
Navicula	Second cuneiform
Greater multangular bone	Third cuneiform
Lesser multangular bone	Navicula
5 distal phalangeal epiphyses	Epiphysis of calcaneus
4 middle phalangeal epiphyses	5 distal phalangeal epiphyses
5 proximal phalangeal epiphyses	4 middle phalangeal epiphyses
5 metacarpal epiphyses	5 proximal phalangeal epiphyses
	5 metatarsal epiphyses

TABLE 4B–2.

Mean Total Number of Centers on the Left Side of Body Ossified at Given Age Levels

	Boys		Girls	
Age (in Mo)	Mean No.	SD	Mean No.	SD
1	4.11	1.41	4.58	1.76
3	6.63	1.86	7.78	2.16
6	9.61	1.95	11.44	2.53
9	11.88	2.66	15.36	4.92
12	13.96	3.96	22.40	6.93
18	19.27	6.61	34.10	8.44
24	29.21	8.10	43.44	6.65
30	37.59	7.40	48.91	6.50
36	43.42	5.34	52.73	5.48
42	47.06	5.26	56.61	3.98
48	51.24	4.59	57.94	3.91
54	53.94	4.35	59.89	3.36
60	56.24	4.07	61.52	2.69

*Ref: Sontag LW, Snell D, Anderson M: *Am J Dis Child* 1939; 58:949.

SKELETAL MATURATION: METHOD OF SONTAG, SNELL, AND ANDERSON

Technique

Roentgenograms are taken of the following areas of the left side of the body: shoulder, elbow, wrist and hand, hip, knee (anteroposterior; lateral after 24 months), ankle and foot (anteroposterior; lateral after 48 months).

Measurements (Tables 4B–1 and 4B–2)

The total number of ossification centers in the left half of the body is counted. A center is counted as soon as it casts a small shadow on the roentgenogram.

Source of Material

These data have been taken from roentgenograms made at regular intervals of all the bones and joints of the left upper and lower extremities of 149 normal children during their first 5 years of life. The children came from the rural and metropolitan area near Yellow Springs, Ohio. There were 75 boys and 74 girls, and they represented a fair economic cross-section. Three black children (1 boy and 2 girls) were included.

150

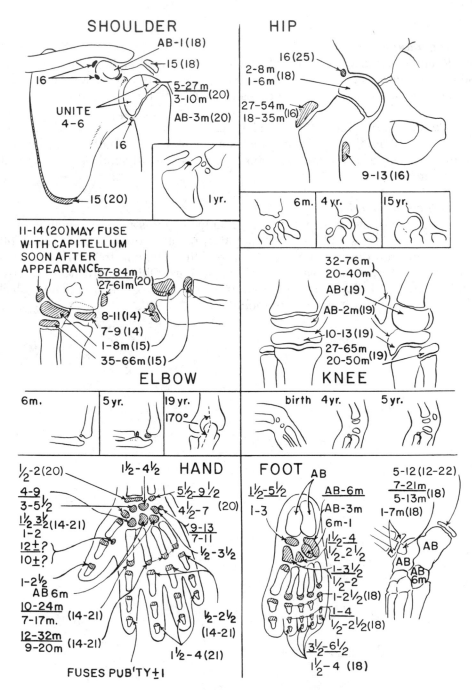

FIG 4B–1.
(From Girdany BR, Golden R: *AJR* 1952; 68:922. Used by permission.)

SKELETAL MATURATION: METHOD
OF GIRDANY AND GOLDEN*

Technique
Conventional technique for each body part.

Measurements
The numbers on Figures 4B–1 and 4B–2 indicate the range from the 10th to the 90th percentile in appearance time of centers of ossification, obtained from the studies on bone growth available in 1950. Statistically significant studies of the time of appearance of ossification centers have been made of relatively few portions of the skeleton after the 6th year of life. Figures followed by m mean months; otherwise all numbers indicate years. Where two sets of numbers are given for one center of ossification, the upper figures refer to males and the lower figures refer to females. A single set of figures applies to both sexes. *AB* indicates that the ossification center is visible at birth. Figures in parentheses give approximate time of fusion.

Source of Material
The figures giving the range of time of appearance of the most important ossification centers have been adapted from multiple sources, including:

Scammon RE, in (Scnaeffer JP (ed): *Morris' Human Anatomy*, ed 11. Philadelphia, Blakiston Co, 1953, p 11.
Vogt EC, Vickers VS: *Radiology* 1938; 31:441.
Milman DH, Bakwin H: *J Pediatr* 1950; 36:617.
Buehl CC, Pyle SI: *J Pediatr* 1942; 21:331.
Ruckensteiner E: *Die normale Entwicklung des Knochensystems im Roentgenbilg.* Leipzig, Georg Thieme, 1931.
Bailey W: AJR 1939; 42:85.

Ref: Girdany BR, Golden R: *AJR* 1952; 68:922.

SKELETAL MATURATION: METHOD
OF GIRDANY AND GOLDEN

VERTEBRA

OSSIFY FROM 3 PRIMARY CENTERS AND 9 SECONDARY CENTERS — ANY OF THESE
SECONDARY CENTERS, EXCEPT FOR ANNULAR EPIPHYSES, MAY FAIL TO FUSE.

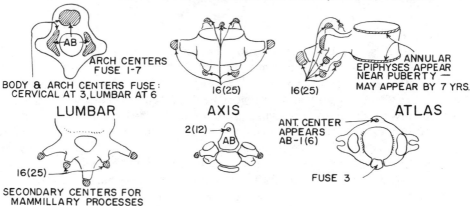

ARCH CENTERS
FUSE 1-7

BODY & ARCH CENTERS FUSE:
CERVICAL AT 3, LUMBAR AT 6

16(25)

16(25)

ANNULAR
EPIPHYSES APPEAR
NEAR PUBERTY —
MAY APPEAR BY 7 YRS.

LUMBAR

AXIS

ATLAS

2(12)

ANT. CENTER
APPEARS
AB-1(6)

FUSE 3

16(25)

SECONDARY CENTERS FOR
MAMMILLARY PROCESSES

SACRUM & COCCYX

LOWER SACRAL BODIES FUSE
AT 18 ⋯ ALL FUSE BY 30

INNOMINATE

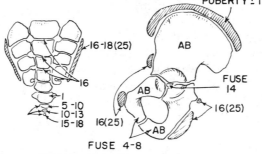

PUBERTY ± 1

16-18(25)

AB

16

FUSE
14

AB

1
5-10
10-13
15-18

16(25)

16(25)

AB

FUSE 4-8

PRIMARY CENTERS AB, SECONDARY
CENTERS APPEAR NEAR PUBERTY,
FUSE 16-30 YRS. — OCCASIONAL CENTERS
AT PUBIC TUBERCLE, ANGLE, & CREST

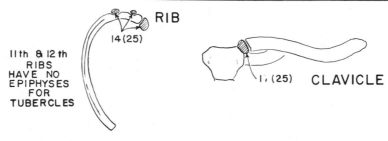

RIB

14(25)

11th & 12th
RIBS
HAVE NO
EPIPHYSES
FOR
TUBERCLES

17(25)   CLAVICLE

FIG 4B-2.
From Girdany BR, Golden R: *AJR* 1952; 68:922. Used by permission.)

SKELETAL MATURATION: METHOD
OF GRAHAM*

FIG 4B–3.
Suggested films for determination of
osseous maturation at various ages. (From
Graham CB: *Radiol Clin North Am* 1972;
10:185. Used by permission.)

Technique

Central ray: Perpendicular to plane of film.
Position: Anteroposterior and lateral.
Target-film distance: Immaterial.

Measurements

The selected examinations that yield the most data at various ages are
shown in Figure 4B–3. The age-at-appearances for selected ossification centers is shown in Table 4B–3. This table is derived from Garn et al.† and modified to be more useful. Important "happenings" at various age levels are bold-
faced. These data are based on a Caucasian population. American black and
Hong Kong Chinese infants are relatively slightly advanced.

Source of Material

Data derived by Garn et al. in the Fels Research Institute Program of Human Development were based on a study of 143 healthy, middle-class Ohio-
born children of Northwestern European ancestry.

*Ref: Graham CB: *Radiol Clin North Am* 1972; 10:185.
†Ref: Garn et al: *Med Radiogr Photogr* 1967; 43:45.

SKELETAL MATURATION: METHOD OF GRAHAM

TABLE 4B–3.

Age-at-Appearance (years, months) Percentiles for Selected Ossification Centers*†

Centers	Boys			Girls		
	5th	50th	95th	5th	50th	95th
Humerus, head	—	0–0	0–4	—	0–0	0–4
Tibia, proximal	—	0–0	0–1	—	0–0	0–0
Coracoid process of scapula	—	0–0	0–4	—	0–0	0–5
Cuboid	—	0–1	0–4	—	0–1	0–2
Capitate	**—**	**0–3**	**0–7**	**—**	**0–2**	**0–7**
Hamate	**0–0**	**0–4**	**0–10**	**—**	**0–2**	**0–7**
Capitellum of humerus	**0–1**	**0–4**	**1–1**	**0–1**	**0–3**	**0–9**
Femur, head	**0–1**	**0–4**	**0–8**	**0–0**	**0–4**	**0–7**
Cuneiform 3	**0–1**	**0–6**	**1–7**	**—**	**0–3**	**1–3**
Humerus, greater tuberosity	**0–3**	**0–10**	**2–4**	**0–2**	**0–6**	**1–2**
Toe phalanx 5M	—	1–0	3–10	—	0–9	2–1
Radius, distal	0–6	1–1	2–4	0–5	0–10	1–8
Toe phalanx 1 D	0–9	1–3	2–1	0–5	0–9	1–8
Toe phalanx 4 M	0–5	1–3	2–11	0–5	0–11	3–0
Finger phalanx 3 P	0–9	1–4	2–2	0–5	0–10	1–7
Toe phalanx 3 M	0–5	1–5	4–3	0–3	1–0	2–6
Finger phalanx 2 P	0–9	1–5	2–2	0–5	0–10	1–8
Finger phalanx 4 P	0–10	1–6	2–5	0–5	0–11	1–8
Finger phalanx 1 D	0–9	1–6	2–8	0–5	1–0	1–9
Toe phalanx 3 P	0–11	1–7	2–6	0–6	1–1	1–11
Metacarpal 2	0–11	1–7	2–10	0–8	1–1	1–8
Toe phalanx 4 P	0–11	1–8	2–8	0–7	1–3	2–1
Toe phalanx 2 P	1–0	1–9	2–8	0–8	1–2	2–1
Metacarpal 3	0–11	1–9	3–0	0–8	1–2	1–11
Finger phalanx 5 P	1–0	1–10	2–10	0–8	1–2	2–1
Finger phalanx 3 M	1–0	2–0	3–4	0–8	1–3	2–4
Metacarpal 4	1–1	2–0	3–7	0–9	1–3	2–2
Toe phalanx 2 M	0–11	2–0	4–1	0–6	1–2	2–3
Finger phalanx 4 M	1–0	2–1	3–3	0–8	1–3	2–5
Metacarpal 5	1–3	2–2	3–10	0–10	1–4	2–4
Cuneiform 1	**0–11**	**2–2**	**3–9**	**0–6**	**1–5**	**2–10**
Metatarsal 1	1–5	2–2	3–1	1–0	1–7	2–3
Finger phalanx 2 M	1–4	2–2	3–4	0–8	1–4	2–6
Toe phalanx 1 P	1–5	2–4	3–4	0–11	1–7	2–6
Finger phalanx 3 D	1–4	2–5	3–9	0–9	1–6	2–8
Triquetrum	0–6	2–5	5–6	0–3	1–8	3–9
Finger phalanx 4 D	1–4	2–5	3–9	0–9	1–6	2–10
Toe phalanx 5 P	1–6	2–5	3–8	1–0	1–9	2–8
Metacarpal 1	1–5	2–7	4–4	0–11	1–7	2–8

*Adapted from Garn et al: *Med Radiogr Photogr* 1967; 43:45.
†P = proximal; M = middle; D = distal.

SKELETAL MATURATION: METHOD OF GRAHAM

TABLE 4B – 3 (cont.).

Centers	Boys			Girls		
	5th	50th	95th	5th	50th	95th
Cuneiform 2	**1 – 2**	**2 – 8**	**4 – 3**	**0 – 10**	**1 – 10**	**3 – 0**
Metatarsal 2	1 – 11	2 – 10	4 – 4	1 – 3	2 – 2	3 – 5
Femur, greater trochanter	1 – 11	3 – 0	4 – 4	1 – 0	1 – 10	3 · 0
Finger phalanx 1 P	1 – 10	3 – 0	4 – 7	0 – 11	1 – 9	2 – 10
Navicular of foot	**1 – 1**	**3 – 0**	**5 – 5**	**0 – 9**	**1 – 11**	**3 – 7**
Finger phalanx 2 D	1 – 10	3 – 2	5 – 0	1 – 1	2 – 6	3 – 3
Finger phalanx 5 D	2 – 1	3 – 3	5 – 0	1 – 0	2 – 0	3 – 5
Finger phalanx 5 M	1 – 11	3 – 5	5 – 10	0 – 11	2 – 0	3 – 6
Fibula, proximal	**1 – 10**	**3 – 6**	**5 – 3**	**1 – 4**	**2 – 7**	**3 – 11**
Metatarsal 3	2 – 4	3 – 6	5 – 0	1 – 5	2 – 6	3 – 8
Toe phalanx 5 D	2 – 4	3 – 11	6 – 4	1 – 2	2 – 4	4 – 1
Patella	**2 – 7**	**4 – 0**	**6 – 0**	**1 – 6**	**2 – 6**	**4 – 0**
Metatarsal 4	2 – 11	4 – 0	5 – 9	1 – 9	2 – 10	4 – 1
Lunate	1 – 6	4 – 1	6 – 9	1 – 1	2 – 7	5 – 8
Toe phalanx 3 D	3 – 0	4 – 4	6 – 2	1 – 4	2 – 9	4 – 1
Metatarsal 5	3 – 1	4 – 4	6 – 4	2 – 1	3 – 3	4 – 11
Toe phalanx 4 D	2 – 11	4 – 5	6 – 5	1 – 4	2 – 7	4 – 1
Toe phalanx 2 D	3 – 3	4 – 8	6 – 9	1 – 6	2 – 11	4 – 6
Radius, head	**3 – 0**	**5 – 3**	**8 – 0**	**2 – 3**	**3 – 10**	**6 – 3**
Navicular of wrist	3 – 7	5 – 8	7 – 10	2 – 4	4 – 1	6 – 0
Greater multangular	3 – 6	5 – 10	9 – 0	1 – 11	4 – 1	6 – 4
Lesser multangular	3 – 1	6 – 3	8 – 6	2 – 5	4 – 2	6 – 0
Medial epicondyle of humerus	**4 – 3**	**6 – 3**	**8 – 5**	**2 – 1**	**3 – 5**	**5 – 1**
Ulna, distal	5 – 3	7 – 1	9 – 1	3 – 3	5 – 4	7 – 8
Calcaneal apophysis	**5 – 2**	**7 – 7**	**9 – 7**	**3 – 6**	**5 – 4**	**7 – 4**
Olecranon of ulna	**7 – 9**	**9 – 8**	**11 – 11**	**5 – 7**	**8 – 0**	**9 – 11**
Lateral epicondyle of humerus	**9 – 3**	**11 – 3**	**13 – 8**	**7 – 2**	**9 – 3**	**11 – 3**
Tibial tubercle	**9 – 11**	**11 – 10**	**13 – 5**	**7 – 11**	**10 – 3**	**11 – 10**
Adductor sesamoid of thumb	11 – 0	12 – 9	14 – 7	8 – 8	10 – 9	12 – 8
Os acetabulum	11 – 11	13 – 6	15 – 4	9 – 7	11 – 6	13 – 5
Acromion	**12 – 2**	**13 – 9**	**15 – 6**	**10 – 4**	**11 – 11**	**13 – 9**
Iliac crest	**12 – 0**	**14 – 0**	**15 – 11**	**10 – 10**	**12 – 9**	**15 – 4**
Coracoid apophysis	**12 – 9**	**14 – 4**	**16 – 4**	**10 – 4**	**12 – 3**	**14 – 4**
Ischial tuberosity	**13 – 7**	**15 – 3**	**17 – 1**	**11 – 9**	**13 – 11**	**16 – 0**

SKELETAL MATURATION: METHOD OF GREULICH-PYLE

MALE

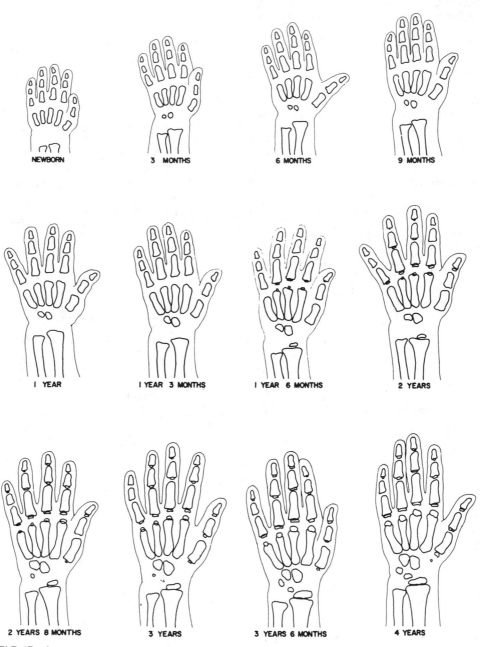

FIG 4B–4.
(Adapted from Greulich WW, Pyle SI: *Radiographic Atlas of Skeletal Development of the Hand and Wrist,* ed 2. Stanford, Calif, Stanford University Press, 1959.)

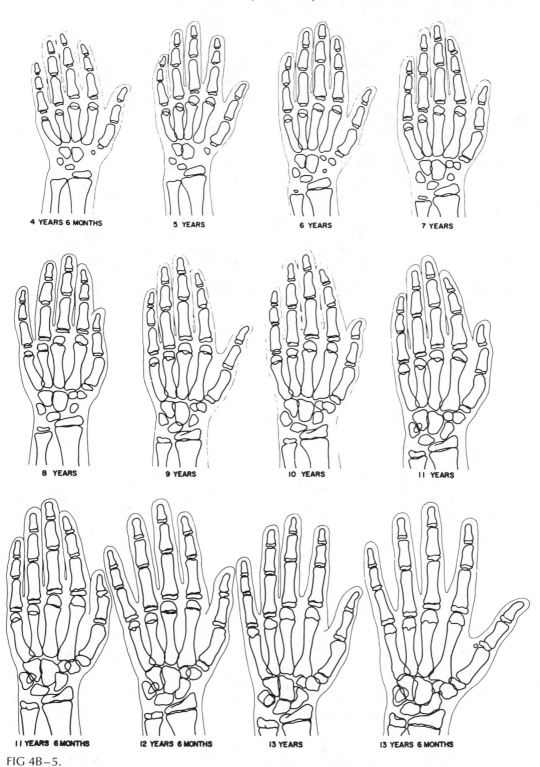

FIG 4B–5.
(Adapted from Greulich WW, Pyle SI: *Radiographic Atlas of Skeletal Development of the Hand and Wrist,* ed 2. Stanford, Calif, Stanford University Press, 1959.)

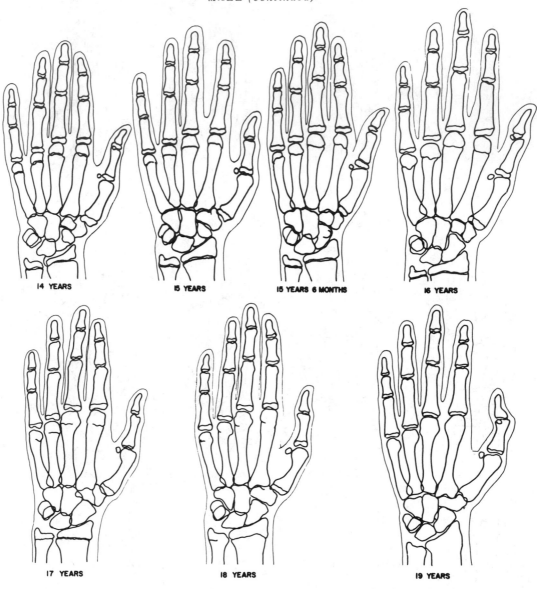

FEMALE

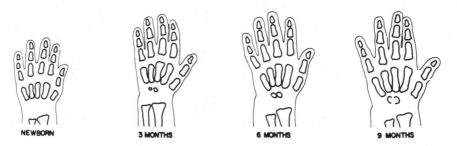

FIG 4B–6.
(Adapted from Greulich WW, Pyle SI: *Radiographic Atlas of Skeletal Development of the Hand and Wrist,* ed 2. Stanford, Calif, Stanford University Press, 1959.)

SKELETAL MATURATION: METHOD OF GREULICH-PYLE

FEMALE

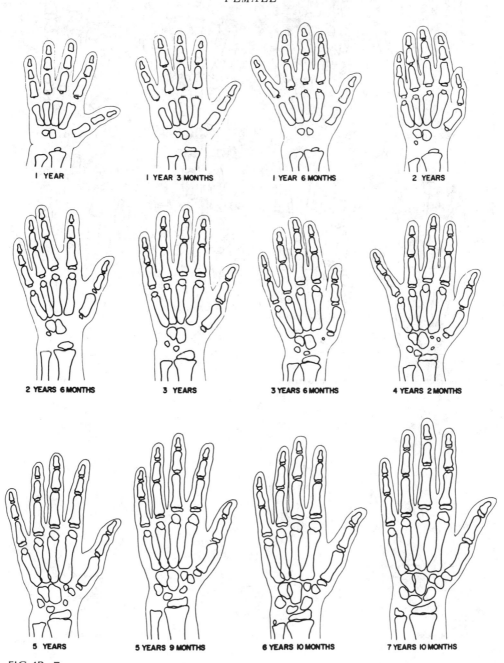

FIG 4B–7.
(Adapted from Greulich WW, Pyle SI: *Radiographic Atlas of Skeletal Development of the Hand and Wrist,* ed 2. Stanford, Calif, Stanford University Press, 1959.)

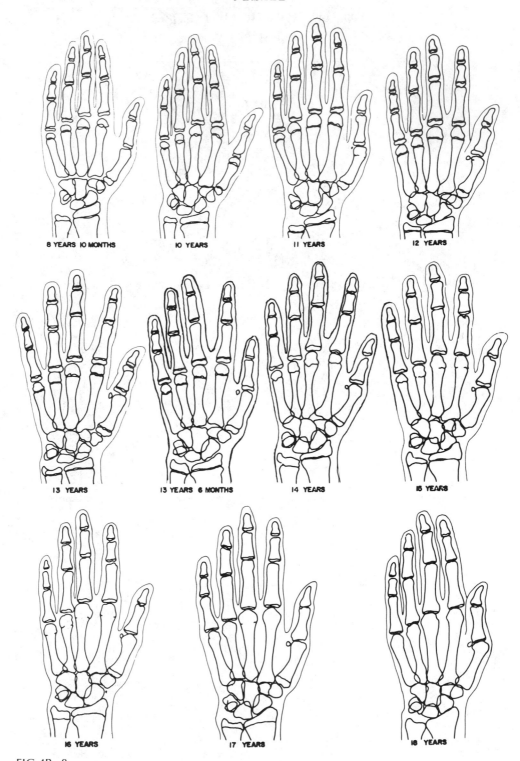

FIG 4B–8.
(Adapted from Greulich WW, Pyle SI: *Radiographic Atlas of Skeletal Development of the Hand and Wrist*, ed 2. Stanford, Calif, Stanford University Press, 1959.)

SKELETAL MATURATION: METHOD OF GREULICH-PYLE

Technique
   Central ray: Perpendicular to plane of film and centered halfway be-
   tween tips of fingers and distal end of radius.
   Position: Posteroanterior.
   Target-film distance. Immaterial.

Measurements (Figs 4B−4 to 4B−8)
The patient's film is compared with the standard of the same sex and
nearest chronologic age. It is next compared with adjacent standards, both
older and younger than the one that is of the next chronologic age. For a more
detailed comparison, select the standard that superficially appears to resem-
ble the patient's film most closely.

Source of Material
Each of the standards was selected from 100 films of children of the same
sex and age. The film chosen was selected as the most representative of the
central tendency of the group. All children were white; all were born in the
United States; almost all were of North European ancestry. The entire group
included 1,000 children.
   Note: Pyle, Waterhouse, and Greulich* published in 1971 a radiographic
reference standard for the assessment of skeletal age from hand-wrist films of
children and youths. The reference standard is based in part on the 1959
Greulich and Pyle Atlas that contains one series of reference films for males
and another series for females. The new reference standard uses a single series of reference films. The osseous features indicating one and the same skeletal maturity level of each hand-wrist bone appear in the male and female at
different chronologic ages. The films in the single film series are calibrated to
show the natural chronologic differences between the appearance of the osseous features in males and females.
   Studies of skeletal age assessments by research workers using left hand-
wrist films and the bone-specific Greulich and Pyle method showed intraob-
server differences ranging from 0.25 to 0.47 years. Observer training improves
reliability of assessments.†

---

*Ref: Pyle SI, Waterhouse AM, Greulich WW: *A Radiographic Standard of Reference for the
Growing Hand and Wrist.* Cleveland, The Press of Case Western Reserve University, 1971.
   †Ref: Roche AF, et al: *AJR* 1970; 108:511; Johnson GF, et al: *AJR* 1973; 118:320.

DETERMINATION OF NEONATAL MATURATION BY TOOTH APPEARANCE ON THE CHEST RADIOGRAPH*

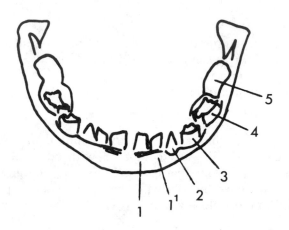

FIG 4B–9.
Tracing of an anteroposterior view of the mandible of a hypothyroid newborn infant. Deciduous teeth are labeled: *1* = central incisors, *1'* = lateral incisor, *2* = lateral incisor (canine), *3* = first molar, *4* = second molar, *5* = follicle of the first permanent molar, the enamel of which is not yet visibly mineralized. (From Kuhns LR, Sherman MP, Poznanski AK: *Radiology* 1972; 102:597. Used by permission.)

Technique
Central ray: Perpendicular to plane of film centered over midchest.
Position: Anteroposterior and lateral.
Target-film distance: Immaterial.

Measurements (Figs 4B–9 and 4B–10)

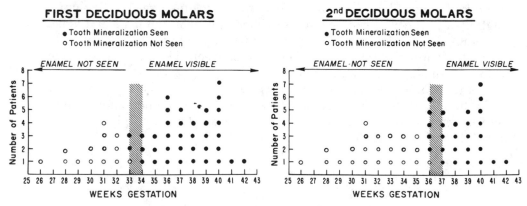

FIG 4B–10.
Summary of first and second deciduous molar mineralization. (From Kuhns LR, Sherman MP, Poznanski AK: *Radiology* 1972; 102:597. Used by permission.)

*Ref: Kuhns LR, Sherman MP, Poznanski AK: *Radiology* 1972; 102:597.

DETERMINATION OF NEONATAL MATURATION BY TOOTH APPEARANCE ON THE CHEST RADIOGRAPH

No second deciduous molar appeared prior to 36 to 37 weeks of gestational age. No first deciduous molar was visibly mineralized before 33 to 34 weeks of gestational age. Tooth age appears to correlate more closely with gestational age than with bone age.

Source of Material

Based on study of 51 white infants of both sexes. All films were taken within 2 days of birth. No difference in tooth development exists between races.

HUMERAL HEAD OSSIFICATION IN THE NEWBORN FOR ASSESSMENT OF GESTATIONAL AGE*

Technique
   Central ray: Perpendicular to plane of film centered over midchest.
   Position: Anteroposterior.
   Target-film distance: Immaterial.

Measurements
The humeral head is almost never present before 38 weeks of gestational age. It is seen in 15% of newborns at 38 to 39 weeks, in 40% of infants at 40 to 41 weeks, and in 82% of newborns at 42 weeks or more gestational age.

Source of Material
Based on a study of 309 newborns of both sexes.

*Ref: Kuhns LR, et al. *Radiology* 1973; 107:145.

OSSIFICATION AND FUSION OF THE STERNUM (Fig 4B−11)*

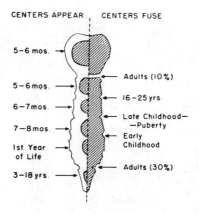

FIG 4B−11.

Ossification and fusion of the sternum. (From Currarino G, Silverman FN: *Radiology* 1958; 70:532. Used by permission.)

*Ref: Currarino G, Silverman FN, *Radiology* 1958; 70:532.

STANDARDS FOR LIMB BONE LENGTH
RATIOS IN CHILDREN*

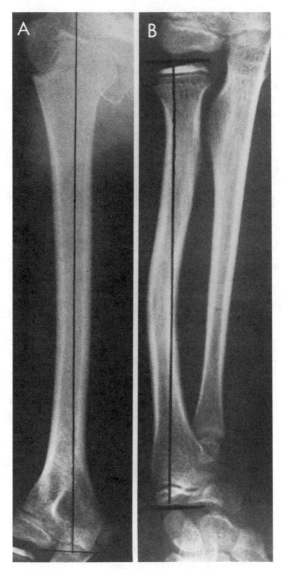

FIG 4B–12.
Guidelines for measuring total bone lengths in humerus **(A)** and radius **(B)**. (From Robinow M, Chumlea WC: *Radiology* 1982; 143:433. Used by permission.)

Ref: Robinow M, Chumlea WC: *Radiology* 1982; 143:433.

STANDARDS FOR LIMB BONE LENGTH
RATIOS IN CHILDREN

Technique
  Central ray: Perpendicular to plane of film centered over midlimb.
  Position: Anteroposterior or posteroanterior.
  Target-film distance: 7½ feet (228.6 cm) to eliminate magnification.

Measurement (Fig 4B–12)
  From age 0–2 months to 12 years, the length was measured parallel to the long axis of the most proximal edge to the most distal edge of the diaphysis. From 10 years through adolescence, length measurements were made from the most proximal edge of the epiphysis at the opposite end. From 10 through 12 years there are, therefore, two sets of measurements.

TABLE 4B–4.

Diaphyseal Bone Length Ratios*

| | | | | | Percentile | | | | |
Bone Ratio	Age (yr)	No.	Mean	SD	5	10	50	90	95
Radius	0.2–0.49	134	0.82	0.04	0.77	0.78	0.82	0.87	0.89
Humerus	0.5–0.99	132	0.79	0.03	0.74	0.75	0.78	0.83	0.85
	1.0–1.49	45	0.77	0.03	0.73	0.74	0.77	0.81	0.82
	1.5–1.99	123	0.76	0.02	0.72	0.73	0.76	0.79	0.80
	2.0–9.99	218	0.75	0.02	0.71	0.72	0.74	0.77	0.78
	10.0–15.0	170	0.75	0.02	0.71	0.72	0.75	0.78	0.78
Tibia	0.2–0.49	133	0.81	0.04	0.75	0.77	0.82	0.86	0.87
Femur	0.5–0.99	132	0.81	0.03	0.76	0.77	0.81	0.84	0.85
	1.0–1.49	45	0.81	0.02	0.78	0.78	0.81	0.83	0.83
	1.5–1.99	124	0.81	0.02	0.78	0.78	0.81	0.84	0.84
	2.0–9.99	218	0.81	0.02	0.78	0.78	0.81	0.84	0.85
	10.0–15.0	170	0.82	0.02	0.78	0.79	0.82	0.85	0.86
Humerus	0.2–0.49	133	0.83	0.05	0.75	0.76	0.83	0.90	0.92
Femur	0.5–0.99	132	0.79	0.03	0.73	0.74	0.79	0.82	0.83
	1.0–1.49	45	0.77	0.02	0.73	0.74	0.77	0.80	0.80
	1.5–1.99	124	0.76	0.02	0.73	0.73	0.76	0.79	0.80
	2.0–9.99	218	0.71	0.03	0.67	0.68	0.71	0.75	0.75
	10.0–15.0	170	0.69	0.02	0.65	0.66	0.69	0.71	0.72
Radius	0.2–0.49	134	0.84	0.05	0.77	0.78	0.83	0.90	0.94
Tibia	0.5–0.99	132	0.77	0.03	0.72	0.73	0.77	0.81	0.82
	1.0–1.49	45	0.74	0.02	0.69	0.70	0.74	0.77	0.78
	1.5–1.99	123	0.71	0.03	0.67	0.68	0.71	0.75	0.76
	2.0–9.99	218	0.65	0.03	0.61	0.62	0.65	0.69	0.70
	10.0–15.0	170	0.63	0.02	0.59	0.60	0.62	0.65	0.66

*From Robinow M, Chumlea WC: *Radiology* 1982; 143:433. Used by permission.

STANDARDS FOR LIMB BONE LENGTH
RATIOS IN CHILDREN

TABLE 4B−5.

Total Bone Length Ratios*

Bone Ratio	Age (yr)	No.	Mean	SD	Percentile				
					5	10	50	90	95
Radius Humerus	10.0−15.0	174	0.75	0.02	0.72	0.72	0.74	0.77	0.78
Tibia Femur	10.0−15.0	174	0.84	0.02	0.80	0.81	0.84	0.87	0.88
Humerus Femur	10.0−15.0	174	0.67	0.02	0.64	0.65	0.67	0.69	0.70
Radius Tibia	10.0−15.0	174	0.59	0.02	0.57	0.57	0.60	0.62	0.62

*From Robinow M, Chumlea WC: *Radiology* 1982; 143:433. Used by permission.

Tables 4B−4 and 4B−5 show the means and standard deviations for each ratio and respective percentiles. These data are useful in evaluating disproportional limb growth in various types of short-limb dwarfing.

Source of Material

Radiographs made at regular intervals from 2 months to 18 years of all children enrolled in the Child Research Council study, Denver, between 1935 and 1967. All children were white. See Tables 4B−4 and 4B−5 for breakdown of numbers and ages.

HAND MEASUREMENTS FOR DETECTION OF GONADAL DYSGENESIS

Metacarpal Sign*

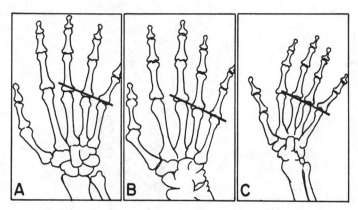

FIG 4B–13.
The metacarpal sign: **A,** negative; **B,** borderline; **C,** positive.

The Carpal Sign†

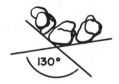

NORMAL **TURNER'S SYNDROME**

FIG 4B–14.
(From Keats TE, Burns TW: *Radiol Clin North Am* 1964; 2:297. Used by permission.)

*Ref: Archibald RM, et al: *J Clin Endocrinol* 1959; 19:1312.
†Ref: Kosowicz J: *J Clin Endocrinol* 1962; 22:949.

HAND MEASUREMENTS FOR DETECTION OF GONADAL DYSGENESIS

Phalangeal Sign*

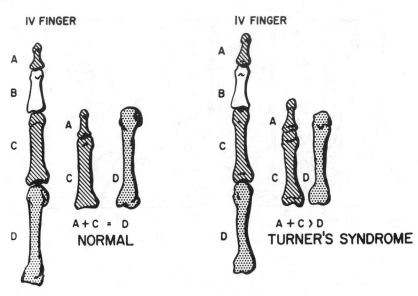

FIG 4B–15.
(From Keats TE, Burns TW: *Radiol Clin North Am* 1964; 2:297. Used by permission.)

Technique
  Central ray: Perpendicular to plane of film centered over palm.
  Projection: Posteroanterior.
  Target-film distance: Immaterial.

Measurements
Metacarpal sign (Fig 4B–13): A line drawn tangentially to the distal end of the heads of the fifth and fourth metacarpals extends distally to the head of the third metacarpal. A positive sign is present when the line passes through the head of the third metacarpal. When the line is tangential to the head of the third metacarpal, the sign is considered borderline. A positive metacarpal sign, while not diagnostic in itself, is an accessory sign of gonadal dysgenesis to be correlated with other radiographic and clinical findings. It has no significance when detectable in more than one generation.

The *carpal sign* (Fig 4B–14): Two tangents are drawn, the first touching the proximal contour of the navicular and lunate bones and the second touching the triangular and lunate bones. In normal subjects, a value of 131.5° is obtained. In patients with gonadal dysgenesis, the carpal angle is 117° or less.

The *phalangeal sign* (Fig 4B–15): Comparison of the length of the fourth metacarpal with the total length of the distal plus proximal phalanges of the

*Ref: Kosowicz J: *AJR* 1965, 93:354.

HAND MEASUREMENTS FOR DETECTION OF GONADAL DYSGENESIS

fourth finger in normal subjects indicates equal dimensions of these bones; the differences do not exceed 2 mm. In some cases of gonadal aplasia, the total height of the distal and proximal phalanges exceeds by 3 mm or more the height of the fourth metacarpal.

Source of Material

The metacarpal sign is based on a study of 2,594 unselected patients. The carpal and phalangeal signs of Kosowicz are based on measurements of 466 normal subjects.

The Spine

MEASUREMENT OF ATLAS-ODONTOID DISTANCE

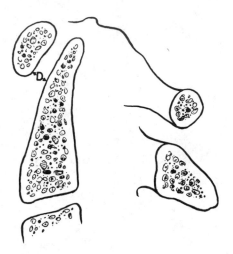

FIG 4C–1.

This measurement is useful in the diagnosis of minimum atlantoaxial subluxation. Normal range:

1. Adult (average normal in mm)*:

    Female: $D_F = 1.238 - (0.0074 \times$ age in years) $\pm$ 0.900 mm.
    Between ages of 20 and 80 years.

    Male: $D_M = 2.052 - (0.0192 \times$ age in years) $\pm$ 1.00 mm.
    Between ages of 30 and 80 years.

2. Children (average normal in mm)†:

    $D = 2.0$; 99% of patients will be between 1 mm and 4 mm. Maximum distance found in a normal patient was 5 mm.

Technique

Central ray: Perpendicular to plane of film centered at level of thyroid cartilage.

Position: Lateral. Patient sitting with head in "neutral" position.

Target-film distance: 72 inches.

Measurements (Fig 4C–1)

Measurement is made between the posteroinferior margin of the anterior arch of the atlas and the anterior surface of the odontoid process.

There is a significant difference between measurements in extension and in neutral position, but there is a negligible difference between flexion and

*Ref: Hinck VC, Hopkins CE: AJR 1960; 84:945.
†Ref: Locke GR, Gardner JI, Van Epps EF: AJR 1966; 97:135.

MEASUREMENT OF ATLAS-ODONTOID DISTANCE*

neutral position.* Ninety-five percent of normal adults will have an atlas-odontoid distance in flexion between 0.3 and 1.8 mm, in neutral position between 0.4 mm and 2.0 mm, and in extension between 0.3 and 2.2 mm.* Neutral position is recommended for children.

Source of Material

Hinck studied 25 adult males (aged 30–80 years) and 25 adult females (aged 20–80 years).

Locke studied 200 children whose ages ranged from 3 to 15 years. Lateral roentgenograms were made in neutral, flexion, and extension positions at target-film distances of 72 inches (patient sitting) and 40 inches (patient supine). Neutral position is recommended because flexion at both 72- and 40-inch distances tends to increase the atlas-odontoid distance, as does extension at a 40-inch distance.

*Ref: Hinck VC, Hopkins CE: AJR 1960; 84:945.

DETECTION OF ANTERIOR
ATLANTO-OCCIPITAL DISLOCATION*

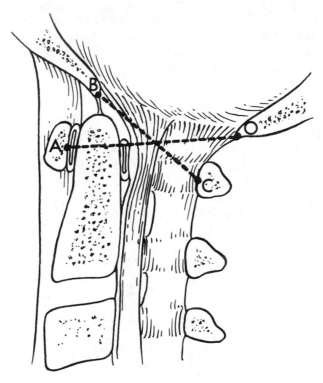

FIG 4C–2.
Normal relationship between the occipital and atlas vertebra. (From Powers B, et al: *Neurosurgery* 1979; 4:12. Used by permission.)

Technique

　　Central ray: Perpendicular to plane of film centered over midcervical spine.
　　Position: True lateral.
　　Target-film distance: Immaterial.

　　Measurement (Fig 4C–2)

B = basion
O = opisthion of the occipital bone
A = anterior arch of the atlas
C = posterior arch of the atlas

*Ref: Powers B, et al: *Neurosurgery* 1979; 4:12.

DETECTION OF ANTERIOR ATLANTO-OCCIPITAL DISLOCATION

The ratio BC/OA is used to determine anterior atlanto-occipital dislocation. BC/OA is equal to or greater than 1 in all cases of atlanto-occipital dislocation. Ratios less than 1 are normal. This relationship is valid only in the absence of associated fractures of the atlas.

Source of Material

Normal criteria were determined from a series of 100 normal adult and 50 pediatric normal cervical spine examinations. Criteria were tested against four cases of dislocation.

DIFFERENTIATION BETWEEN TRUE AND PSEUDOSUBLUXATION OF C2 ON C3 IN CHILDREN: THE POSTERIOR CERVICAL LINE*

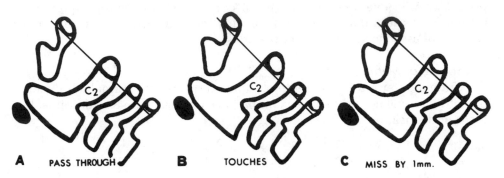

A PASS THROUGH   **B** TOUCHES   **C** MISS BY 1mm.

FIG 4C–3.
Normal positions of the posterior cervical line. (From Swischuk LE: *Radiology* 1977; 122:759. Used by permission.)

Technique
    Central ray: Perpendicular to plane of film centered over cervical spine.
    Position: True lateral.
    Target-film distance: Immaterial.

Measurements (Fig 4C–3)
    The line is drawn through the anterior cortex of the posterior arches of C1, C2, and C3. In the normal situation, or in pseudosubluxation, the line is normal if it: (1) passes through or just behind the anterior cortex of the posterior arch of C2; (2) touches the anterior aspect of the cortex of C2; or (3) comes within 1 mm of the cortex of C2.
    In pathologic dislocation of C2 on C3, the posterior cervical line misses the posterior arch of C2 by 2 mm or more. If the line misses the arch by 1.5 mm, one should be suspicious, but if the distance is 2 mm or more, true dislocation should be assumed unless further tests show that there is no dislocation.

Source of Material
Based on a study of 500 children up to the age of 14 years.

*Ref: Swischuk LE: Radiology 1977; 122:759.

MEASUREMENT OF THE INTERSPINOUS DISTANCE FOR THE DETECTION OF ANTERIOR CERVICAL DISLOCATION IN THE SUPINE FRONTAL PROJECTION*

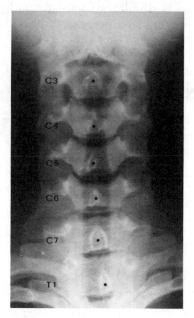

FIG 4C–4.
Measurement of the interspinous distances in a normal supine frontal projection. (From Naidich JB, et al: *Radiology* 1977; 123:113. Used by permission.)

Technique
Central ray: *Perpendicular to plane of film centered over midcervical spine.*
Position: Anteroposterior projection, supine.
Target-film distance: Immaterial.

Measurements (Fig 4C–4)
The interspinous distance (ISD) is measured from the center of the spinous process above to the center of the spinous process below. A widened interspinous distance, which measures more than 1½ times the ISD above and more than 1½ times the ISD below, indicates the presence of an anterior cervical dislocation at the level of the abnormal widening.

Ref: Naidich JB, et al: *Radiology* 1977; 123:113.

MEASUREMENT OF THE INTERSPINOUS DISTANCE FOR THE DETECTION OF ANTERIOR CERVICAL DISLOCATION IN THE SUPINE FRONTAL PROJECTION

This measurement is particularly useful in patients in whom the lower cervical spine cannot be visualized because of obscuration by the shoulders.

Source of Material
Based on a study of 500 patients with normal cervical spines and 14 patients with documented anterior cervical dislocations.

MEASUREMENT OF THE SAGITTAL DIAMETER OF THE CERVICAL SPINAL CANAL IN INFANTS*

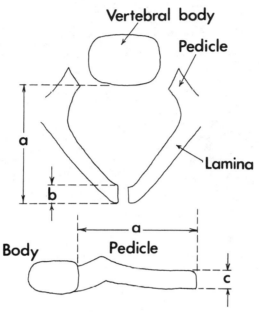

FIG 4C–5.
Cervical spinal canal in infants. a = Distance from posterior border of vertebral body to tip of the spinous process; b = thickness (in dissected specimen) of the spinous process; c = height (on lateral radiograph) of the spinous process. At this age b = c. (Adapted from Naik DR: *Clin Radiol* 1970; 21:323. Used by permission.)

Technique
   Central ray: Projected to the seventh cervical vertebra.
   Position: True lateral.
   Target-film distance: 90 cm.

Measurements (Fig 4C–5 and Table 4C–1)
   The sagittal diameter can be determined by measuring from the posterior border of the vertebral body to the posterior end of the laminae (distance *a*) and subtracting the height (*c*) of the laminae. Sagittal diameter of the spinal canal = *a-c*.

*Ref: Naik DR: *Clin Radiol* 1970; 21:323.

MEASUREMENT OF THE SAGITTAL DIAMETER
OF THE CERVICAL SPINAL CANAL IN INFANTS

TABLE 4C–1.

Sagittal Diameter of Spinal Canal*†

Vertebral Level	Mean Diameter (mm)
C_2	12.5
C_3	11.5
C_4	11.5
C_5	12.2
C_6	12.6
C_7	12.1

*From Naik DR: *Clin Radiol* 1970; 21:323. Used by permission.
†Standard deviation is 0.7 mm.

Source of Material

Twenty-five normal spines in infants under 12 months of age were studied postmortem.

MEASUREMENT OF THE SAGITTAL DIAMETER OF THE CERVICAL SPINAL CANAL IN CHILDREN*

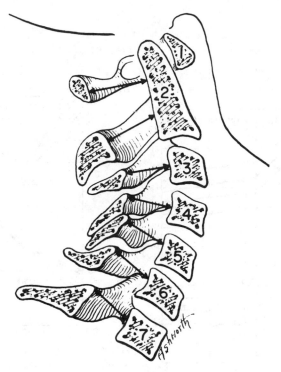

FIG 4C–6.
(From Hinck VC, Hopkins CE, Savara BS: *Radiology* 1962; 79:97. Used by permission.)

Technique
  Central ray: Projected through the fourth cervical vertebra.
  Position: True lateral. Patient seated with the head in neutral position.
  Target-film distance: 5 feet distance from target to midsagittal plane of spine. Distance from midplane to cassette varied up to 2.5 cm.

Measurements (Figs 4C–6 to 4C–8)
  The sagittal diameter was measured from the middle of the posterior surface of the ventral body to the nearest point on the ventral line of the cortex seen at the junction of spinous processes and laminae (*arrows*).
  Gradual widening of the lower cervical canal and even ballooning of the midcanal may be seen in normal children 10 years old or younger and occasionally in persons up to 18 years of age.†

---

  *Ref: Hinck VC, Hopkins CE, Savara BS: *Radiology* 1962; 79:97.
  †Ref: Yousefzadeh DK, et al: *Radiology* 1982; 144:319.

MEASUREMENT OF THE SAGITTAL DIAMETER
OF THE CERVICAL SPINAL CANAL IN CHILDREN

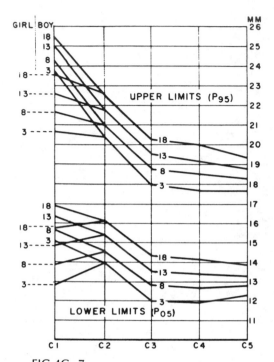

FIG 4C–7.

Ninety percent tolerance limits for sagittal diameters of C1–C5 in boys and girls from 3 to 18 years of age. (From Hinck VC, Hopkins CE, Savara BS: *Radiology* 1962; 79:97. Used by permission.)

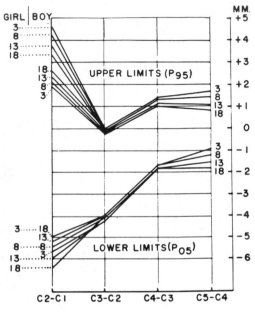

FIG 4C–8.

Ninety percent tolerance limits for sagittal diameter differences between adjacent vertebrae, C1–C5, in boys and girls from 3 to 18 years of age. (From Hinck VC, Hopkins CE, Savara BS: *Radiology* 1962; 79:97. Used by permission.)

Source of Material

Measurements were made on 333 films, using the Bolton-Broadbent cephalometer, on 48 white children aged 3 to 18 years, at annual intervals.

MEASUREMENT OF THE SAGITTAL DIAMETER OF THE CERVICAL SPINAL CANAL IN ADULTS*

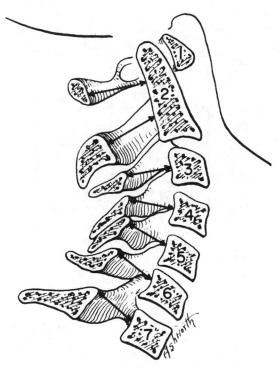

FIG 4C–9.
(From Hinck VC, Hopkins CE, Savara BS: *Radiology* 1962; 79:97. Used by permission.)

Technique

Central ray: Projected through the fourth cervical vertebra.
Position: True lateral. Patient seated with the head in neutral position.
Target-film distance: 73.8 inches. Target–table top distance was 72 inches, and table top to film in Bucky tray was 1.8 inches.

Measurements (Fig 4C–9 and 4C–10)

The sagittal diameter was measured from the middle of the posterior surface of the ventral body to the nearest point on the ventral line of the cortex seen at the junction of spinous processes and laminae *(arrows).*

Ref: Wolf BS, Khilnani M, Malis L: *J Mt Sinai Hosp* 1956; 23:283.

MEASUREMENT OF THE SAGITTAL DIAMETER OF THE CERVICAL SPINAL CANAL IN ADULTS*

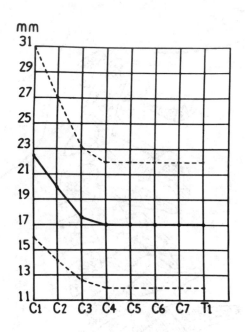

FIG 4C–10.
Curves for average, maximal, and minimal sagittal measurements of cervical spinal canal in adults. Plotted values are uncorrected measurements from lateral neck films taken at 72-inch target–table top distance. True measurements are 1.5 mm less than those shown. (From Wolf BS, Khilnani M, Malis L: *J Mt Sinai Hosp* 1956; 23:283. Used by permission.)

Source of Material

Measurements were made on 200 adults with no known neurological disturbances and showing no obvious bone or joint changes on the films.

*Ref: Wolf BS, Khilnani M, Malis L: *J Mt Sinai Hosp* 1956; 23:283.

CERVICAL SPINAL STENOSIS: DETERMINATION BY VERTEBRAL BODY RATIO METHOD*

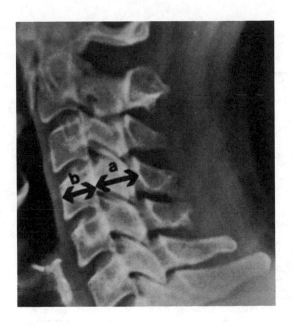

FIG 4C–11.
The sagittal diameter of the spinal canal *(a)* is measured from the posterior surface of the vertebral body to the nearest point of the corresponding spinal laminar line. The sagittal diameter of the vertebral body *(b)* is measured at the midpoint, from the anterior surface to the posterior surface. The spinal canal/ vertebral body ratio is determined with the formula *a/b*. The normal ratio is approximately 1.00. (From Pavlov H, et al: *Radiology* 1987; 164:771–775. Used by permission.)

Technique
   Central ray: Perpendicular to plane of film.
   Position: Lateral.
   Target-film distance: Immaterial.

Measurement (Fig 4C–11)
The ratio values for normal individuals are given in Table 4C–2.

*Ref: Pavlov H, et al: *Radiology* 1987; 164:771–775.

CERVICAL SPINAL STENOSIS: DETERMINATION BY VERTEBRAL BODY RATIO METHOD

TABLE 4C–2.

Cervical Spinal Canal Values*†

Method	Male Controls ($n = 49$)	Female Controls ($n = 25$)
Conventional		
C3	19.24 ± 0.188 (13.7–23.5)‡	17.19 ± 0.151 (13.3–20.0)‡
C4	18.56 ± 0.195 (14.3–23.5)§	16.92 ± 0.134 (13.7–20.4)§
C5	18.71 ± 0.183 (14.7–23.5)¶	17.04 ± 0.138 (14.8–19.6)¶
C6	19.03 ± 0.193 (15.0–23.5)#	17.52 ± 0.144 (15.2–20.1)#
Ratio		
C3	1.008 ± 0.118 (0.69–1.27)**	1.018 ± 0.106 (0.81–1.25)**
C4	0.973 ± 0.110 (0.76–1.19)**	1.011 ± 0.071 (0.85–1.18)**
C5	0.975 ± 0.091 (0.80–1.17)**	1.016 ± 0.057 (0.89–1.15)**
C6	0.978 ± 0.104 (0.80–1.23)**	1.016 ± 0.078 (0.87–1.26)**

*From Pavlov H, et al: *Radiology* 1987; 164:771–775. Used by permission.
†Note.—Values expressed as mean ± standard deviation, with range in parentheses. For conventional method, values represent sagittal spinal canal diameter in millimeters. For ratio method, values represent ratio of sagittal spinal canal diameter to sagittal diameter of corresponding vertebral body.
‡Difference between values for male and female controls, $P = .0001$.
§Difference between values for male and female controls, $P = .0005$.
¶Difference between values for male and female controls, $P = .0002$.
#Difference between values for male and female controls, $P = .001$.
**Difference between value for male and female controls was not significant.

Source of Material

Normal ratios were obtained from radiographs of 49 men and 25 women aged 15 to 38 years.

MEASUREMENT OF THE NORMAL SPINAL
CORD IN CHILDHOOD*

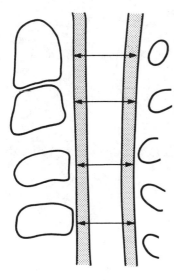

FIG 4C–12.
Measurement of the sagittal width of the subarachnoid space. (From Boltshauser E, Hoare RD: *Neuroradiology* 1976; 10:235. Used by permission.)

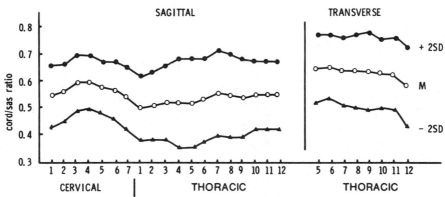

FIG 4C–13.
Mean and two standard deviations of cord subarachnoid space ratio in sagittal and transverse planes. (From Boltshauser E, Hoare RD: *Neuroradiology* 1976; 10:235. Used by permission.)

Technique
Air myelography with tomography.
   Central ray: Perpendicular to plane of film.
   Position: Anteroposterior and lateral.
   Target-film distance: Immaterial.

Ref: Boltshauser E, Hoare RD: *Neuroradiology* 1976; 10:235.

MEASUREMENT OF THE NORMAL SPINAL
CORD IN CHILDHOOD

Measurements (Fig 4C–12)

The spinal cord and subarachnoid space are measured in the sagittal diameter of the midvertebral level, at right angles to the long axis of the cord, and in the transverse diameter at interpedicular level. The cord/subarachnoid space (cord/sas) ratio is calculated.

Normal values are given in Figure 4C–13. The values are independent of sex. These measurements are of use in evaluating cord atrophy.

Source of Material

Based on a study of 110 normal air myelograms in children aged 1 month to 15 years.

MEASUREMENT OF NORMAL SPINAL CORD IN INFANTS AND CHILDREN BY CT METRIZAMIDE MYELOGRAPHY*

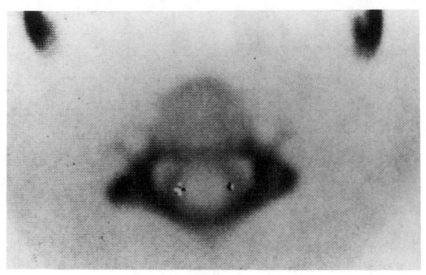

FIG 4C–14.
Diameter of the cervical cord. Transverse diameter, 11.1 mm. (From Resjo IM, et al: *Radiology* 1979; 130:691. Used by permission.)

Technique

1. Technicare Delta 50 scanner with 256 matrix and scan circles of 20 to 40 cm. Thirteen-millimeter slice collimation and table indexing 26 mm.
2. Scan localization with radiopaque ruler and anteroposterior radiograph. Most patients were scanned in the supine position.
3. Two to 16 ml metrizamide (140 to 250 mg iodine/ml). Head flexion and Trendelenburg position for a few minutes improved visualization about the upper cord. For CT without routine myelogram filming, a smaller amount of metrizamide is better.

Measurement (Fig 4C–14 and Table 4C–3)

Sagittal and transverse measurements of cord were performed with electronic calipers.

It is important to use high window width settings and low concentration of metrizamide to obtain the true size of the cord. Low window settings and dense metrizamide underestimate cord size.

*Ref: Resjo IM, et al: *Radiology* 1979; 130:691.

MEASUREMENT OF NORMAL SPINAL CORD IN INFANTS AND CHILDREN BY CT METRIZAMIDE MYELOGRAPHY

TABLE 4C–3.

Range of Cord Measurements by Age Group (Millimeters)*

Age Group	Cervical		Midthoracic		Conus	
	Sagittal Diameter	Transverse Diameter	Sagittal Diameter	Transverse Diameter	Sagittal Diameter	Transverse Diameter
0–3 mo	4.5–5	4.5–7	2.5–5	3–4	4	5
3–18 mo	5–7	7–12	4.5–6	5–7.5	5.5–7	6.5–7
1½–6 yr	7–7.5	10.5–12	5–6.5	6–7	6.5–7	6.5–9
Older than 6 yr	7.5–9	10–14	5–6.5	7–8.5	6.5–9	8–11

*From Resjo IM, et al: *Radiology* 1979; 130:691.

Source of Material

Measurements were taken from normal cords in 25 infants and children and from 4 children with well-localized abnormality at a distance from the normal measurements.

MEASUREMENT OF THE SAGITTAL DIAMETER
OF THE CERVICAL SPINAL CORD IN ADULTS*

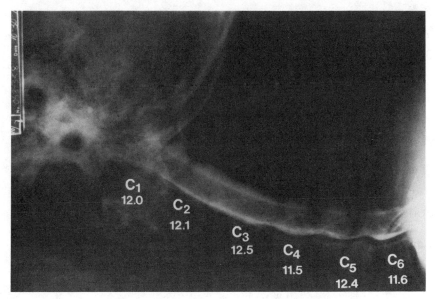

FIG 4C–15.
Myelogram indicating cord atrophy, especially at C4. (From Devkota J, et al: *South Med J* 1982; 75:1363. Used by permission.)

Technique
Metrizamide myelography:
   Central ray: Centered to midcervical spine.
   Position: Prone: cross table lateral.
   Target-film distance: 40 inches.

Measurements (Fig 4C–15 and Table 4C–4)
Measurment of the anteroposterior diameters of the cervical cord were made at the middle of the posterior aspect of each vertebral body.

Ref: Devkota J, et al: *South Med J* 1982; 75:1363.

MEASUREMENT OF THE SAGITTAL DIAMETER
OF THE CERVICAL SPINAL CORD IN ADULTS

TABLE 4C—4.

Anteroposterior Diameter of Normal Cervical Spinal Cord

	Mean (2:1 Magnification)	Variance	Corrected (1.1:1 Magnification)	Variance	No. Patients
C1	15.94 mm	1.94	8.767 mm	.587	100
C2	15.72 mm	2.21	8.646 mm	.669	100
C3	15.07 mm	2.48	8.288 mm	.750	100
C4	14.54 mm	3.90	7.997 mm	1.180	100
C5	14.33 mm	2.94	7.881 mm	.889	55
C6	14.02 mm	2.13	7.711 mm	.774	55

Source of Material

Measurements based on 100 selected cervical myelograms of patients without long-tract signs.

MEASUREMENT OF THE WIDTH OF THE CERVICAL SPINAL CORD IN ADULTS*

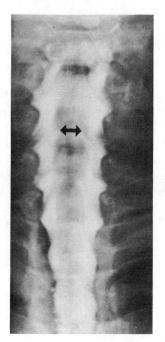

FIG 4C–16.
Normal cervical myelogram demonstrating method of measurement. (From Porter EC: *AJR* 1956; 76:270. Used by permission.)

Technique
Central ray: Centered over midportion of the cervical spine.
Position: Posteroanterior.
Target-film distance: Measurements from spot films were made at fluoroscopy, and the anode-to-spine and the spine-to-film distance varied to some extent. The average target-film distance was 33 inches.

Measurements (Fig 4C–16)
Measurements were made at the level of the fourth and sixth cervical vertebrae when possible. The distance between the "inner" shadow of the true cord was measured rather than the entire central shadow, which includes the nerve roots. Average width = 1.4 cm; minimum width = 1.0 cm; maximum width = 1.7 cm.

Source of Material
The measurements were based on cervical myelograms of 63 patients who showed either ruptured intervertebral discs or no pathology at operation.

*Ref: Porter EC: *AJR* 1956; 76:270.

MEASUREMENT OF NORMAL THORACIC SPINAL CORD AND SUBARACHNOID SPACE IN ADULTS BY CT METRIZAMIDE MYELOGRAPHY*

Technique

1. GE 8000 CT/T scanner. Slice thickness not stated.
2. Scan localization with scout view film. Supine or prone position for scanning.
3. Unstated volume of metrizamide (170 to 300 mg iodine/ml). Time delay between injection and scanning not critical as long as it does not exceed 6 hours. Trendelenburg position at some time before scanning to opacify the thoracic region.

Measurements (Figs 4C−17 and 4C−18; Table 4C−5)

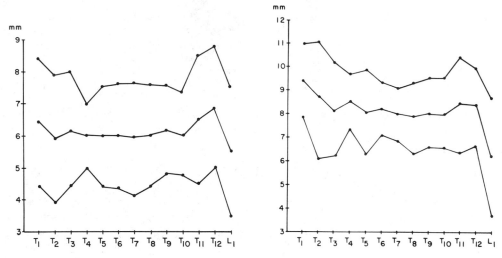

FIG 4C−17.
CT sagittal *(left)* and coronal *(right)* diameters of normal thoracic spinal cord in vivo (*n* = 28). *Center line* = plot of mean values at each level; *upper line* = mean = 2 SD; *lower line* = mean − 2 SD. (From Gellad F, et al: *AJNR* 1983; 4:614. Used by permission.)

Ref: Gellad F, et al: *AJNR* 1983; 4:614.

MEASUREMENT OF NORMAL THORACIC SPINAL CORD AND SUBARACHNOID SPACE IN ADULTS BY CT METRIZAMIDE MYELOGRAPHY

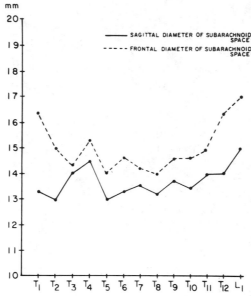

FIG 4C–18.

Mean CT sagittal and frontal diameters of normal subarachnoid space in vivo (*n* = 28). (From Gellad F, et al: *AJNR* 1983; 4:614. Used by permission.)

TABLE 4C–5.

CT Diameters (Mean ± 2SD) of Normal Thoracic Cord and Subarachnoid Space In Vivo (*n* = 28)*

	Thoracic Cord		Subarachnoid Space	
	Sagittal Diameter	Frontal Diameter	Sagittal	Frontal
T_1	6.4±2	9.4±1.6	13.3±2.5	16.4±1.8
T_2	5.9±2	8.7±2.5	13.0±2.4	14.9±2.5
T_3	6.2±1.8	8.2±2	14.0±2.8	14.1±2.4
T_4	6.0±1	8.5±1.2	14.5±2.2	15.7±2.5
T_5	6.0±1.6	8.1±1.8	13.0±3.4	13.9±2.8
T_6	6.0±1.7	8.2±1.1	13.3±3.2	14.6±2.2
T_7	5.9±1.8	8.0±1.2	13.5±3.0	14.2±3.3
T_8	6.0±1.6	7.8±1.5	13.2±2.6	13.9±2.7
T_9	6.2±1.4	8.0±1.5	13.7±2.8	14.5±2.6
T_{10}	6.0±1.3	8.0±1.5	13.4±2.8	14.4±2.8
T_{11}	6.5±2	8.4±2	14.0±3.4	14.9±3.1
T_{12}	6.8±1.8	8.3±1.7	14.0±3.5	16.3±3.4
L_1	5.5±2	6.2±2.5	15.0±3.6	17.0±3.2

*From Gellad F. et al: *Am J Neuroradiol* 1983; 4:614. Used by permission.

MEASUREMENT OF NORMAL THORACIC SPINAL CORD AND SUBARACHNOID SPACE IN ADULTS BY CT METRIZAMIDE MYELOGRAPHY

Sagittal and transverse measurements of cord and subarachnoid space with electronic calipers.

Window width of 1,000 HU and window level set so that densities of cord and metrizamide lie within the gray-scale range of the viewer.

Source of Material

Measurements were taken from 28 patients with symptoms related to the cervical or lumbar spine. The mean dimensions correlate well with postmortem measurements obtained from 10 patients dying from illnesses other than spinal disease.

MEASUREMENT OF NORMAL CERVICAL SPINAL CORD IN ADULTS BY CT METRIZAMIDE MYELOGRAPHY*

Technique

1. Technicare Delta 50 F. S. with 13-mm slice collimation and the gantry angulation perpendicular to the longitudinal axis of the spinal column.
2. Localization with radiopaque catheters and AP radiograph made before scanning. Patients scanned in supine position.
3. Nineteen millimeters of metrizamide (170 mg iodine/ml) in the lumbar subarachnoid space. After completion of the myelogram, the patient is placed in lateral decubitus position for 1 hour to mix the cervical region.

Measurement (Table 4C–6 and Fig 4C–19)

TABLE 4C–6.

Normal Mean Frontal and Sagittal Diameter
(± 2 SD) of Cervical Cord*

	Frontal Diameter (mm)	Sagittal Diameter (mm)
C_1	10.4 ± 1.7	7.2 ± 1.6
C_2	10.9 ± 2.2	6.5 ± 2.0
C_3	11.3 ± 2.0	6.2 ± 2.2
C_4	11.7 ± 1.9	6.0 ± 1.5
C_5	11.8 ± 2.7	6.2 ± 2.3
C_6	10.5 ± 2.3	6.4 ± 2.7
C_7	9.3 ± 2.5	6.8 ± 2.5

*From Thijssen HOM, et al: *Neuroradiology* 1979; 18:57. Used by permission.

*Ref: Thijssen HOM, et al: *Neuroradiology* 1979; 18:57.

MEASUREMENT OF NORMAL CERVICAL SPINAL CORD IN ADULTS BY CT METRIZAMIDE MYELOGRAPHY

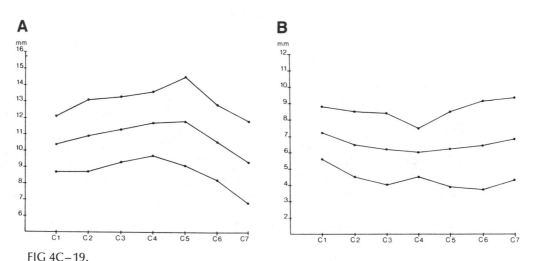

FIG 4C–19.
A, Normal frontal diameter of cervical cord. Mean value ± 2 SD; $n = 20$. **B,** normal sagittal diameter of cervical cord. Mean value ± 2 SD; $n = 20$. (From Thijssen HOM, et al: *Neuroradiology* 1979; 18:57. Used by permission.)

Transverse and sagittal diameters are measured with electronic calipers. Window level of 200 HU and window widths of 400 to 600 HU.

Source of Material
Measurements were taken on 20 patients undergoing lumbar myelography because of suspected herniated disc. There was no clinical suspicion of cervical pathology.

MEASUREMENT OF THE SAGITTAL DIAMETER OF THE THORACIC SPINAL CORD IN ADULTS*

Technique
Pantopaque myelography:
  Central ray: Lateral thoracic myelogram.
  Position: Cross table lateral.
  Target-film distance: Variable with myelogram.

Measurements
Diameters given at vertebral body level (Table 4C–7).

TABLE 4C–7.
Anteroposterior Diameters of Normal Thoracic Spinal Cord

Vertebral Levels	Minimum (mm)	Average (mm)	Maximum (mm)
D3		6.0	
D4	5.6	6.2	7.3
D5	3.7	6.1	7.2
D6	3.7	6.1	7.8
D7	5.3	6.3	7.9
D8	3.4	6.3	7.8
D9	3.7	6.2	8.0
D10	6.0	6.5	7.0
D11	4.5	6.9	10.5
D12	3.8	7.4	9.3

Source of Material
Measured on all myelograms for disc pathology from 1953 to 1965 at Neuroligische Klinik, Prague.

*Ref: Jirout J: Fortschr Geb Roentgenstr 1966; 104:89.

MEASUREMENT OF THORACIC SPINE LENGTH ON CHEST FILMS OF NEWBORN INFANTS*

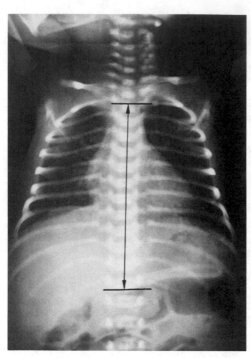

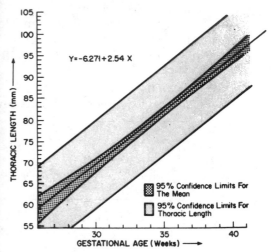

FIG 4C–21.
Plot of linear regression model of spine length and gestational age. (From Kuhns LR, Holt JF: *Radiology* 1975; 116:395. Used by permission.)

FIG 4C–20.
Measurement of thoracic spine length. (From Kuhns LR, Holt JF: *Radiology* 1975; 116:395.

Technique
Central ray: Perpendicular to plane of film centered over midchest.
Position: Anteroposterior, supine.
Target-film distance: 40 inches (102 cm).

Measurements (Fig 4C–20)
The length of the thoracic spine is taken as the distance from the superior edge of the first thoracic vertebra to the inferior edge of the twelfth thoracic vertebral body. Normal dimensions are shown in Figure 4C–21. If the gestational age is known, a markedly lengthened thoracic spine suggests that the mother is diabetic, while a markedly shortened thoracic spine suggests retarded intrauterine growth.

Source of Material
Data based on a study of 88 normal newborns.

Ref: Kuhns LR, Holt JF: *Radiology* 1975; 116:395.

MEASUREMENT OF THORACIC SPINE LENGTH ON CHEST FILMS FROM BIRTH TO 16 YEARS*

Technique

Central ray: Perpendicular to plane of film.

Position: Children under 2 years: supine, AP projection. Children over 2 years: upright, PA projection.

Target-film distance: Under 2 years: 100 cm; over 2 years: 180 cm.

Measurement

The length of the thoracic spine was measured in the frontal projection from the superior edge of the first thoracic vertebral body to the lower edge of the twelfth vertebral body.

The results of the statistical analysis of these data are shown in Fig 4C–22.

*Ref: Currarino G, et al: *Skeletal Radiol* 1986; 15:628–630.

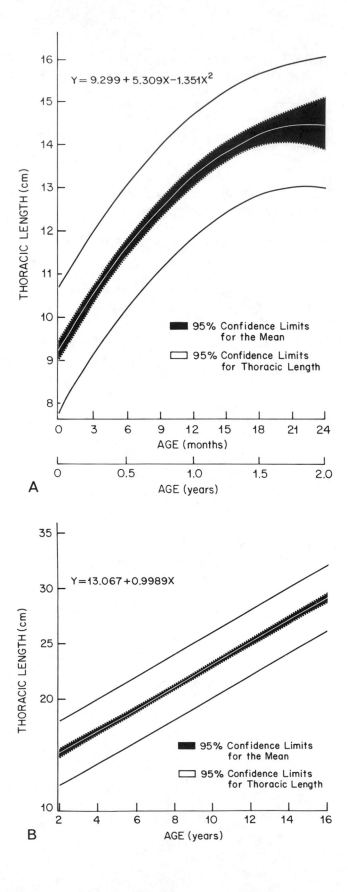

$Y = 9.299 + 5.309X - 1.351X^2$

■ 95% Confidence Limits
for the Mean

□ 95% Confidence Limits
for Thoracic Length

AGE (months)

AGE (years)

A

$Y = 13.067 + 0.9989X$

■ 95% Confidence Limits
for the Mean

□ 95% Confidence Limits
for Thoracic Length

AGE (years)

B

MEASUREMENT OF THORACIC SPINE LENGTH
ON CHEST FILMS FROM BIRTH TO 16 YEARS

Source of Material

Data based on a study of 331 children from birth to 16 years without thoracic or vertebral anomalies.

←FIG 4C–22.

Results of statistical analysis in children from birth to 2 years (**A**), and children from 2 to 16 years (**B**). The predicted values for the mean are indicated by the *center curve,* and the 95% confidence limits for the mean by the *shaded area.* The boundaries of the *unshaded area* (outside curves) denote the calculated 95% confidence limits for thoracic length for an individual child. In the equations shown in these figures Y is the thoracic length in centimeters, and X is the age in years. (From Currarino G, Williams B, Reisch JS: *Skeletal Radiol* 1986; 15:628–630. Used by permission.)

MEASUREMENT OF THE SAGITTAL DIAMETER
OF THE LUMBAR SPINAL CANAL IN CHILDREN
AND ADULTS*

Technique
   Central ray: Perpendicular to plane of film centered at level of third
   lumbar vertebral body.
   Position: Lateral lumbar spine.
   Target-film distance: 40 inches.

Measurements (Fig 4C–23 and Table 4C–8)
   The sagittal diameter of the spinal canal is measured at the level of each
lumbar vertebra. The sagittal diameter is the shortest midline perpendicular
distance from the posterior surface of the vertebral body to the inner surface
of the neural arch.

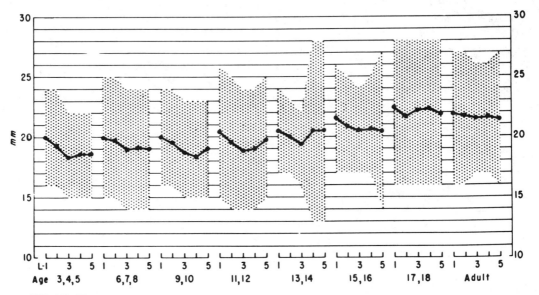

FIG 4C–23.
Age group means and 90% tolerance limits for the sagittal diameter of the spinal canal of each lumbar
vertebra, male and female combined. (From Hinck VC, Hopkins CE, Clark WM: *Radiology* 1965;
85:929. Used by permission.)

Ref: Hinck VC, Hopkins CE, Clark WM: *Radiology* 1965; 85:929.

MEASUREMENT OF THE SAGITTAL DIAMETER OF THE LUMBAR SPINAL CANAL IN CHILDREN AND ADULTS

TABLE 4C–8.

Age-Group Means and Standard Deviations by Sex (mm)*

Vertebra	Male No.	Male Mean	Male SD	Female No.	Female Mean	Female SD	Male No.	Male Mean	Male SD	Female No.	Female Mean	Female SD
		Age 3, 4, 5 yrs						*Age 6, 7, 8 yrs*				
L1	15	20.3	1.8	9	19.8	1.2	14	20.3	1.9	10	19.3	2.6
2	15	19.6	1.2	9	18.9	1.4	15	19.9	1.7	9	19.5	1.6
3	15	18.4	1.4	9	18.1	1.4	15	19.1	1.8	10	18.4	1.6
4	15	18.8	1.1	9	18.0	1.5	15	19.0	1.7	10	19.1	1.8
5	14	19.0	1.6	9	17.5	1.4	15	19.0	2.4	10	19.1	2.3
		Age 9, 10 yrs						*Age 11, 12 yrs*				
L1	8	20.1	1.0	4	19.8	1.9	5	22.6	2.0	11	19.6	1.1
2	8	19.6	1.0	5	19.6	1.7	5	21.2	2.7	11	18.9	1.7
3	8	18.8	1.6	5	18.9	1.3	5	19.9	2.9	11	18.4	1.4
4	8	18.6	1.7	5	18.6	1.2	5	18.8	3.0	11	19.1	1.7
5	8	19.1	1.9	5	18.9	1.1	5	19.7	2.7	11	19.8	2.4
		Age 13, 14 yrs						*Age 15, 16 yrs*				
L1	14	20.5	1.5	10	20.8	1.4	10	21.6	2.2	18	21.6	2.2
2	14	19.7	1.4	10	20.1	0.9	11	20.8	2.1	18	20.9	1.8
3	14	18.9	1.7	10	20.0	1.3	11	20.5	1.6	18	20.7	1.6
4	14	20.4	4.1	10	20.2	2.5	11	20.0	1.7	18	21.0	2.1
5	14	20.8	4.2	10	20.1	3.2	10	20.1	2.9	18	20.8	3.4
		Age 17, 18 yrs						*Adult*				
L1	11	23.9	1.9	17	21.7	1.7	22	22.2	3.1	25	21.3	2.3
2	11	22.4	2.3	17	21.3	1.9	23	22.3	2.7	26	21.2	2.1
3	12	22.6	2.3	18	22.0	3.1	23	21.7	2.6	26	21.3	2.1
4	12	22.9	2.8	18	21.9	2.6	23	21.8	2.4	26	21.3	1.9
5	12	22.6	3.4	18	21.4	2.2	21	22.6	2.7	25	20.4	2.4

*Hinck VC, Hopkins CE, Clark WM: *Radiology* 1965; 85:929. Used by permission.

Source of Material

Films were selected on the basis of readability, and an attempt was made to eliminate subjects who showed significant anomalies and other problems likely to influence growth and development. The number of subjects in each group is shown in Table 4C–8.

NORMAL INTERPEDICULATE DISTANCES
IN CHILDREN AND ADULTS

Technique
  Central ray: Perpendicular to plane of film centered over midportion of
    segment of spine being examined.
  Position: Anteroposterior.
  Target-film distance: 40 inches.

Measurements (Figs 4C–24 to 4C–32)
Interpediculate distance is the shortest distance between the medial surfaces of the pedicles of a given vertebra.

Figures 4C–25 to 4C–32 from Hinck and associates* contain a shaded
area for each graph, which indicates the 90% tolerance range. These tolerance
ranges are the high and low limits within which the central 90% of "normals"
may be expected to fall.

Figure 4C–24 from Schwarz† shows the "extreme upper limits" for the
normal spinal canal in newborns to adults.

Source of Material
Hinck used 474 radiographs, including 353 children (under age 19 years)
and 121 adults. Radiographs were selected from the files of the University of
Oregon Medical School, and an attempt was made to eliminate subjects with
significant anomalies and problems likely to influence growth and development.

Schwarz used radiographs of 200 patients.

*Ref: Hinck VC, et al: *AJR* 1966; 97:141.
†Ref: Schwarz GS: *AJR* 1956; 76:476.

NORMAL INTERPEDICULATE DISTANCES
IN CHILDREN AND ADULTS

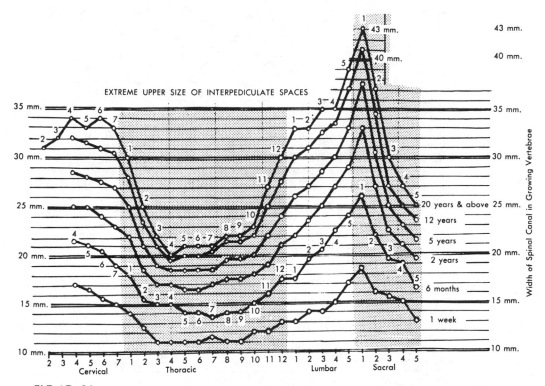

FIG 4C–24.
Newborn through 20 years. All curves delineate the maximum measurement observed for a given vertebra at the age designated. (Adapted from Schwarz GS: *AJR* 1956; 76:476.)

NORMAL INTERPEDICULATE DISTANCES
IN CHILDREN AND ADULTS

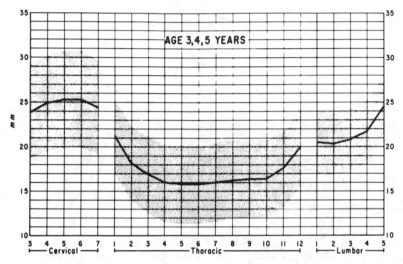

FIG 4C–25.
(From Hinck VC, et al: *AJR* 1966; 97:141. Used by permission.)

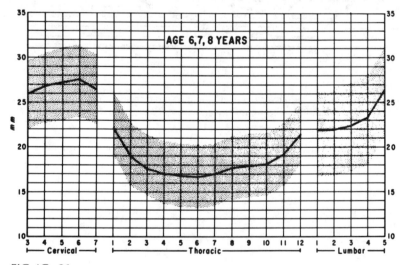

FIG 4C–26.
(From Hinck VC, et al: *AJR* 1966; 97:141. Used by permission.)

NORMAL INTERPEDICULATE DISTANCES
IN CHILDREN AND ADULTS

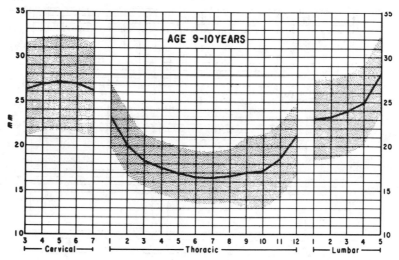

FIG 4C–27.
(From Hinck VC, et al: *AJR* 1966; 97:141. Used by permission.)

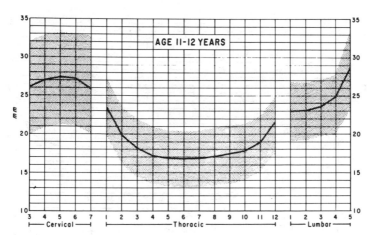

FIG 4C–28.
(From Hinck VC, et al: *AJR* 1966; 97:141. Used by permission.)

NORMAL INTERPEDICULATE DISTANCES
IN CHILDREN AND ADULTS

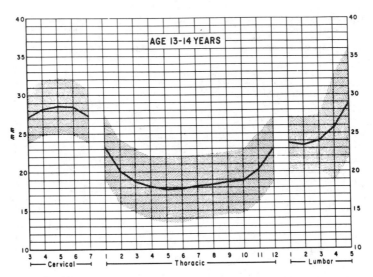

FIG 4C–29.
(From Hinck VC, et al: *AJR* 1966; 97:141. Used by permission.)

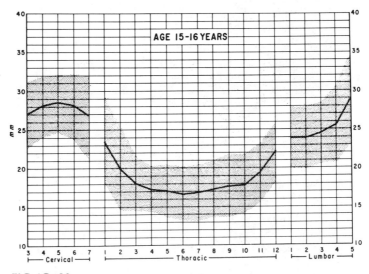

FIG 4C–30.
(From Hinck VC, et al: *AJR* 1966; 97:141. Used by permission.)

NORMAL INTERPEDICULATE DISTANCES
IN CHILDREN AND ADULTS

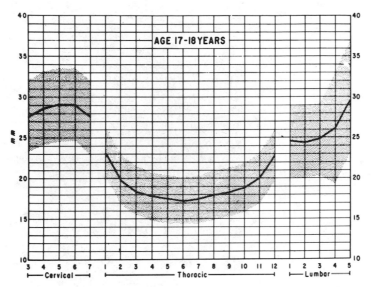

FIG 4C–31.
(From Hinck VC, et al: *AJR* 1966; 97:141. Used by permission.)

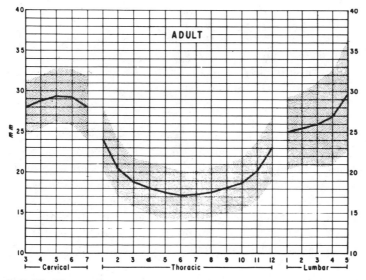

FIG 4C–32.
(From Hinck VC, et al: *AJR* 1966; 97:141. Used by permission.)

MEASUREMENT OF THE LUMBAR SPINAL CANAL
FOR DETECTION OF THE NARROW SPINAL CANAL*

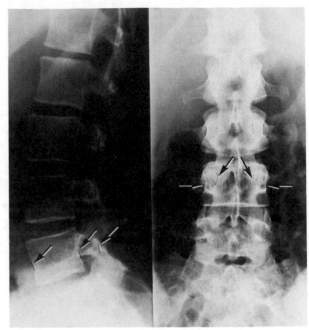

FIG 4C–33.
Measurement of the normal lumbar spinal canal (From Williams RM: *Australas Radiol* 1975; 19:356. Used by permission.)

Technique
Central ray: Perpendicular to plane of film centered over the midlumbar spine.
Position: Anteroposterior and lateral.
Target-film distance: Immaterial.

Measurements (Fig 4C–33)
Measurements of the canal are related proportionately to the size of the adjacent vertebra. The AP measurement of the canal is made on the lateral projection and is taken from the middle of the posterior edge of the vertebral body to the base of the spinous process. The transverse measurement, taken from the frontal film, is the interpedicular distance.

Measurement of the vertebral body is made from the midpoint of the lateral margin of the vertebral body in the AP film and between the midpoints of the anterior and posterior surfaces of the vertebral body in the lateral projection.

The AP canal measurement is multiplied by the interpedicular distance

*Ref: Williams RM: *Australas Radiol* 1975; 19:356.

MEASUREMENT OF THE LUMBAR SPINAL CANAL
FOR DETECTION OF THE NARROW SPINAL CANAL

and is used as the numerator in a ratio with product of AP and transverse diameters of the vertebral body as the denominator.

The total range of normals was found to be:

L3 and L4: 1:3.0 to 1:6.0
L5: 1:3.2 to 1:6.5

The higher values represent narrower lumbar spine canals.

Source of Material
Data based on a study of 100 Australian patients.

MEASUREMENTS OF LUMBAR SPINAL CANAL BY CT IN NORMAL ADULTS*

Technique

1. CT was performed on Ohio Nuclear 50 FS with 18-second scan time, 13-mm collimation, and 36- or 42-cm scan circle diameter displayed on 256 × 256 matrix.
2. *Measurements:* Directly on the CT video display using computer functions. Images were enlarged four times for cursor placement.

Measurement (Figs 4C–34 and 4C–35)

Each vertebral level was divided into four major zones: upper, middle, and lower vertebral body, and disc space.

Anteroposterior spinal cord and interpedicular diameters were measured with typical window of 800 HU and the lower window limit at the bone-soft tissue interface value of 115 HU. Electronic calipers measure the diameter.

Spinal canal cross-sectioned areas were outlined with an irregular region of interest, using the windows set in paragraph 2. Windows were reset with upper limit of 115 HU and number of pixels within the ROI less than upper limit totaled. Multiplying this total by known area per pixel yields the cross-sectional area of the spinal canal.

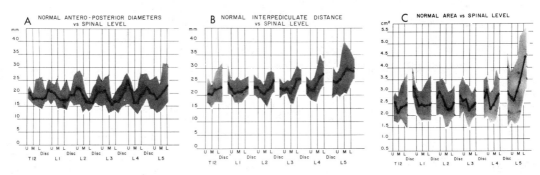

FIG 4C–34.
(From Ullrich CG, et al: *Radiology* 1980; 134:137. Used by permission.)

Figure 4C–34 gives normal spinal canal measurements. Note that cross-sectional area measurements are directly related to setting of the upper window limits, and 115 HU gave a "true canal area" on a spinal phantom.

Ref: Ullrich CG, et al: *Radiology* 1980; 134:137.

MEASUREMENTS OF LUMBAR SPINAL CANAL
BY CT IN NORMAL ADULTS

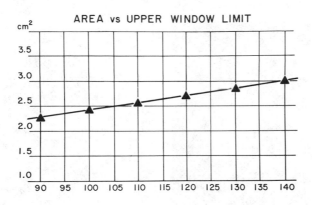

FIG 4C–35.

Variation of calculated cross-sectional area with change in upper window limit. By selecting progressively higher upper window limits, progressively larger calculated areas are obtained. This is because the higher upper window limit allows more pixels to fall within the window and be counted. Data from four different images of the same vertebral body were plotted, and the best straight line was drawn using the least squares linear regression method (correlation coefficient: 0.84). (From Ullrich CG, et al: *Radiology* 1980; 134:137. Used by permission.)

Source of Material

Thirty men 18 to 74 years of age and 30 women 27 to 74 years of age undergoing abdominal CT studies for other reasons. Anteroposterior radiographs and CT scans were normal. Minor degenerative changes were allowed if there was no encroachment upon the spinal cord.

MEASUREMENT OF DEPTH OF THE LATERAL RECESSES OF LUMBOSACRAL SPINE*

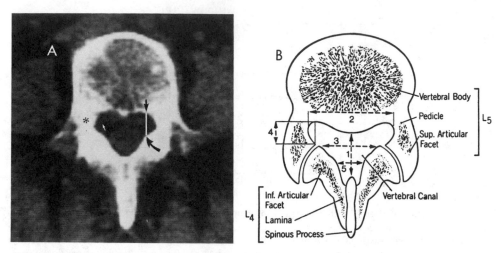

FIG 4C–36.
(From Mikhael MA, et al: *Radiology* 1981; 140:97. Used by permission.)

Technique

1. Anteroposterior measurements corrected for magnification.
2. Measured on plain lateral radiographs, polytomograms, CT scans, and myelograms.

*Ref: Mikhael MA, et al: *Radiology* 1981; 140:97.

MEASUREMENT OF DEPTH OF THE LATERAL RECESSES OF LUMBOSACRAL SPINE

Measurement (Figs 4C−36 and 4C−37).

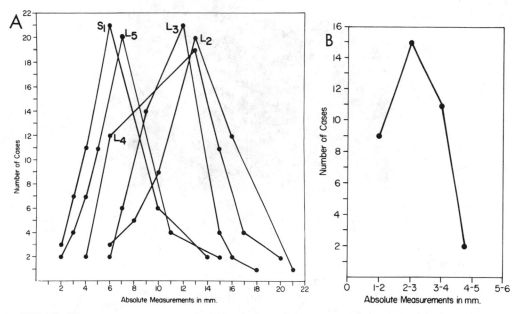

FIG 4C−37.
A, normal range of the absolute depth of the lateral recess as measured on CT scans and polytomograms at L2-L5 and S1 in 50 asymptomatic patients. **B,** absolute depth of the lateral recess as measured on CT scans and polytomograms in 35 patients with surgically proved lateral recess syndrome. (From Mikhael MA, et al: *Radiology* 1981; 140:97. Used by permission.)

The normal lateral recess reduces in size proceeding from L2 to S1. The lateral recess syndrome occurred most frequently at L5-S1.

Source of Material
Measurements on 50 asymptomatic patients and 35 with lateral recess syndrome surgically confirmed.

MEASUREMENT OF THE NORMAL
SACRAL SAC IN ADULTS*

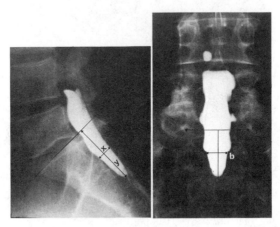

FIG 4C–38.
Points of measurement of sacral sac. (From Evison G, et al: *Br J Radiol* 1979; 52:777. Used by permission.)

Technique
Myelography with oily contrast agent:
   Central ray: Perpendicular to plane of film.
   Position: Anteroposterior and lateral erect.
   Target-film distance: 45 cm. Magnification for lateral views is 1.25 to 1.30 and for AP views is 1.30 to 1.36.

Measurement (Fig 4C–38 and Table 4C–9)
An interpedicular line was drawn between the midpoints of the medial borders of the pedicles of the first sacral segment. A line at right angles to this was taken as perpendicular. The width of the sac was measured at the midpoint between the interpedicular line and the tip of the sac *(b).*

On the lateral view, the upper margin of the body of the first sacral segment was projected backward to the posterior margin of the vertebral canal. A line was drawn at right angles to the tip of the sac. Measurements were made of the distance along this line from the upper border of the sacrum to the tip of the sacral sac *(Y).* The sagittal diameter was measured at the midpoint of the line between the upper border of the sacrum and the tip of the sac *(X).*

Ref: Evison G, et al: *Br J Radiol* 1979; 52:777.

MEASUREMENT OF THE NORMAL
SACRAL SAC IN ADULTS

TABLE 4C–9.

Measurements of Sacral Sac*

	AP View: Width at the Midpoint			Lateral View: Sagittal Diameter			Sacral Level of Termination			
	<1 cm	1–2 cm	>2 cm	<1 cm	1–2 cm	>2 cm	S1	S2	S3	S4
n	1	99	60	6	137	17	28	111	20	1
%	0.6	61.9	37.5	3.8	85.6	10.6	17.5	69.4	12.5	0.6

*From Evison G, et al: *Br J Radiol* 1979; 52:777. Used by permission.

Source of Material

Based on myelograms of 335 patients.

VERTEBRAL BODY AND INTERVERTEBRAL DISC INDEX (TWELFTH THORACIC TO THIRD LUMBAR)*

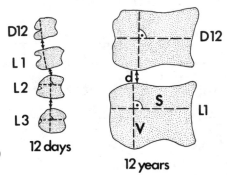

FIG 4C–39.
(Adapted from Brandner ME: *AJR* 1970; 110:618.)

Technique
    Central ray: Projected through first lumbar vertebra.
    Position: True lateral projection with Bucky table.
    Target-film distance: 110 cm. However, indices are independent of target-film distance.

Measurements (Fig 4C–39; Tables 4C–10 and 4C–11)

$$I_{vb} = \text{Vertebral body index} = \frac{v}{s} = \frac{\text{Height of vertebral body}}{\text{Sagittal diameter of vertebral body}}$$

Height is the largest vertical measurement of the body. Sagittal diameter is the smallest anteroposterior measurement of the body.

$$I_{d} = \text{Intervertebral disc index} = \frac{d}{v} = \frac{\text{Intervertebral disc thickness}}{\text{Height of vertebral body}}$$

Upper disc and lower vertebral body are compared.
Note: Additional work by Brandner† based on a study of adults indicates that the intervertebral disc index d/v in adults is comparable to the results obtained in children.

*Ref: Brandner ME: *AJR* 1970; 110:618.
†Ref: Brandner ME: *AJR* 1972; 114:411.

VERTEBRAL BODY AND INTERVERTEBRAL DISC INDEX IN CHILDREN (TWELFTH THORACIC TO THIRD LUMBAR)

TABLE 4C–10.

I_{vb} *(v/s)* of Vertebral Bodies*†

Vertebral Body	Age Group	No.	Mean v/s
D12	0–1 mo	13	0.81
	2–18 mo	26	0.91
	19–36 mo	22	0.86
	4–12 yrs (F)	18	0.86
	4–12 yrs (M)	35	0.78
	13 yrs and over (F)	7	0.93
	13 yrs and over (M)	20	0.84
L1	0–1 mo	16	0.87
	2–18 mo (F)	11	1.02
	2–18 mo (M)	16	0.96
	2–18 mo (M & F)	27	0.98
	19–36 mo	23	0.89
	4–12 yrs (F)	20	0.87
	4–12 yrs (M)	40	0.80
	13 yrs and over (F)	19	1.03
	13 yrs and over (M)	27	0.87
L2	0–1 mo	10	0.92
	2–18 mo	21	1.01
	19–36 mo	20	0.91
	4–12 yrs	49	0.82
	13 yrs and over (F)	15	1.03
	13 yrs and over (M)	25	0.88
L3	0–1 mo	11	0.95
	2–18 mo	17	0.98
	19–36 mo	16	0.88
	4–12 yrs	35	0.79
	13 yrs and over (F)	11	1.00
	13 yrs and over (M)	17	0.87

*Adapted from Brandner ME: *AJR* 1970; 110:618.
†F = female; M = male.

VERTEBRAL BODY AND INTERVERTEBRAL DISC INDEX IN CHILDREN (TWELFTH THORACIC TO THIRD LUMBAR)

TABLE 4C–11.

I_d (d/v) of Intervertebral Disc
and Vertebral Body*

Vertebral Segment	Age Group	No.	Mean d/v
D 11/12	0–1 mo	12	0.37
	2–18 mo	26	0.30
	19–36 mo	19	0.25
	4–12 yrs	49	0.24
	13 yrs and over	21	0.18
D 12/L1	0–1 mo	17	0.35
	2–18 mo	27	0.28
	19–36 mo	20	0.26
	4–12 yrs	53	0.25
	13 yrs and over	37	0.19
L 1/2	0–1 mo	15	0.35
	2–18 mo	26	0.26
	19–36 mo	19	0.27
	4–12 yrs	44	0.28
	13 yrs and over	37	0.20
L 2/3	0–1 mo	9	0.38
	2–18 mo	18	0.28
	19–36 mo	15	0.30
	4–12 yrs	32	0.30
	13 yrs and over	22	0.21

*Adapted from Brandner ME: *AJR* 1970; 110:618.

Source of Material

Brandner studied 187 roentgenograms of dorsal and lumbar spines from newborns to adolescents.

MEASUREMENT OF VERTEBRAL BODY HEIGHT AND INTERVERTEBRAL DISC WIDTH: DORSAL AND LUMBAR REGIONS IN FEMALES*

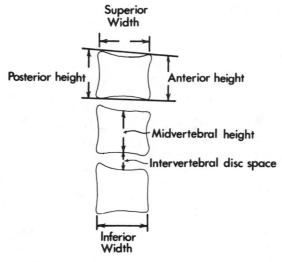

FIG 4C–40.

Technique

    Central ray: Dorsal spine: projected through ninth dorsal vertebra, lumbar spine: projected through third lumbar vertebra.

    Position: True lateral. Patient lying on left side.

    Target-film distance: 40 inches.

Ref: Hurxthal LM: *AJR* 1968; 103:635.

MEASUREMENT OF VERTEBRAL BODY HEIGHT AND INTERVERTEBRAL DISC WIDTH: DORSAL AND LUMBAR REGIONS IN FEMALES

Measurements (Fig 4C−40 and Table 4C−12)

TABLE 4C−12.*

Inter-vertebral Disc or Vertebra Level	Mean Inter-vertebral Disc Space (mm)	Mean Height of Anterior Vertebral Border (mm)	Mean Height of Posterior Vertebral Border (mm)	Mean Midline Height of Vertebra (mm)	Mean Width of Superior Border of Vertebra (mm)	Mean Width of Inferior Border of Vertebra (mm)	Range in Disc Space (mm)
L5-4 + L5	11.0	35.4	32.2	31.0	37.8	39.6	8-14
L4-3 + L4	10.2	35.1	33.7	28.0	39.0	38.3	7-17
L3-2 + L3	10.2	34.7	34.3	34.0	37.0	37.6	6-16
L2-1 + L2	7.9	32.9	33.7	29.0	34.9	36.5	3-10
L1-D12 + L1	6.9	31.7	32.4	31.0	35.8	33.3	5-12
D12-11 + D12	6.4	28.7	28.5	31.5	35.5	34.0	4-12
D11-10 + D11	4.7	26.7	27.1	28.5	35.2	35.2	4-8
D10-9 + D10	4.4	26.5	26.0	25.0	35.0	35.1	4-7
D9-8 + D9	4.4	24.8	24.9	25.0	33.8	33.8	4-5
D8-7 + D8	4.4	23.3	24.0	23.0	31.1	31.7	4-1
D7-6 + D7	4.0	23.5	23.7	22.0	29.6	31.4	3-8
Totals in mm (to nearest integral)							
Younger group	75	323	321	308	386	388	3-17
Older group	84	321	337	316	386	395	3-14

Mean age
  Younger group   22 years
                  (15−30)
  Older group   62 years
                  (47−75)

*From Hurxthal LM: *AJR* 1968; 103:635. Used by permission.

Source of Material

Hurxthal measured 220 vertebrae on 20 lateral roentgenograms of dorsal and lumbar spines selected from ambulatory women in good health. Ten subjects were between ages 15 years and 30 years, and 10 subjects were between ages 47 years and 75 years.

MEASUREMENTS IN SPONDYLOLISTHESIS*†

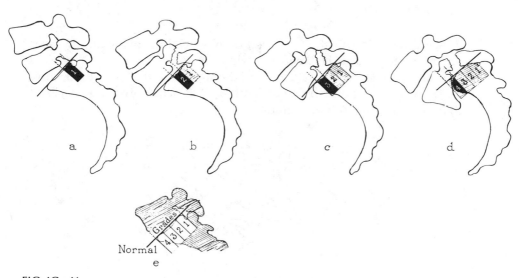

FIG 4C–41.
Meyerding's method of classifying the degree of spondylolisthesis. (From Meyerding HW: *Surg Gynecol Obstet* 1932; 54:374. Used by permission.)

Technique

Central ray: Centered over lumbosacral junction perpendicular to plane of film.

Position: True lateral. Upright and horizontal positions may be necessary to demonstrate spondylolisthesis.

Target-film distance: Immaterial. Distance of at least 36 inches desirable.

Measurements

1. Meyerding's classification scheme* (Fig 4C–41) is not based on actual measurements but on the position of the posterior aspect of the body of the fifth lumbar vertebra in relation to the superior surface of the first sacral segment, which is divided into quarters.
2. Garland and Thomas's vertical line† (Fig 4C–42) is drawn perpendicular to the upper surface of the first sacral body at its anterior superior margin. In all normal individuals the anterior inferior margin of the fifth lumbar body lay from 1 to 8 mm behind this line.

*Ref: Meyerding HW: *Surg Gynecol Obstet* 1932; 54:374.
†Ref: Garland LH, Thomas SF: *AJR* 1946; 55:275.

MEASUREMENTS IN SPONDYLOLISTHESIS

Source of Material

1. Meyerding's classification is based on observations made of 207 cases of spondylolisthesis between 1918 and 1931.
2. Garland and Thomas's data are based on a study of 170 cases. Twenty of these had neural arch defects; of the 20, 8 has showed spondylolisthesis, according to their criteria.

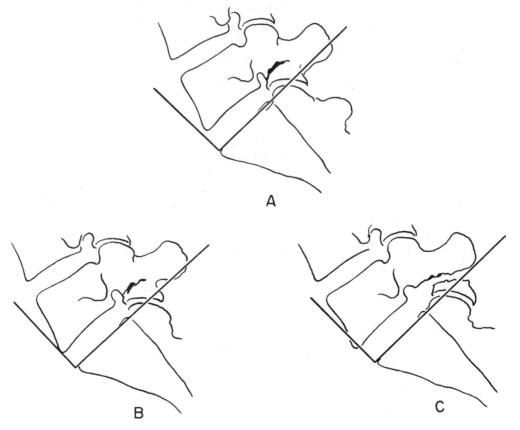

FIG 4C–42.
Diagram illustrating use of the right-angle test line for diagnosis of anterior spondylolisthesis. **A,** neural arch defects without slip. Note that the anterior margin of the fifth lumbar body lies about 3 mm behind the test line. **B,** neural arch defects without definite slip. The body of the fifth lumbar vertebra does touch the test line, but its posterior edge is not significantly out of line, and none of the other findings of spondylolisthesis are present. Occasionally, defects of this type can be shown to slip slightly in the erect position. **C,** spondylolisthesis, partial grade 1. The anterior margin of the fifth lumbar body crosses the test line. (Adapted from Garland LH, Thomas SF: *AJR* 1946; 55:275.)

MEASUREMENT OF NORMAL INTERVERTEBRAL DISC HEIGHTS*

Technique
 Central ray: Perpendicular to plane of film.
 Position: Upright in neutral position.
 Target-film distance: Measurements corrected for magnification.

Measurements (Fig 4C–43)

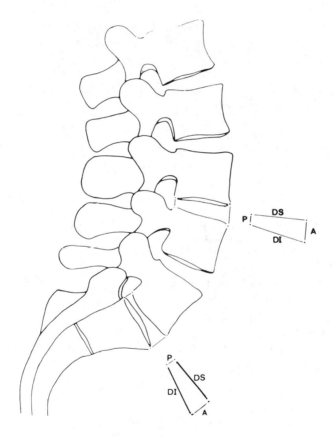

FIG 4C–43.
Tracing of a lateral radiograph of a lumbar spine in the upright position showing the position of the marks used for taking measurements. *A* = anterior disc height; *P* = posterior disc height; *DS* = superior disc depth; *DI* = inferior disc depth. (From Tibrewal SB, Pearcy MJ: *Spine* 1984; 10:452–454. Used by permission.)

Ref: Tibrewal SB, Pearcy MJ: *Spine* 1984; 10:452–454.

MEASUREMENT OF NORMAL INTERVERTEBRAL DISC HEIGHTS

A nondimensional index of disc shape was calculated from the height and depth measurements to indicate how the wedged shape of the disc varied at different levels. This index was calculated as:

$$\frac{\text{anterior disc height} - \text{posterior disc height} \times 100\%}{\text{Disc depth}}$$

The individual measurements and disc shapes are shown in Table 4C–13.

TABLE 4C–13.

True Mean Disc Heights, Depths, and Shapes for Each Level of the Lumbar Spine in the Upright Position for the 11 Normal Subjects*†

Level	Anterior Disc Height		Posterior Disc Height		Disc Depth		Disc Shape	
	Mean	Range (mm)	Mean	Range (mm)	Mean	Range (mm)	Mean	Range (%)
L1-L2	8	6–11	4	2–6	34	29–37	12	3–25
L2-L3	11	8–13‡	4.5	2–6	34	29–38	19	8–25‡
L3-L4	12.5	11–15	4.5	3–6	33	29–36§	23	18–29
L4-L5	14	11–16§	5.5	3–8	33	29–36	26	19–38
L5-S1	13	9–16	4.5	3–6§	31	27–34‡	27	14–46

*From Tibrewal SB, Pearcy MJ: *Spine* 1984; 10:452–454. Used by permission.
†Statistically significant differences between one level and the next superior level.
‡ = $P < 0.01$.
§ = $P < 0.05$.

Source of Material

Data based on a study of 11 normal men, ranging in age from 25 to 36 years.

MEASURED HEIGHT OF THE LUMBOSACRAL DISC WITH AND WITHOUT TRANSITIONAL VERTEBRAE*

Technique
  Central ray: Perpendicular to plane of film.
  Position: Anteroposterior and lateral horizontal.
  Target-film distance: Disregarded because of differences in pelvic width.

Measurement (Fig 4C−44)

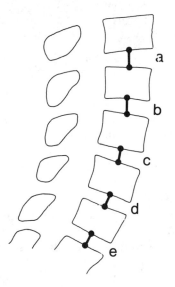

FIG 4C−44.
Disc height measurements. In the two groups of patients studied, the 95% confidence limits were derived from the formula (average e/average (a + b + c + d)) × 100. (From Nicholson AA, et al: *Br J Radiol* 1988; 61:454−455. Used by permission.)

The average disc height was measured at each lumbar level between adjacent end-plates at the midpoint between the anterior and posterior margins of the vertebra. The height of the lumbosacral intervertebral disc was expressed as a proportion of the sum of the disc heights of the other four levels and the differences presented as 95% confidence limits.

The results are given in Table 4C−14.

Ref: Nicholson AA, et al: *Br J Radiol* 1988; 61:454−455.

MEASURED HEIGHT OF THE LUMBOSACRAL DISC WITH AND WITHOUT TRANSITIONAL VERTEBRAE

TABLE 4C–14.

Disc Height Measurements (mm) in Normal and Transitional Lumbar Spines (mean ± sem)*

	Normal (46)	Transitional (48)	Significance
L1:L2	11.13±1.78	10.4±2	NS
L2:L3	12.21±1.84	13.0±2.5	NS
L3:L4	12.93±2.01	12.5±2	NS
L4:L5	12.98±2.11†	12.0±2.5	NS
L5:S1	10.37±2.05†	8.2±2.5	$P < 0.001$

*From Nicholson AA, et al: *Br J Radiol* 1988; 61:454–455. Used by permission.
†Significant difference: $P < 0.001$.

The lumbosacral intervertebral disc is significantly narrower than its counterpart in nontransitional spines. Even in normal spines the lumbosacral disc is significantly narrower than discs at higher levels. This narrowing does not imply disc degeneration.

Source of Material

Data are based on radiographic examination of 46 young adults with transitional vertebrae and 48 age- and sex-matched subjects without transitional segmentation. All subjects were under age 40 years.

MEASUREMENT OF THE NORMAL WEDGING OF THE DORSOLUMBAR VERTEBRAE*

Technique
Central ray: Perpendicular to plane of film.
Position: Lateral.
Target-film distance: Immaterial.

Measurement (Fig 4C–45)

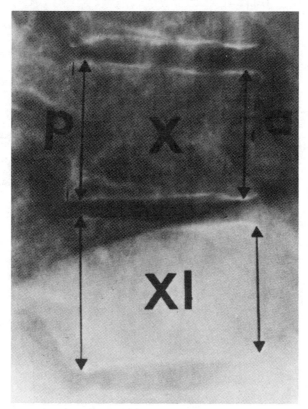

FIG 4C–45.
Degree of wedging measured as the ratio between the heights of the anterior *(a)* and the posterior *(p)* aspects. (From Lauridsen KN, De Carvalho A, Andersen AH: *Acta Radiol Diagn* 1984; 25:29–32, 1984. Used by permission.)

Ref: Lauridsen KN, et al: *Acta Radiol Diagn* 1984; 25:29–32.

MEASUREMENT OF THE NORMAL WEDGING OF THE DORSOLUMBAR VERTEBRAE

The heights of the anterior (a) and posterior (p) aspects were measured at a distance of 2 mm from the midpoint of the vertebral margins to avoid the edges, which are difficult to define. The mean a/p ratios were calculated and are shown in Table 4C–15.

TABLE 4C–15.

Degree of Vertebral Wedging in the Male and Female Groups*

Vertebrae	Confidence limits				Total
	80%	90%	95%	97.5%	
Males					
Th8	0.81	0.77	0.75	0.72	62
Th9	0.84	0.81	0.78	0.76	67
Th10	0.86	0.83	0.80	0.78	67
Th11	0.85	0.81	0.79	0.76	66
Th12	0.84	0.81	0.79	0.77	63
L1	0.86	0.84	0.82	0.80	68
L2	0.90	0.88	0.86	0.84	68
L3	0.95	0.92	0.90	0.88	67
Females					
Th8	0.86	0.84	0.82	0.80	94
Th9	0.90	0.88	0.85	0.84	95
Th10	0.91	0.89	0.87	0.85	95
Th11	0.87	0.85	0.82	0.80	94
Th12	0.89	0.87	0.85	0.84	96
L1	0.90	0.88	0.86	0.84	95
L2	0.94	0.92	0.90	0.89	95
L3	0.96	0.94	0.92	0.90	95

*From Lauridsen KN, De Carvalho A, Andersen AH: *Acta Radiol Diagn* 1984; 25:29–32. Used by permission.

Source of Material

Data based on a study of 164 persons, 96 women aged 25 to 59 years and 68 men aged 17 to 59 years. Subjects selected at random and those with fractures were excluded.

MEASUREMENT OF THE LUMBOSACRAL ANGLE*

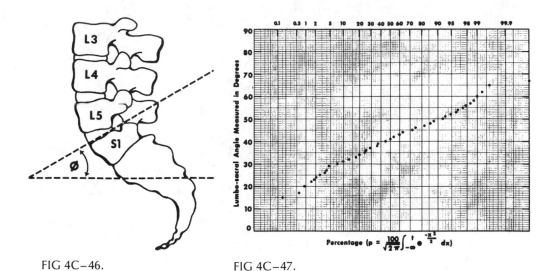

FIG 4C–46.   FIG 4C–47.

Technique
Central ray: Perpendicular to plane of film. Upright spot films of L5-S1 intervertebral space centered 1 inch below iliac crest.
Position: True lateral with patient standing.
Target-film distance: 40 inches.

Measurements (Figs 4C–46 and 4C–47)
Line of inclination in Figure 4C–46 is the plane of the 1st sacral surface. Line of horizontal is drawn parallel to the bottom margin of the film.
Lumbrosacral angle is ϕ. Mean lumbosacral angle = 41.1°. SD = 7.7°. Ninety-five percent of all values will lie between 25.7° and 56.5°.
Values in the study approximated a normal distribution.
By using the graph (Fig 4C–47) it is possible to find the percentage of individuals above or below a given value. For example, an angle of 50° shows 92% of individuals less than that angle and 8% greater.
When supine and standing views are compared, there is usually an increase in the lumbosacral angle of 8° to 12° in the standing position.

Source of Material
Hellems and Keats used 319 normal males ranging in age from 17 to 58 years who had lumbosacral spine films made as part of a routine preemployment examination.

Ref: Hellems HK, Keats TE: *AJR* 1971; 113:642.

MEASUREMENT OF SCOLIOSIS

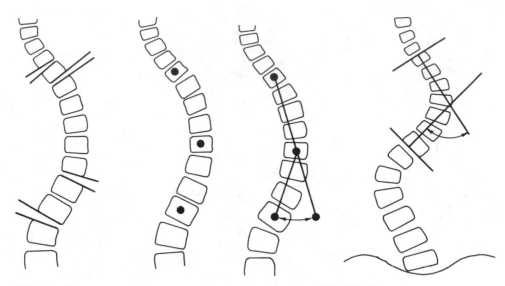

FIG 4C–48.
Method of Ferguson. (Adapted from Kittleson AC, Lim LW: *AJR* 1970; 108:775.)

FIG 4C–49.
Method of Cobb. (Adapted from Kittleson AC, Lim LW: *AJR* 1970; 108:775.)

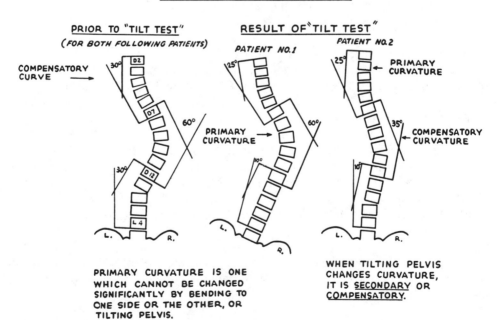

FIG 4C–50.
(From Meschan I: *Roentgen Signs in Clinical Diagnosis.* Philadelphia, WB Saunders Co, 1956, p 453.)

MEASUREMENT OF SCOLIOSIS*†

Technique
  Central ray: Perpendicular to plane of film centered over dorsolumbar junction.
  Position: Anteroposterior.
  Target-film distance: Immaterial.

Measurements (Figs 4C–48 and 4C–49)

The secondary curvatures function to bring the head erect over the pelvis and keep the body in balance in the erect posture. When the primary curve is not definitely identified, examination is made with the patient seated with the pelvis elevated 4 inches (by sandbag or otherwise) on the side of the convexity of the lumbar curve. No support is allowed the patient. In this posture the muscles at the convex aspect of the lumbar curve cause marked straightening throughout that curve if it is compensatory but little or no straightening (except possibly at the end of the curve) if it is primary (Fig 4C–50).

The Ferguson and Cobb methods are two systems for measurement of scoliosis. The Scoliosis Research Society has selected the Cobb system as the standard method of measurement.‡ The Ferguson method should be used for curves under 50°. The Cobb method should be used for curves over 50°.

Method of Ferguson (Fig 4C–48).

1. Locate the end vertebrae: the vertebra at each end of a curve that is the least rotated and lies between the two curves.
2. Locate the apex vertebra: the most rotated vertebra at the peak of the curve.
3. In each of these three vertebrae, the *center* of the *outline* of the *body* is marked with a dot.
4. Lines are drawn from the apex to each end vertebra. The angle of the curve is the divergence of these two lines from 180°.

Method of Cobb (Fig 4C–49).

1. Locate the top vertebra of the curve: the highest one whose superior surface tilts to the side of the concavity of the curve to be measured.
2. Locate the bottom vertebra: the lowest one whose inferior surface tilts to the side of the concavity of the curve to be measured.
3. Erect intersecting perpendiculars from the superior surface of the top and the inferior surface of the bottom vertebrae of the curve. The selection of the end vertebrae and the top and bottom vertebrae is aided

*Ref: Cobb JR: Am Acad Orthop Surg 1948; 5:261–275.

†Ref: Ferguson AB: Roentgen Diagnosis of Extremities and Spine. New York, Paul B Hoeber Inc, 1949.

‡Ref: Kittelson AC, and Lim LW: Am J Roentgenol 1970; 108:775.

by a study of the disc spaces. All of the vertebrae in a given curve will show widening of the disc space on the convex side of the curve.
4. The angle formed by these perpendiculars is the angle of the curve.

Source of Material
Original observations from the clinical work of Ferguson and from Cobb.

MEASUREMENT OF VERTEBRAL ROTATION*

Technique
   Central ray: Perpendicular to plane of film.
   Position: Anteroposterior.
   Target-film distance: Immaterial.

Measurement (Fig 4C 51 and Table 4C–16)

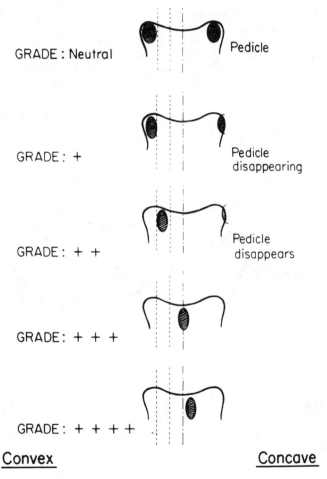

GRADE : Neutral — Pedicle

GRADE : + — Pedicle disappearing

GRADE : + + — Pedicle disappears

GRADE : + + +

GRADE : + + + +

Convex   Concave

FIG 4C–51.
Pedicle method of determining vertebral rotation. (From Nash CL, Moe JH: *J Bone Joint Surg* 1969; 51A:223–229. Used by permission.)

Ref: Nash CL, Moe JH: *J Bone Joint Surg* 1969; 51A: 223–229.

MEASUREMENT OF VERTEBRAL ROTATION

TABLE 4C–16.
Pedicle Method of Determining Vertebral Rotation*

	Pedicle	
Grade	Convex	Concave
Neutral	No asymmetry	No asymmetry
+	Migrates within first segment	May start disappearing
	Early distortion	Early distortion
++	Migrates to second segment	Gradually disappears
+++	Migrates to middle segment	Not visible
++++	Migrates past midline to concave side of vertebral body	Not visible

*From Nash CL, Moe JH: *J Bone Joint Surg* 1969; 51A:223–229. Used by permission.

Figure 4C–52 summarizes a simplified technique for describing vertebral rotation and estimating the degree of rotation present.

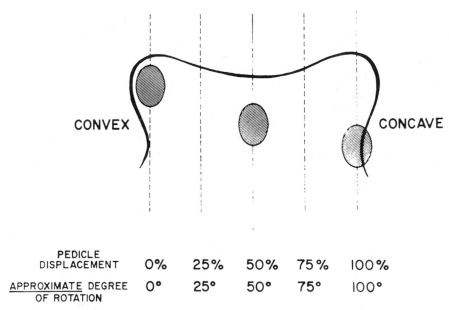

PEDICLE DISPLACEMENT	0%	25%	50%	75%	100%
APPROXIMATE DEGREE OF ROTATION	0°	25°	50°	75°	100°

FIG 4C–52.
(From Nash CL, Moe JH: *J Bone Joint Surg* 1969; 51A:223–229. Used by permission.)

Source of Material
Data derived from a study of a dessicated normal young adult spine.

MEASUREMENT OF THORACIC KYPHOSIS*

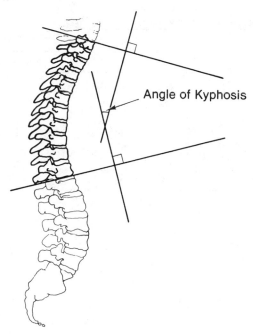

Angle of Kyphosis

FIG 4C–53.
Method of measuring kyphosis. (From Fon GT, et al: *AJR* 1980; 134:979. Used by permission.)

Technique
   Central ray: Perpendicular to plane of film centered over midchest.
   Position: True lateral standing with arms above shoulders.
   Target-film distance: Immaterial.

Measurement (Fig 4C–53; Tables 4C–17 and 4C–18)
   The upper and lower vertebral bodies defining the curve were selected and lines drawn extending along the superior border of the upper end vertebra, as well as along the inferior border of the lower end vertebra. Perpendiculars were drawn from these two lines, and the angle was measured at the intersection.

Ref: Fon GT, et al: *AJR* 1980; 134:979.

MEASUREMENT OF THORACIC KYPHOSIS

TABLE 4C–17.

Degree of Normal Kyphosis in Males by Age

Age (yr)	No. Cases	Kyphosis (Degree)			
		Mean	SD	Minimum	Maximum
2–9	26	20.88	7.85	5	40
10–19	28	25.11	8.16	8	39
20–29	37	26.27	8.12	13	48
30–39	26	29.04	7.93	13	49
40–49	20	29.75	6.93	17	44
50–59	10	33.00	6.46	25	45
60–69	9	34.67	5.12	25	62
70–79	3	40.67	7.57	32	66

TABLE 4C–18.

Degree of Normal Kyphosis in Females by Age

Age (yr)	No. Cases	Kyphosis (Degree)			
		Mean	SD	Minimum	Maximum
2–9	23	23.87	6.67	8	36
10–19	22	26.00	7.43	11	41
20–29	24	26.83	7.98	7	40
30–39	26	28.42	8.63	10	42
40–49	32	32.66	6.72	21	50
50–59	17	40.71	9.88	22	53
60–69	7	44.86	7.80	34	54
70–79	6	41.67	9.00	30	56

Source of Material

Thoracic kyphosis was measured in 316 normal subjects, 159 males and 157 females, ranging in age from 2 to 77 years.

The Upper Extremity

AXIAL RELATIONSHIPS OF THE SHOULDER AND MEASUREMENT OF THE JOINT SPACE*

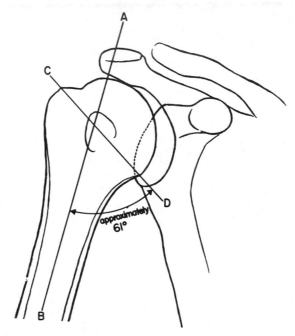

FIG 4D–1.
Axial angle. Average for adult females, 62°. Average for adult males, 60°.

Technique
   Central ray: Perpendicular to the plane of the film centered over the shoulder.
   Position: Anteroposterior: external rotation (anatomic position) for axial angle; internal or external rotation for joint space.
   Target-film distance: 36–40 inches for joint space. Immaterial for axial angle.

Measurements (Fig 4D–1)
Axial angle:

AB Axis of the shaft is drawn between 2 points, each measured to lie in the midline of the diaphysis.
CD Axis of the head is drawn between the apex of the greater tuberosity to the junction of the shaft with the distal extremity of the articular surface of the head (the point where the medial cortex changes from a band to a line).

*Ref: Keats TE, et al: Radiology 1966; 87:904.

AXIAL RELATIONSHIPS OF THE SHOULDER AND MEASUREMENT OF THE JOINT SPACE*

Source of Material

Data on the axial angle were derived from a study of 50 normal subjects, equally divided between males and females ranging in age from 17 to 72 years.

MEASUREMENT OF THE JOINT SPACE OF THE SHOULDER*

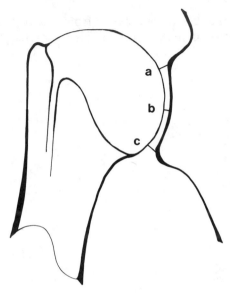

FIG 4D–2.
Measuring technique. (From Petersson CJ, Redlund-Johnell I: *Acta Orthop Scand* 1983; 54:274. Used by permission.)

Technique
Central ray: Perpendicular to plane of the film centered over the shoulder.
Position: Anteroposterior with patient supine, arm in zero adduction and outward rotation.
Target-film distance: 110 cm.

Measurement (Fig 4D–2)
The projection of the joint surface of the humeral head forms a half-circle, the diameter of which is the line joining the two terminal points of the joint surface projection. The midpoint of this line is determined with a ruler. With the ruler aimed at this point and perpendicular to the joint surface of the head of the humerus, the joint space is measured at three sites, *a*, *b*, and *c*. Point *a* is the superior edge of the glenoid surface and point *c* the inferior edge. Point *b* is the midpoint. The three measurements are averaged.

Ref: Petersson CJ, Redlund-Johnell I: *Acta Orthop Scand* 1983; 54:274.

MEASUREMENT OF THE JOINT SPACE
OF THE SHOULDER

The average was found to be between 4 and 5 mm. The value does not change with age, except in women, in whom it increases slightly.

Source of Material

A total of 175 images were reviewed, 88 of men and 87 of women. There were 10 to 11 patients in each 10-year age group between 10 and 90.

MEASUREMENT OF THE ACROMIOHUMERAL DISTANCE*

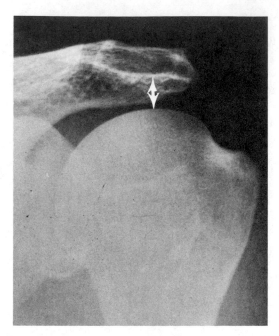

FIG 4D–3.
(From Alexander C: *Proc Coll Radiol Aust* 1959; 3:102. Used by permission.)

Technique
Central ray: Perpendicular to the plane of the film centered over the humeral head.
Position: Anteroposterior: arm in adduction and neutral rotation.
Target-film distance: 36 inches.

Measurement (Fig 4D–3)
The measured distance is the minimum one between the inferior surface of the acromion tangential to the x-ray beam and the articular cortex of the humerus.

The range of normal measurement is 7 to 11 mm; the mean distance is 9.3 mm. A reduction of distance below 7 mm is believed to be a reliable indication of degenerative disease of the supraspinatus tendon.

Source of Material
Measurements were made in 53 shoulders that showed no clinical evidence of rotator cuff abnormality or bursitis.

*Ref: Alexander C: *Proc Coll Radiol Aust* 1959; 3:102.

MEASUREMENT OF THE ACROMIOCLAVICULAR JOINT*

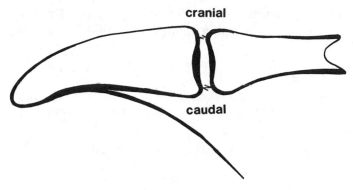

FIG 4D–4.
Cranial and caudad measuring sites for the acromioclavicular joint. (From Petersson CJ, Redlund-Johnell I: *Acta Orthop Scand* 1983; 54:431. Used by permission.)

Technique
Central ray: Perpendicular to plane of film centered over the shoulder.
Position: Anteroposterior with the patient supine.
Target-film distance: 110 cm.

Measurement (Fig 4D–4)
The joint space is measured at the superior and inferior borders and an average of the two measurements made. Normal measurements are shown in Table 4D–1.

TABLE 4D–1.

Acromioclavicular Joint Space in Various Measuring Sites*†

	Cranial	Caudal	Integral
Men	3.8 ± 1.0	2.7 ± 0.6	3.3 ± 0.8
Women	3.5 ± 1.0	2.4 ± 0.6	2.9 ± 0.8
Common	3.7 ± 1.0	2.6 ± 0.6	3.1 ± 0.8

*From Petersson CJ, Redlund-Johnell I: *Acta Orthop Scand* 1983; 54:431. Used by permission.
†Measurements in millimeters, average ± 1 SD.

*Ref: Petersson CJ, Redlund-Johnell I: *Acta Orthop Scand* 1983; 54:431.

MEASUREMENT OF THE ACROMIOCLAVICULAR JOINT

There is no right-left difference in either sex. The joint space is wider in men than in women, and in both men and women there is a reduction in joint space with age.

Source of Material

One hundred fifty-one images were reviewed, 75 of men and 76 of women. There were 10 to 11 patients in each 10-year group between ages 20 and 90 years.

MEASUREMENT OF THE AXIAL ANGLES AT THE ELBOW*

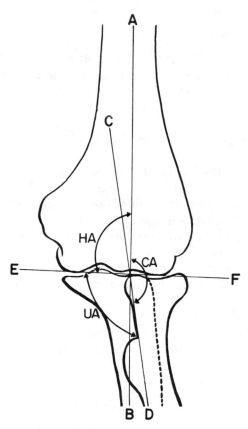

FIG 4D–5.

TABLE 4D–2.*

Angle	Min	Max	Average
Males			
CA	154°	178°	169°
HA	77°	95°	85°
UA	74°	99°	84°
Females			
CA	158°	178°	167°
HA	72°	91°	83°
UA	72°	93°	84°

*From Keats TE, et al: *Radiology* 1966; 87:904. Used by permission.

*Ref: Keats TE, et al: *Radiology* 1966; 87:904.

MEASUREMENT OF THE AXIAL ANGLES
AT THE ELBOW*

Technique
   Central ray: Perpendicular to plane of film.
   Position: Arm fully extended with the two epicondyles perfectly flat with respect to the film.
   Target-film distance: Immaterial.

Measurements (Fig 4D–5 and Table 4D–2)

AB = Line of axis of the shaft of the humerus.
CD = Line of axis of the shaft of the ulna.
 EF = Transverse line drawn tangentially to the most distal points of the articular surfaces of the trochlea and capitellum.
CA = The carrying angle formed by the intersection of AB and CD, measured on the radial side.
HA = The humeral angle formed by the intersection of AB and EF.
UA = The ulnar angle formed by the intersection of CD and EF.

Source of Material
   The data have been derived from a study of 50 normal subjects, equally divided between males and females ranging in age from 21 to 66 years.

*Ref: Keats TE, et al: *Radiology* 1966; 87:904.

DETECTION OF SUPRACONDYLAR FRACTURES
OF THE HUMERUS*

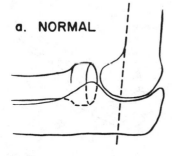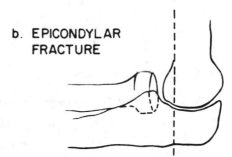

FIG 4D−6.
Use of anterior humeral cortical line in detection of supracondylar fracture. (From Nelson SW: *Radiol Clin North Am* 1966; 4:241. Used by permission.)

Technique
Central ray: Perpendicular to plane of film.
Position: True lateral with elbow flexed.
Target-film distance: Immaterial.

Measurements (Fig 4D−6)
In the normal lateral projection, a line drawn along the anterior cortex of the humerus and extended through its condyles will intersect a substantial portion of the condyles anteriorly and only a small portion posteriorly. When a supracondylar fracture is present, the anterior cortical line will intersect only a small portion of the condyles anteriorly and a larger portion posteriorly.

Source of Material
None given. Based on Nelson's extensive experience in this field.

*Ref: Nelson SW: *Radiol Clin North Am* 1966; 4:241.

DETECTION OF DISLOCATION OF
THE RADIAL HEAD*

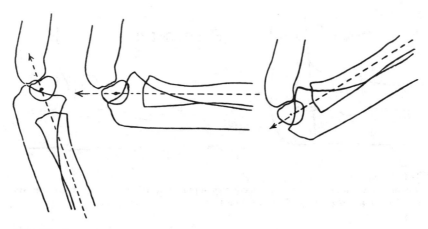

FIG 4D–7.
(From Storen G: *Acta Chir Scand* 1959; 116:144. Used by permission.

Technique
Central ray: Perpendicular to plane of film centered over joint.
Position: Lateral with elbow flexed.
Target film-distance: Immaterial.

Measurements (Fig 4D–7)
In the lateral projection, a line extending the radial axis should pass through the center of the capitellum in all stages of flexion of the elbow. This relationship is particularly useful in children, in whom the epiphyseal ossification centers have not yet appeared, the gap between the bone ends is wide, and the relationships between the bone ends are difficult to determine.

Source of Material
The data are based on the study of approximately 40 patients.

*Ref: Storen G: *Acta Chir Scand* 1959; 116:144.

MEASUREMENT OF THE AXIAL ANGLES
AT THE WRIST*

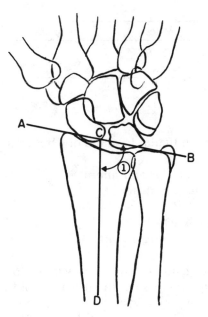

FIG 4D–8.

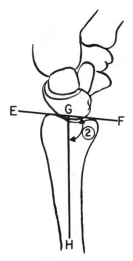

FIG 4D–9.

*Ref: Keats TE, et al: *Radiology* 1966; 87:904.

MEASUREMENT OF THE AXIAL ANGLES
AT THE WRIST*

TABLE 4D–3.

	Males	Females	Average
Angle *1*	72°–93°	73°–95°	83°
Angle 2	79°–93°	80°–94°	85.5°

Technique
    Central ray: Perpendicular to plane of film projected over the navicular bone.
    Position: Posteroanterior and lateral.
    Target-film distance: Immaterial.

Measurements (Table 4D–3)
1. Posteroanterior view (Fig 4D–8):

AB = Line drawn tangentially from the distal tip of the radial styloid process through the base of the ulnar styloid process.
CD = Line drawn along the midshaft of the radius.
Angle *1* = The angle of intersection of *AB* and *CD* measured on the ulnar side.

  2. Lateral view (Fig 4D–9):

EF = Line drawn tangentially across the most distal points of the articular surface of the radius.
GH = Line drawn through the midshaft of the radius.
Angle *2* = The angle of intersection of *EF* and *GH* measured anteriorly.

Source of Material
    The data are based on a study of 50 normal adult subjects, equally divided between males and females ranging in age from 18 to 75 years.

Ref: Keats TE, et al: *Radiology* 1966; 87:904.

MEASUREMENT OF WRIST FLEXION
AND EXTENSION*

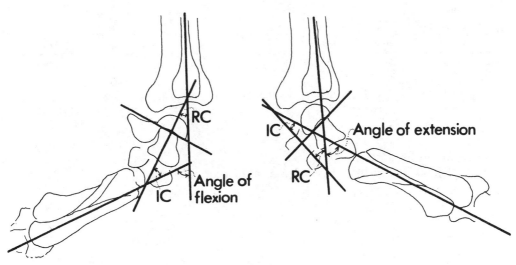

FIG 4D–10.
(Adapted from Brumfield RH, Nickel VL, Nickel E: *South Med J* 1966; 59:909. Used by permission.)

Technique
   Central ray: Perpendicular to plane of film projected over the navicular bone.
   Position: True lateral in full flexion, neutral and full extension.
   Target-film distance: Immaterial.

Measurements (Fig 4D–10 and Table 4D–4)

1. The longitudinal axes of the radius and second metacarpal are drawn. The angles are measured as shown in Figure 4D–10. Total wrist motion is flexion plus extension.
2. The main axes of the lunate are determined by a line on the intercarpal face and a second line drawn at 90° to the first line.
3. The radiocarpal angle (RC) and intercarpal angle (IC) are drawn as shown in Figure 4D–10.

Ref: Brumfield RH, Nickel VL, Nickel E: *South Med J* 1966; 59:909.

MEASUREMENT OF WRIST FLEXION
AND EXTENSION

TABLE 4D–4.

Average Values*

	Extension	Flexion	Total Motion	Radiocarpal	Intercarpal
Males	72°	79°	151°	60°	77°
Females	72°	84°	156°	65°	82°

*From Brumfield RH, Nickel VL, Nickel E: *South Med J* 1966; 59:909. Used by permission.

Source of Material
Ten healthy adults between 25 and 35 years of age.

MEASUREMENT OF THE CARPAL ANGLE*

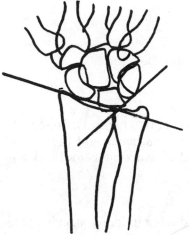

FIG 4D–11.
Measurement of the carpal angle.

TABLE 4D–5.

Age Trends, Sex, and Race Differences in Carpal Angle Percentiles*

		Carpal Angle in Degrees						
		Percentiles				Percentiles		
Age Groups	Sample Size	5th	50th	95th	Sample Size	5th	50th	95th
		White Males				White Females		
4–6	10	116.0	122.0	132.5	13	120.0	126.5	143.0
6–8	36	111.0	124.0	153.5	25	115.0	130.5	147.5
8–10	25	122.0	133.5	147.0	15	115.5	129.5	139.5
10–12	24	155.5	133.0	143.0	19	123.0	134.0	152.5
12–14	24	117.0	132.0	142.5	24	116.0	130.0	143.0
14–24	49	119.0	134.0	149.5	58	115.0	129.0	139.5
24–40	30	114.0	136.0	145.5	42	112.0	130.5	142.5
40–83	33	113.5	134.0	146.5	34	113.0	130.5	149.0
		Black Males				Black Females		
4–6	9	124.0	131.0	143.0	16	116.5	130.5	140.5
6–8	32	119.0	128.5	147.5	22	121.0	133.0	145.6
8–10	31	128.0	139.0	142.0	16	125.0	139.5	155.0
10–12	28	121.0	138.0	152.5	23	125.5	138.5	151.0
12–14	32	125.5	141.0	143.0	28	123.0	141.0	153.5
14–24	52	125.0	146.0	139.5	67	123.0	139.0	150.0
24–40	14	128.0	136.0	142.5	18	127.0	136.5	151.0
40–83	32	125.5	140.0	149.0	46	126.5	140.5	153.5

*From Harper HAS, et al: *Invest Radiol* 1974; 9:217. Used by permission.

*Ref: Harper HAS, et al: *Invest Radiol* 1974; 9:217.

MEASUREMENT OF THE CARPAL ANGLE

Technique
  Central ray: Perpendicular to plane of film.
  Position: Posteroanterior with hand in neutral position.
  Target-film distance: Immaterial.

Measurements (Fig 4D–11)
The carpal angle is defined by the intersection of two tangents, one touching the proximal contour of the navicular and lunate bones and the second touching the triangular and lunate bones. Normal measurements for black and white populations are given in Table 4D–5.

Source of Material
Data derived from hand films of 928 individuals randomly selected. The age distributions are given in Table 4D–5.

MEASUREMENT OF THE CARPAL AXES
FOR THE DETECTION OF LIGAMENTOUS
INSTABILITIES OF THE WRIST*

Technique
   Central ray: Perpendicular to plane of film.
   Position: True lateral, neutral position, and extremes of flexion and extension.
   Target-film distance: Immaterial.

Measurement (Fig 4D–12)
   A line parallel to the center of the radial shaft is its axis. The lunate axis is a line drawn perpendicular to the anterior and posterior distal lunate poles. The scaphoid axis is determined by a line drawn connecting the proximal and distal ventral convexities of the bone. The capitate axis is identified by passing a line from the center of its head through the center of its distal articular surface or the third metacarpal base.
   The application of these data for the detection of ligamentous instabilities is shown in Figure 4D–13.

Ref: Gilula LA, Weeks PM: *Radiology* 1978; 129:641.

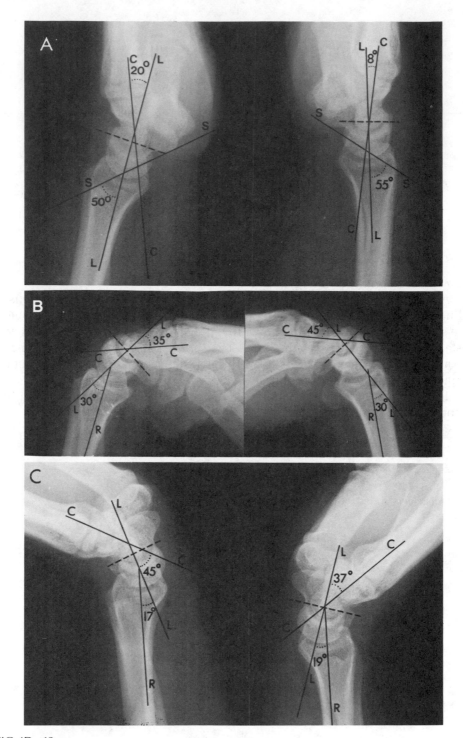

FIG 4D–13.
A, lateral views of the "instability series." Scaphoid (navicular) *(S),* lunate *(L),* and capitate *(C)* axes are drawn on these lateral neutral views. **B,** lateral flexion and **C,** lateral extension (dorsiflexion) views. The right wrist is to the reader's right. (From Gilula LA, Weeks PM: *Radiology* 1978; 129:641. Used by permission.)

MEASUREMENT OF THE CARPAL AXES
FOR THE DETECTION OF LIGAMENTOUS
INSTABILITIES OF THE WRIST

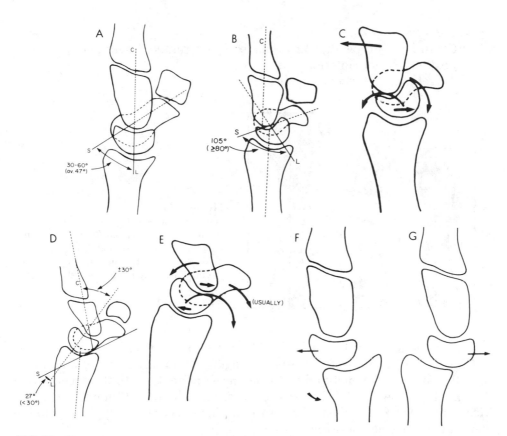

FIG 4D–13.

The axes of the carpal bone. **A,** the axes of the capitate *(C),* lunate *(L),* and scaphoid *(S)* bones are represented by the *solid* and *dashed* straight lines. A normal scapholunate angle is 30° to 60° with an average angle of 47°. The radius, capitate, and lunate axes in this diagram coincide. **B,** dorsiflexion instability can be diagnosed radiographically when the scapholunate angle is 80° or more. **C,** in dorsiflexion instability, the lunate has rotated or tilted so that its distal articular surface faces dorsally and the capitate is dorsal to the midplane of the radius. The scaphoid (navicular) stays in normal position, or its distal palmar tip moves toward the radius (tilts palmarly or ventrally). *Curved arrows* show the path of the carpal bone rotary motion. The *straight arrows* indicate the direction of bone movement or displacement. **D,** palmar flexion instability is diagnosed when the capitolunate angle is 30° or more or when the scapholunate angle is less than 30°. **E,** with palmar flexion instability, the distal articular surface of the lunate faces palmarly (ventrally) and the scaphoid usually tilts palmarly with the lunate. The central axis of the capitate lies palmar to the central radial axis, and the capitate may tilt dorsally. The *curved arrows* represent carpal bone rotation. *Straight arrows* indicate direction of bone movement or displacement. **F,** dorsal carpal subluxation exists when all the carpal bones lie dorsal to the center of the distal radial articular surface. The *curved arrow* indicates an impacted fracture deformity of the distal dorsal radius; the *straight arrow* indicates dorsal movement of the carpus (carpal bones). **G,** palmar carpal subluxation would exist when the lunate and other carpal bones lie palmar to the central axis of the radius. The *arrow* indicates palmar movement of the carpal bones. (From Gilula LA, Weeks PM: *Radiology* 1978; 129:641. Used by permission.)

METACARPOPHALANGEAL LENGTH IN THE
EVALUATION OF SKELETAL MALFORMATION*

Technique
   Central ray: Perpendicular to plane of film centered over palm.
   Position: Posteroanterior.
   Target-film distance: 36 inches.

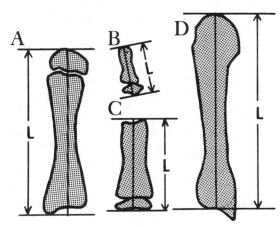

FIG 4D–14.
Length measurements of metacarpals *(A)*, distals *(B)*, and proximals *(C)*, made at right angles to the long axis and including the epiphysis, when separate. The exception is the third metacarpal, excluding the styloid process as in *(D)*. (From Garn SM, et al: *Radiology* 1972; 105:375. Used by permission.)

Measurements (Fig 4D–14 and Tables 4D–6 and 4D–7)
   All measurements were total bone lengths, including epiphyses and representing simple proximal-to-distal axial measurements, with the exception of the "hook" at the base of the third metacarpal, which is difficult to resolve. Measurements taken to the nearest 0.1 mm. The data are also applicable to the 39.37 inch (1 meter) focal film distance.
   These dimensions are useful in the construction of metacarpophalangeal pattern profiles for the evaluation of skeletal malformations, as described by Poznanski et al.†

Ref: Garn SM, et al: *Radiology* 1972; 105:375.
†*Ref:* Poznanski AK, et al: *Radiology* 1972; 104:1.

METACARPOPHALANGEAL LENGTH IN THE EVALUATION OF SKELETAL MALFORMATION

TABLE 4D–6.

Standards for Metacarpal and Phalangeal Lengths and Variability (Age 2–10)*†

Bones		2 Mean	SD	3 Mean	SD	4 Mean	SD	5 Mean	SD	6 Mean	SD	7 Mean	SD	8 Mean	SD	9 Mean	SD	10 Mean	SD
MALES																			
Distal	5	8.8	...	8.4	0.6	9.0	0.7	9.9	0.6	10.7	0.6	11.4	0.8	12.2	0.9	12.6	1.0	13.5	0.9
	4	9.2	0.7	9.9	0.8	10.5	0.8	11.5	0.9	12.3	0.9	13.1	1.0	13.9	1.0	14.4	1.0	15.3	1.2
	3	8.7	0.9	9.5	0.8	10.2	0.8	11.1	0.8	11.8	0.9	12.7	1.0	13.4	1.0	14.0	1.0	14.8	1.2
	2	8.2	0.5	8.8	1.1	9.1	0.8	10.1	0.9	10.8	0.9	11.6	1.0	12.4	1.0	13.0	1.0	13.7	1.1
	1	11.1	0.6	12.3	0.8	13.2	1.0	14.4	0.9	15.4	0.9	16.5	1.0	17.4	1.0	17.9	1.2	19.0	1.2
Middle	5	8.8	0.9	9.8	0.8	10.6	1.0	11.2	1.0	12.0	1.0	12.7	1.1	13.5	1.1	14.3	1.2	15.0	1.2
	4	13.5	0.9	14.5	1.0	15.8	0.9	16.7	0.9	17.7	1.0	18.7	1.1	19.8	1.1	20.9	1.3	21.6	1.4
	3	14.1	0.8	15.1	1.1	16.5	1.0	17.6	1.0	18.7	1.1	19.8	1.2	20.9	1.2	22.0	1.4	22.9	1.4
	2	11.2	0.8	12.3	1.1	13.5	1.0	14.4	0.9	15.3	1.0	16.1	1.1	17.1	1.1	18.1	1.2	18.8	1.2
Proximal	5	16.1	0.7	17.8	0.9	19.2	1.0	20.6	1.0	21.8	1.0	23.0	1.1	24.2	1.3	25.2	1.5	26.4	1.5
	4	20.5	0.9	22.8	1.0	24.7	1.2	26.4	1.2	27.9	1.3	29.5	1.4	31.0	1.6	32.3	1.9	33.9	1.8
	3	21.8	1.0	24.2	1.1	26.3	1.4	28.1	1.4	29.8	1.4	31.5	1.6	33.2	1.8	34.7	2.2	36.1	1.9
	2	19.5	1.0	21.9	1.2	23.7	1.3	25.4	1.4	26.8	1.5	28.3	1.6	29.7	1.8	31.4	1.9	32.5	1.9
	1	15.2	...	15.9	1.1	17.2	1.1	18.3	1.2	19.6	1.2	20.8	1.3	21.8	1.3	23.1	1.5	24.2	1.4
Metacarpal	5	23.9	1.0	26.3	1.5	28.9	1.9	32.1	2.2	34.6	2.2	36.7	2.1	38.8	2.5	40.6	2.5	42.7	2.9
	4	25.5	1.1	28.9	1.5	31.7	2.1	35.0	2.5	37.9	2.7	40.1	2.5	42.2	3.1	44.1	2.8	46.5	3.5
	3	28.6	1.3	32.3	1.8	35.6	2.3	39.3	2.8	42.6	2.9	45.3	2.8	47.6	3.5	49.8	3.0	52.3	3.7
	2	30.6	1.5	34.5	1.7	37.9	2.3	41.6	2.7	44.9	2.9	47.7	2.8	50.2	3.4	52.6	3.0	55.0	3.9
	1	19.6	1.3	22.0	1.2	24.1	1.6	26.7	1.6	29.0	1.7	30.9	1.8	32.7	2.1	34.4	2.1	36.3	2.3
FEMALES																			
Distal	5	7.8	0.6	8.4	0.6	9.1	0.7	9.9	0.7	10.6	0.8	11.4	0.9	12.1	1.0	12.7	1.1	13.5	1.2
	4	9.1	0.7	9.9	0.7	10.6	0.8	11.5	0.9	12.4	1.0	13.2	1.1	14.0	1.1	14.4	1.2	15.5	1.4
	3	8.8	0.7	9.9	0.8	10.2	0.7	11.1	0.9	12.2	1.3	12.7	1.1	13.5	1.1	14.1	1.1	15.0	1.4
	2	8.0	0.8	8.6	0.7	9.4	0.7	10.1	0.8	10.9	0.9	11.7	1.0	12.3	1.1	13.1	1.1	13.8	1.4
	1	11.3	0.8	12.5	0.8	13.2	0.8	14.4	1.0	15.4	1.1	16.3	1.2	17.3	1.3	17.8	1.3	19.0	1.6
Middle	5	9.0	1.2	9.8	1.1	10.5	1.1	11.2	1.1	12.2	1.2	12.9	1.3	13.6	1.4	14.2	1.4	15.2	1.6
	4	13.5	0.9	14.9	1.0	15.8	1.1	16.9	1.2	18.1	1.3	19.1	1.4	20.1	1.4	20.9	1.5	22.2	1.7
	3	14.2	0.9	15.6	1.1	16.6	1.2	17.9	1.2	19.2	1.3	20.3	1.4	21.4	1.4	22.1	1.6	23.6	1.8
	2	11.6	0.9	12.8	1.0	13.6	1.1	14.8	1.1	16.0	1.2	16.8	1.3	17.8	1.4	18.1	1.5	19.6	1.7
Proximal	5	16.3	1.0	17.9	1.1	19.1	1.1	20.6	1.3	22.0	1.4	23.1	1.6	24.4	1.6	25.2	1.6	27.1	2.0
	4	20.7	1.1	22.9	1.3	24.6	1.3	26.3	1.5	28.2	1.7	29.7	1.9	31.2	2.0	32.4	2.0	34.5	2.4
	3	22.2	1.2	24.5	1.3	26.4	1.4	28.3	1.8	30.4	1.8	32.1	2.0	33.7	2.2	35.0	2.2	37.3	2.6
	2	20.1	1.2	22.3	1.3	24.0	1.8	25.8	1.7	27.7	1.7	29.2	1.9	30.7	2.0	31.5	2.4	34.0	2.4
	1	14.9	1.0	16.3	1.1	17.2	1.3	18.8	1.3	20.2	1.3	21.4	1.5	22.7	1.6	23.5	2.0	25.5	2.1
Metacarpal	5	23.7	1.5	26.9	2.1	29.4	1.8	32.6	2.0	35.1	2.1	37.2	2.4	39.4	2.5	40.8	2.5	43.8	2.8
	4	26.0	1.9	29.6	2.7	32.2	2.0	35.6	2.5	38.4	2.7	40.5	2.8	43.1	3.0	44.3	2.8	47.5	3.5
	3	29.4	2.1	33.4	2.9	36.3	2.2	40.3	2.7	43.3	3.1	45.8	3.1	48.7	3.2	49.9	3.2	53.6	3.8
	2	31.3	1.9	35.2	2.7	38.2	2.3	42.2	2.7	45.6	3.2	48.1	3.3	51.2	3.3	52.6	3.4	56.6	4.1
	1	19.9	1.6	22.7	1.6	24.8	1.7	27.3	1.8	29.6	1.9	31.5	2.0	33.5	2.1	34.8	2.4	37.4	2.6

*From Garn SM, et al: *Radiology* 1972; 105:375. Used by permission.
†For each sex *n* ≅ 150 at age 4, 124 at age 9, 78 in adulthood, and 30–85 at intermediate ages. All values are in mm.

METACARPOPHALANGEAL LENGTH IN THE EVALUATION OF SKELETAL MALFORMATION*

TABLE 4D–7.

Standards for Metacarpal and Phalangeal Lengths and Variability (Age 11–Adult)*†

Bones		11 Mean	SD	12 Mean	SD	13 Mean	SD	14 Mean	SD	15 Mean	SD	16 Mean	SD	17 Mean	SD	18 Mean	SD	Adults Mean	SD
MALES																			
Distal	5	14.2	0.9	15.0	0.9	15.8	0.9	16.8	1.0	17.6	1.1	17.9	1.0	18.1	1.0	18.1	1.2	18.7	1.3
	4	16.1	1.2	17.0	1.3	17.8	1.4	18.8	1.3	19.6	1.4	20.0	1.3	20.3	1.3	20.0	1.3	20.5	1.2
	3	15.6	1.2	16.4	1.2	17.1	1.3	18.2	1.3	19.0	1.4	19.3	1.4	19.5	1.3	19.4	1.3	20.1	1.2
	2	14.3	1.1	15.0	1.0	15.7	1.4	16.7	1.2	17.5	1.2	17.8	1.3	18.2	1.3	18.1	1.3	18.8	1.4
	1	19.7	1.2	20.6	1.3	21.7	1.4	22.8	1.3	24.1	1.4	24.5	1.4	24.9	1.4	24.8	1.5	25.2	1.4
Middle	5	15.7	1.4	16.5	1.5	17.5	1.5	18.9	1.6	19.9	1.4	20.5	1.4	20.6	1.4	21.0	1.4	21.6	1.6
	4	22.6	1.5	23.6	1.5	24.8	1.7	26.5	1.6	27.7	1.5	28.4	1.5	28.7	1.4	29.1	1.5	29.6	1.6
	3	24.0	1.4	24.9	1.4	26.3	1.6	28.0	1.5	29.2	1.5	30.0	1.6	30.2	1.6	30.6	1.8	31.1	1.8
	2	19.8	1.8	20.4	1.3	21.6	1.6	23.2	1.5	24.3	1.5	25.0	1.5	25.3	1.4	25.6	1.7	26.1	1.6
Proximal	5	27.6	1.7	28.9	2.0	30.5	2.4	32.9	2.4	34.7	2.0	35.6	1.8	36.1	1.8	35.9	2.0	36.3	2.0
	4	35.3	2.0	37.0	2.4	38.8	2.8	41.6	2.8	43.7	2.6	44.9	2.3	45.4	2.2	45.2	2.5	45.5	2.3
	3	37.8	2.3	39.5	2.6	41.5	2.9	44.4	2.8	46.6	2.5	47.8	2.4	48.3	2.3	48.2	2.7	48.5	2.6
	2	33.9	2.1	35.5	2.4	37.2	2.6	39.8	2.6	41.8	2.2	42.8	2.0	43.3	2.1	43.4	2.4	43.7	2.2
	1	25.4	1.6	26.7	2.0	28.5	2.2	30.9	2.2	32.9	1.8	33.8	1.5	34.6	2.6	34.7	1.8	35.0	1.9
Metacarpal	5	44.6	2.8	47.1	3.2	49.1	4.0	52.2	3.9	55.4	3.6	57.1	2.8	57.9	2.5	57.5	2.9	58.0	3.0
	4	48.4	3.1	51.0	3.7	53.1	4.6	56.4	4.5	59.5	4.1	61.5	3.7	62.6	3.1	61.7	3.4	62.1	3.5
	3	54.6	3.4	57.3	4.0	59.5	5.1	63.1	4.9	66.7	4.4	68.7	4.1	69.7	3.3	69.0	3.7	69.0	3.8
	2	57.3	3.5	60.6	3.9	63.3	5.1	67.1	4.8	70.6	4.3	73.2	3.8	74.2	2.9	73.9	3.5	73.7	3.8
	1	38.2	2.4	40.2	2.7	42.5	3.0	45.1	2.8	47.6	2.6	48.8	2.3	49.5	2.1	49.4	2.7	49.6	2.9
FEMALES																			
Distal	5	14.2	1.3	15.0	1.3	15.4	1.3	15.6	1.3	15.9	1.4	15.9	1.4	16.2	1.3	16.0	1.2	16.2	1.2
	4	16.2	1.4	17.1	1.4	17.6	1.2	17.9	1.3	18.0	1.4	18.0	1.3	18.1	1.4	17.9	1.3	18.0	1.3
	3	15.8	1.3	16.6	1.4	17.1	1.4	17.3	1.3	17.6	1.5	17.5	1.4	17.6	1.4	17.4	1.3	17.7	1.3
	2	14.4	1.3	15.2	1.5	15.7	1.5	15.8	1.5	16.1	1.6	16.0	1.6	16.3	1.5	16.2	1.3	16.6	1.3
	1	20.0	1.7	20.9	1.7	21.4	1.6	21.7	1.6	22.0	1.7	22.0	1.7	22.1	1.8	22.0	1.6	22.1	1.6
Middle	5	16.2	1.7	17.2	1.7	17.9	1.8	18.1	1.6	18.4	1.7	18.5	1.7	18.5	1.9	18.6	1.7	18.7	1.7
	4	23.4	1.8	24.7	1.8	25.7	1.9	25.9	1.6	26.3	1.8	26.4	1.8	26.5	1.9	26.3	1.8	26.4	1.7
	3	24.9	1.9	26.2	1.9	27.2	2.0	27.5	1.7	28.1	1.8	28.0	1.9	28.0	1.8	27.8	1.8	27.9	1.7
	2	20.6	1.8	21.8	1.9	22.7	1.8	23.0	1.8	23.5	1.8	23.3	1.9	23.4	1.9	23.1	1.6	23.2	1.6
Proximal	5	28.7	2.1	30.5	2.2	31.9	2.2	32.3	2.1	32.9	2.2	32.8	2.3	32.8	2.3	32.5	2.0	32.5	1.9
	4	36.5	2.5	38.8	2.6	40.3	2.5	40.9	2.3	41.5	2.5	41.6	2.6	41.7	2.6	41.1	2.2	40.8	2.4
	3	39.5	2.7	41.7	2.8	43.5	2.8	44.1	2.4	44.8	2.6	44.8	2.7	44.8	2.5	44.2	2.4	44.0	2.3
	2	35.9	2.6	38.0	2.6	39.5	2.6	39.9	2.4	40.6	2.6	40.6	2.6	40.7	2.6	39.9	2.3	40.0	2.3
	1	27.2	2.3	29.2	2.4	30.6	2.2	31.1	1.9	31.8	2.0	31.7	2.1	31.9	2.2	31.3	1.9	31.4	2.0
Metacarpal	5	46.3	2.9	48.7	2.9	50.8	2.8	52.1	2.8	52.6	3.0	52.8	3.0	53.0	2.7	52.0	2.7	51.9	3.6
	4	50.2	3.8	52.8	3.7	55.1	3.6	56.2	3.6	56.9	3.6	57.2	3.9	57.2	3.5	56.1	2.9	56.0	3.5
	3	56.5	4.0	59.5	4.2	62.1	4.0	63.4	3.9	63.9	3.9	64.3	4.0	64.5	4.0	63.2	3.4	62.6	4.0
	2	59.9	4.3	63.2	4.4	66.2	4.2	67.4	3.9	68.1	4.2	68.6	4.3	68.9	4.1	67.5	3.4	66.9	4.3
	1	39.7	3.0	42.0	3.0	43.8	2.7	44.4	2.5	45.3	2.4	45.0	2.8	45.0	2.6	44.6	2.2	44.2	2.6

*From Garn SM, et al: *Radiology* 1972; 105:375. Used by permission.
†For each sex $n \cong 150$ at age 4, 124 at age 9, 78 in adulthood, and 30–85 at intermediate ages. All values are in mm.

*Ref: Garn SM, et al: *Radiology* 1972; 105:375.

METACARPOPHALANGEAL LENGTH IN THE EVALUATION OF SKELETAL MALFORMATION

Source of Material

Six hundred eighty-four metacarpal and phalangeal lengths were measured at the ages shown in Tables 4D–6 and 4D–7. All subjects were white and of European ancestry.

METACARPAL INDEX IN INFANTS

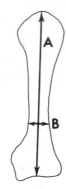
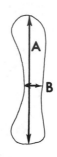

SECOND METACARPAL   FIFTH METACARPAL

FIG 4D–15.

Technique

   Central ray: Perpendicular to plane of film centered over palm.

   Position: Posteroanterior.

   Target-film distance: 30 inches.

Measurements (Fig 4D–15 and Table 4D–8)

1. Axial length: Place a ruler along center line of the shaft of the bone so that the shaft is divided into two equal part measurement *(A)*.
2. Minimal width of shaft measurement *(B)*.
3. Metacarpal index is calculated by measuring the second, third, fourth, and fifth metacarpals. The sum of lengths *(A)* is divided by the sum of widths *(B)*.

TABLE 4D–8.

Metacarpal Index During First 2 Years*

Age (mo)	Sex	Mean	SD
6	M	5.23	0.46
	F	5.60	0.37
12	M	5.30	0.41
	F	5.75	0.41
18	M	5.28	0.40
	F	5.82	0.45
24	M	5.40	0.43
	F	5.84	0.43

*From Joseph MC, Meadow SR: *Arch Dis Child* 1969; 44:515. Used by permission.

Ref: Joseph MC, Meadow SR: *Arch Dis Child* 1969; 44:515.

METACARPAL INDEX IN INFANTS

Patients with Marfan's syndrome had a metacarpal index of 7 or greater. In patients with Down's syndrome the metacarpal index is within normal limits.

Source of Material

Radiographs of both hands of 25 girls and 25 boys were taken at ages 6 months, 12 months, 18 months, and 24 months. The children were examined, were known to be healthy, and had been studied by Dr. Alice Stewart, Oxford University.

MEASUREMENT OF CARPAL LENGTH
IN CHILDREN*

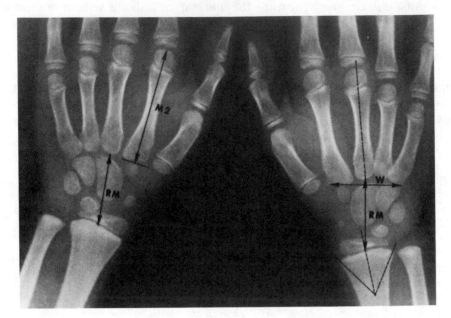

FIG 4D–16.
Measurement used in evaluating carpal and metacarpal size. (From Poznanski AK, et al: *Radiology* 1978; 129:661. Used by permission.)

*Ref: Poznanski AK, et al: *Radiology* 1978; 129:661.

MEASUREMENT OF CARPAL LENGTH
IN CHILDREN

FIG 4D–17.

Nomogram for determining relationships. (From Poznanski AK, et al: *Radiology* 1978; 129:661. Used by permission.)

Technique
Central ray: Perpendicular to plane of film.
Position: Posteroanterior.
Target-film distance: Immaterial.

Measurements (Figs 4D–16 and 4D–17)

RM = A line from the point on the third metacarpal to the midgrowth plate of the radius. The point on the metacarpal is defined as the intersection of the central axis of this bone with the proximal end. The midportion of the distal radius can be determined by observation or by using a bisected triangle superimposed on the distal radial growth plate. The intersection of the bisection of the angle with the growth plate determines the point.

W = A line joining the most radial point on the base of the second metacarpal and the most ulnar point on the base of the fifth metacarpal.

M2 = The maximum length of the second metacarpal.

MEASUREMENT OF CARPAL LENGTH IN CHILDREN

The nomogram (Fig 4D–17) is used for determining relationships between W vs. RM and $M2$ vs. RM. To determine how deviant a specific child is from the mean, a ruler is placed between the two points on the scales that correspond to these measures in the child in question. The intersection of the line with the central scales will give the number of standard deviations that this relationship deviates from the mean. Note that there are separate scales for males and females. For example, in evaluating RM against W, if, in a boy's wrist, W measures 36 mm and RM 28 mm, this wrist is quite small, being 4 standard deviations outside the normal limits. On the other hand, if both W and RM each measured 36 mm in a boy, then this child is exactly at the mean of the normal range.

These measures (or ratios) are useful in evaluating patients with juvenile rheumatoid arthritis and congenital malformation syndromes, because shortening of the carpus occurs in multiple epiphyseal dysplasia, the otopalatodigital syndromes, Turner syndrome, and arthrogryposis.

Source of Material

Five hundred thirty-nine hand radiographs of 280 boys ranging in age from 1.5 to 15.4 years and 259 girls ranging in age from 1.5 to 14.5 years.

METACARPAL INDEX IN ADULTS*

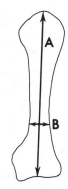 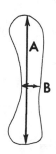

SECOND METACARPAL   FIFTH METACARPAL

FIG 4D–18.

Technique
   Central ray: Perpendicular to plane of film centered
   over palm.
   Position: Posteroanterior.
   Target-film distance: 30 inches.

Measurements (Fig 4D–18; Tables 4D–9 to 4D–12)

1. Axial length: Place a ruler along the center line of the shaft of the
    bone so that the shaft is divided into two equal parts *(A)*.
2. Minimal width of shaft *(B)*.
3. Relative slenderness of each bone = *A/B*.
4. Metacarpal index is calculated by averaging the relative slenderness
    of the second, third, fourth, and fifth metacarpals.

*Ref: Parish JG: Br J Radiol 1966; 39:52.

TABLE 4D—9.

Male Right Hand: Length, Width, and Relative Slenderness of Metacarpals, and Metacarpal Index*

Right Metacarpal		Mean (mm)	Range (mm)	SD	Coefficient of Variability (%)†
1	Length	46.20	41—55	±2.9	6.3
	Width	10.98	8.5—13.0	±1.03	9.4
	Rel. slend.	4.25	3.6—5.2	±0.42	9.9
2	Length	68.60	57—79	±3.8	5.5
	Width	9.47	8.0—11.5	±0.76	8.0
	Rel. slend.	7.29	6.0—8.6	±0.61	8.4
3	Length	66.40	59—75	±3.2	4.8
	Width	9.31	8.0—10.5	±0.68	7.3
	Rel. slend.	7.16	6.3—8.1	±0.50	7.0
4	Length	59.40	51—65	±3.0	5.1
	Width	7.61	6.5—9.0	±0.58	7.6
	Rel. slend.	7.85	6.4—9.2	±0.63	8.0
5	Length	55.30	49—61	±2.7	4.9
	Width	9.01	7.5—10.5	±0.76	8.4
	Rel. slend.	6.18	5.0—7.7	±0.57	9.2
Index		6.86	5.9—8.1	±0.45	6.6

*From Parish JG: *Br J Radiol* 1966; 39:52. Used by permission.
†Coefficient of variability = (SD/Mean) × 100.

TABLE 4D–10.

Male Left Hand: Length, Width, and Relative Slenderness of Metacarpals, and Metacarpal Index*

Left Metacarpal		Mean (mm)	Range (mm)	SD	Coefficient of Variability (%)†
1	Length	46.20	40–54	±3.1	6.7
	Width	10.93	9.5–13.0	±0.88	8.1
	Rel. slend.	4.24	3.5–5.1	±0.36	8.5
2	Length	68.60	63–78	±3.4	5.0
	Width	9.34	8.0–11.0	±0.77	8.2
	Rel. slend.	7.41	6.4–9.1	±0.59	8.0
3	Length	66.50	59–75	±3.2	4.8
	Width	9.22	7.5–10.5	±0.71	7.7
	Rel. slend.	7.25	6.3–9.1	±0.55	7.6
4	Length	59.40	55–66	±3.1	5.2
	Width	7.47	6.5–9.0	±0.56	7.5
	Rel. slend.	7.99	6.9–9.8	±0.60	7.5
5	Length	55.40	49–61	±2.7	4.9
	Width	8.68	7.5–10.0	±0.73	8.4
	Rel. slend.	6.42	5.4–7.7	±0.59	9.2
Index		7.02	6.0–85	±0.49	7.0

*From Parish JG: *Br J Radiol* 1966; 39:52. Used by permission.
†Coefficient of variability = (SD/Mean) × 100.

TABLE 4D–11.

Female Right Hand: Length, Width, and Relative Slenderness of Metacarpals, and Metacarpal Index*

Right Metacarpal		Mean (mm)	Range (mm)	SD	Coefficient of Variability (%)†
1	Length	42.70	37–49	±2.3	5.4
	Width	9.04	7.5–11.0	±0.74	8.2
	Rel. slend.	4.74	3.8–6.1	±0.42	8.9
2	Length	64.40	58–74	±3.2	5.0
	Width	8.02	6.5–9.5	±0.62	7.7
	Rel. slend.	8.06	6.7–9.2	±0.63	7.8
3	Length	62.00	57–69	±3.1	5.0
	Width	8.03	6.5–9.5	±0.62	7.7
	Rel. slend.	7.76	6.4–9.1	±0.62	8.0
4	Length	55.60	50–61	±2.8	5.0
	Width	6.38	5.0–7.5	±0.55	8.6
	Rel. slend.	8.78	7.2–10.7	±0.83	9.5
5	Length	51.50	46–57	±2.5	4.9
	Width	7.35	6.0–9.0	±0.61	8.3
	Rel. slend.	7.05	5.4–8.8	±0.63	8.9
Index		7.60	6.3–8.9	±0.52	6.8

*From Parish JG: *Br J Radiol* 1966; 39:52. Used by permission.
†Coefficient of variability = (SD/Mean) × 100.

METACARPAL INDEX IN ADULTS

TABLE 4D–12.

Female Left Hand: Length, Width, and Relative Slenderness of Metacarpals, and Metacarpal Index*

Left Metacarpal		Mean (mm)	Range (mm)	SD	Coefficient of Variability (%)†
1	Length	42.40	37–49	±2.3	5.4
	Width	9.04	7.5–11.0	±0.71	7.9
	Rel. slend.	4.71	4.0–5.9	±0.42	8.9
2	Length	64.00	58–73	±3.1	4.8
	Width	7.90	6.5–9.0	±0.57	7.2
	Rel. slend.	8.13	6.9–9.7	±0.60	7.4
3	Length	61.70	56–70	±3.1	5.0
	Width	7.87	7.0–9.0	±0.53	6.7
	Rel. slend.	7.87	6.7–9.4	±0.53	6.7
4	Length	55.20	50–61	±2.8	5.1
	Width	6.13	5.0–7.0	±0.51	8.3
	Rel. slend.	9.05	7.6–10.9	±0.80	8.8
5	Length	51.10	46–57	±2.5	4.9
	Width	7.10	6.0–9.0	±0.65	9.2
	Rel. slend.	7.25	5.2–8.7	±0.67	9.2
Index		7.78	6.8–9.0	±0.49	6.3

*From Parish JG: *Br J Radiol* 1966; 39:52. Used by permission.
†Coefficient of variability = (SD/Mean) × 100.

The metacarpal index is above the normal range in arachnodactyly and below normal in Morquio's disease, Weill-Marchesani syndrome, and familial streblodactyly. Parish suggests for arachnodactyly a dividing line between normal and abnormal at the 3 SD level of 8.4 in males and 9.2 in females.

Source of Material

Eighty-two female and 51 male patients between the ages of 21 and 45 years who were seen in the physical medicine department of Dryburn Hospital, Durham, England. Patients exhibiting bone or joint disease or congenital abnormalities of the skeletal system were excluded from the study.

RELATIVE PROPORTIONS OF THE BONES
OF THE THUMB*

Technique
   Central ray: Perpendicular to plane of film projected over palm.
   Position: Posteroanterior.
   Target-film distance: Immaterial.

Measurements (See Fig 4D–18 and Table 4D–13)
Measurements are made along the axis of each bone and the maximum length is used.

The ratio approach is more useful than comparisons with normal standards for length because it is not dependent on the size of the individual and a relative disproportion in length of bones is more easily detected.

Source of Material
Measurements are from the studies of Garn at Fels Research Institute, Yellow Springs, Ohio.

Ref: Poznanski AK, Garn SM, Holt JF: *Radiology* 1971; 100:115.

RELATIVE PROPORTIONS OF THE BONES
OF THE THUMB

TABLE 4D–13.*†

		Males				Females			
		Diaphysis and Epiphysis			Diaphysis	Diaphysis and Epiphysis			Diaphysis
		Adult	9 Yr	4 Yr	1 Yr	Adult	9 Yr	4 Yr	1 Yr
Met 2/Met 1	Mean	1.49	1.53	1.57	1.64	1.52	1.52	1.55	1.60
	SD	0.05	0.05	0.06	0.06	0.07	0.06	0.07	0.09
Met 2/P 1	Mean	2.10	2.28	2.22	2.13	2.13	2.25	2.22	2.15
	SD	0.10	0.12	0.11	0.11	0.12	0.13	0.11	0.13
Met 2/D 1	Mean	2.93	2.93	2.88	2.85	3.02	2.96	2.90	2.89
	SD	0.16	0.15	0.16	0.18	0.20	0.16	0.14	0.19
Met 1/Met 2	Mean	0.67	0.66	0.64	0.61	0.66	0.66	0.65	0.63
	SD	0.02	0.02	0.02	0.02	0.04	0.03	0.03	0.04
Met 1/P 1	Mean	1.41	1.49	1.41	1.31	1.41	1.49	1.44	1.34
	SD	0.06	0.06	0.06	0.06	0.05	0.07	0.06	0.07
Met 1/D 1	Mean	1.97	1.92	1.82	1.74	1.99	1.95	1.88	1.81
	SD	0.12	0.10	0.10	0.10	0.12	0.11	0.11	0.14
P 1/Met 2	Mean	0.48	0.44	0.45	0.47	0.47	0.45	0.45	0.47
	SD	0.02	0.02	0.02	0.02	0.03	0.02	0.02	0.03
P 1/Met 1	Mean	0.71	0.67	0.71	0.77	0.71	0.67	0.70	0.75
	SD	0.03	0.03	0.03	0.04	0.03	0.03	0.03	0.04
P 1/D1	Mean	1.40	1.29	1.30	1.34	1.42	1.32	1.31	1.35
	SD	0.08	0.07	0.07	0.08	0.09	0.08	0.07	0.09
D 1/Met 2	Mean	0.34	0.34	0.35	0.35	0.33	0.34	0.35	0.35
	SD	0.02	0.02	0.02	0.02	0.02	0.02	0.02	0.02
D 1/Met 1	Mean	0.51	0.52	0.55	0.58	0.50	0.51	0.53	0.56
	SD	0.03	0.03	0.03	0.03	0.03	0.03	0.03	0.04
D 1/P 1	Mean	0.72	0.78	0.77	0.75	0.71	0.76	0.77	0.75
	SD	0.04	0.04	0.04	0.04	0.04	0.05	0.04	0.05

*From Poznanski AK, Garn SM, Holt JF: *Radiology* 1971; 100:115. Used by permission.
†Met 1 = metacarpal of the thumb; Met 2 = second metacarpal; P 1 = proximal phalanx of the thumb; D 1 = Distal phalanx of the thumb.

MEASUREMENT OF COMBINED CORTICAL THICKNESS OF METACARPAL* AND HUMERUS† IN CHILDREN AND ADULTS‡

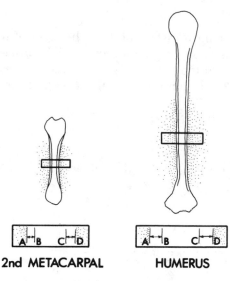

2nd METACARPAL   **HUMERUS**

C.C. T. = AB + CD

FIG 4D–19.

Technique

Central ray: Metacarpal: perpendicular to plane of film projected over palm.

Humerus: perpendicular to plane of film centered over lower third of humerus.

Position: Metacarpal: posteroanterior.

Humerus: anteroposterior.

Target-film distance: Metacarpal: 36 inches.

Humerus: 42 inches.

Measurements

1. Second metacarpal (right or left) (Fig 4D–19 and Table 4D–14). Measurements made at midshaft. C.C.T. = Shaft width (T) − medullary width (M).

2. Female humerus (left) (Fig 4D–19 and Table 4D–15). Measurements

---

*Ref: Garn SM: *The Earlier Gain and the Later Loss of Cortical Bone in Nutritional Perspective.* Springfield, Ill, Charles C Thomas, Publisher, 1970.

†Ref: Bloom RA, Laws JW: *Br J Radiol* 1970; 43:522.

‡Ref: Virtama P, Helelä T: *Acta Radiol* 1969; suppl 293.

MEASUREMENT OF COMBINED CORTICAL THICKNESS OF METACARPAL AND HUMERUS IN CHILDREN AND ADULTS

are made at the most distal point on the shaft of the bone where the endosteal borders of the lateral and medial cortices are parallel to each other and to the outer margins of the cortices. This is usually about 10 to 12 cm from the most distal end of the bone.

The combined cortical thickness (CCT) is the sum of the medial and lateral cortices.

3. Age-dependent variations of CCT of second right metacarpal bone in males (Fig 4D–20).

TABLE 4D–14.

Second Metacarpal Right or Left (See Fig 4D–19)*

Age	Total Width (T) (mm)		Medullary Width (M) (mm)		Cortical Width (C.C.T) (mm)	
	Mean	SD	Mean	SD	Mean	SD
Males						
1	4.50	0.34	3.04	0.45	1.46	0.30
2	5.11	0.44	3.24	0.62	1.85	0.39
4	5.53	0.49	3.04	0.62	2.48	0.37
6	6.05	0.53	3.06	0.66	2.98	0.44
8	6.57	0.54	3.13	0.66	3.43	0.45
10	7.16	0.59	3.28	0.66	3.88	0.49
12	7.73	0.65	3.43	0.72	4.29	0.60
14	8.52	0.77	3.63	0.72	4.89	0.68
16	9.11	0.72	3.81	0.75	5.29	0.51
18	9.31	0.68	3.56	0.90	5.75	0.66
30	9.36	0.68	3.41	0.81	5.94	0.43
40	9.35	0.50	3.72	0.83	5.63	0.60
50	9.65	0.88	3.84	0.93	5.81	0.63
60	9.69	0.62	4.44	0.84	5.24	0.62
70	9.38	0.58	4.61	1.05	4.76	0.73
80	9.07	0.51	4.23	0.62	4.89	0.56

MEASUREMENT OF COMBINED CORTICAL THICKNESS OF METACARPAL AND HUMERUS IN CHILDREN AND ADULTS

TABLE 4D–14 (cont.).

Age	Total Width (T) (mm)		Medullary Width (M) (mm)		Cortical Width (C.C.T) (mm)	
	Mean	SD	Mean	SD	Mean	SD
Females						
1	4.35	0.36	2.87	0.38	1.47	0.31
2	4.91	0.47	3.12	0.53	1.79	0.36
4	5.37	0.49	3.04	0.49	2.32	0.35
6	5.76	0.53	3.01	0.51	2.76	0.43
8	6.26	0.58	3.05	0.58	3.20	0.41
10	6.80	0.63	3.26	0.64	3.53	0.48
12	7.40	0.68	3.25	0.74	4.14	0.57
14	7.77	0.62	2.94	0.68	4.83	0.57
16	7.79	0.61	2.71	0.71	5.08	0.60
18	7.90	0.64	2.71	0.72	5.18	0.68
30	7.94	0.55	2.61	0.80	5.33	0.69
40	8.08	0.65	2.59	0.89	5.45	0.81
50	7.79	0.66	2.27	0.71	5.52	0.75
60	8.12	0.43	3.26	0.88	4.85	0.68
70	8.34	0.70	4.38	0.88	3.99	0.63
80	8.29	0.61	5.00	0.64	3.30	0.51

*From Garn SM, Poznanski AK, Nagy JM: *Radiology* 1971; 100:509. Used by permission.

TABLE 4D–15.

Female Humerus (Left) (See Fig 4D–19)*

Age Group	Mean CCT	SD
Teens	8.65	0.90
20–29	8.60	0.80
30–39	9.00	0.75
40–49	8.90	0.80
50–54	8.35	1.00
55–59	7.95	1.26
60–64	7.25	1.30
65–69	6.60	1.25
70–74	6.50	1.10
75–79	5.75	1.20
80+	5.50	0.75

*From Bloom RA, Laws JW: *Br J Radiol* 1970; 43:522. Used by permission.

MEASUREMENT OF COMBINED CORTICAL THICKNESS OF METACARPAL AND HUMERUS IN CHILDREN AND ADULTS

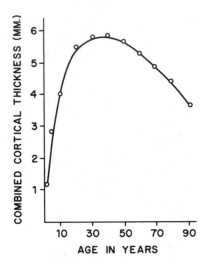

FIG 4D–20.
Dependent variations of CCT of second right metacarpal bone in males. (From Virtama P, Helelä T: *Acta Radiol* 1969; Suppl 293. Used by permission.)

Source of Material

Metacarpal measurements are from 734 patients in Garn's extensive studies on growth.

Humerus measurements are from 254 unselected female patients, King's College Hospital, London.

Note: Virtama and Helelä have published the results of their extensive studies on CCT in which 34 bone sites were measured in females and males between ages 1 year and 90 years who live in southwestern Finland. Figure 4D–20 shows an example of variation in CCT with age. Virtama and Helelä compared their results with those from Fels Research Institute for Human Development, Yellow Springs, Ohio, and concluded that the amount of cortical bone in the Finnish population is lower than that in the Ohio population.

Note: It should be pointed out that rotation of the limb at the time of filming may influence the dimensions of the cortex of the humerus and femur.*

*Ref: Horsman A: *Br J Radiol* 1977; 50:23.

MEASUREMENT OF BONE MINERAL DENSITY*

Technique

1. Single photon absorptiometry utilizes a Na (T1) scintillation detector and a 200-mCi I-125 source, held rigidly in parallel opposed geometry and motor-driven in a direction across the longitudinal axis of the radius.
2. Dual-photon absorptiometry utilizes a dual-photon bone mineral analyzer consisting of a whole-body scanner frame, a 1.5-Ci gadolinium-153 source, and a NaI (T1) detector.

Measurement

Normal bone mineral content of the radius by single photon absorptiometry is given in Figures 4D–21 and 4D–22.

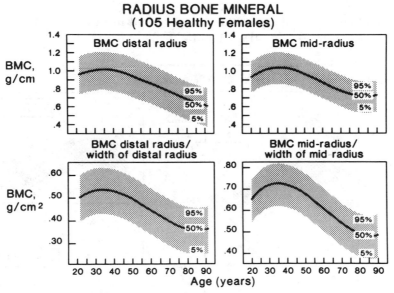

RADIUS BONE MINERAL
(105 Healthy Females)

FIG 4D–21.

Normal bone mineral content *(BMC)* at distal tenth of radius length and at midradius, in women at varying ages, from cross-sectional study performed by Wahner. Data are expressed as gm/cm (bone mineral content) and normalized (gm/cm²). (From Wahner HW, Dunn WL, Riggs BL: *J Nucl Med* 1984; 25:1241–1253. Used by permission.)

*Ref: Wahner HW, Dunn WL, Riggs BL: *J Nucl Med* 1984; 25:1241–1253.

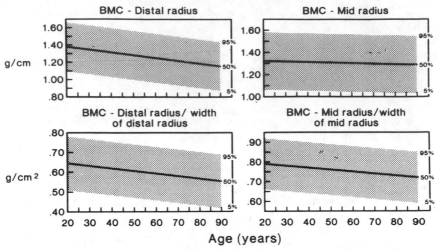

RADIUS BONE MINERAL
(82 Healthy Males)

FIG 4D–22.
Normal bone mineral content *(BMC)* at distal tenth of radius length and at midradius for men. See Figure 4D–21 for more details. (From Wahner HW, Dunn WL, Riggs BL: *J Nucl Med* 1984; 25:1241–1253. Used by permission.)

Normal bone mineral content of the spine and hip by dual photon absorptiometry is given in Figures 4D–23 and 4D–24.

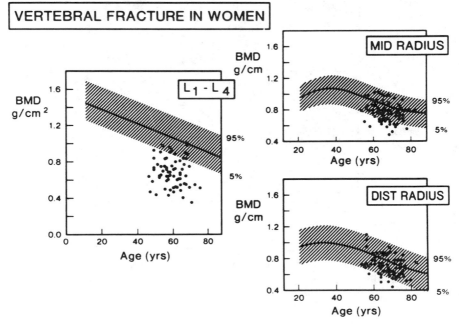

FIG 4D–23.
Bone mineral content in spine by dual-photon absorptiometry: in normal subjects *(shaded area)* and women with osteoporosis *(dots)*. Spinal data have been normalized to correct for loss of vertebral height occurring with lumbar fracture. Bone mineral in radius for comparison. (From Wahner HW, Dunn WL, Riggs BL: *J Nucl Med* 1984; 25:1241–1253. Used by permission.)

MEASUREMENT OF BONE MINERAL DENSITY

BONE MINERAL – HIP NORMAL VALUES

Bone Mineral (BM) g/cm²

Age (years)

FIG 4D–24.
Bone mineral content at three sites in proximal femur in normal subjects, obtained with dual-photon absorptiometry. (From Wahner HW, Dunn WL, Riggs BC: *J Nucl Med* 1984; 25:1241–1253. Used by permission.)

Source of Material

Data for the single photon measurements of the radius were obtained from 105 healthy women and 82 men. The data for the dual-photon absorptiometry of the spine and hip are based on a study of 187 normal subjects, 105 women and 82 men, ranging in age from 20 to 89 years.

The Pelvis and Hip

MEASUREMENT OF THE ADULT SYMPHYSIS PUBIS*

Technique
 Central ray: Perpendicular to plane of film.
 Position: Anteroposterior supine.
 Target-film distance: 40 inches.

Measurements

1. Width of the symphysis: The width of the symphysis was measured in its midthird, representing the width of the joint anteriorly. The mean transverse width was 5.9 ± 1.3 mm in males and 4.9 ± 1.1 mm in females.
2. Superior and inferior margin relationship: The upper margins of the pubic bones at the symphysis pubis were on the same horizontal plane in 97% of males and 89% of females. The lower margins were at the same level in 99.5% of males and 95% of females, which indicates that determination of malalignment is best made at the lower margins.

Source of Material
Data based on a study of 200 adult females and 200 adult males.

*Ref: Vix VA, Ryu CY: AJR 1971; 112:517.

AXIAL RELATIONSHIPS OF THE HIP JOINT*

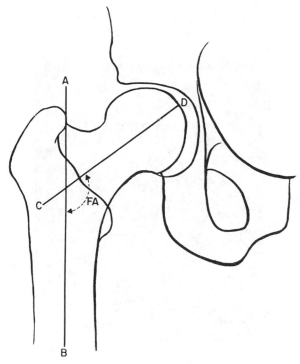

FIG 4E–1.
Angle *FA:* males 128°, females 127°.

Technique
Central ray: Passes through a point 1 inch below the center of the inguinal ligament perpendicular to the plane of the film.
Position: Anteroposterior. The patient is placed flat on his back with the toe of the foot pointing somewhat to the median plane.
Target-film distance: Immaterial.

Measurements (Fig 4E–1)

AB = Line along midaxis of femoral shaft.
CD = Line along midaxis of femoral head and neck.
Angle FA = Angle of the femoral neck at intersection of AB and CD.

Source of Material
The data are based on a study of 50 normal adult subjects, equally divided between men and women ranging in age from 19 to 76 years.

*Ref: Keats TE, et al: *Radiology* 1966; 87:904.

MEASUREMENT OF THE WIDTH
OF THE HIP JOINT SPACE*

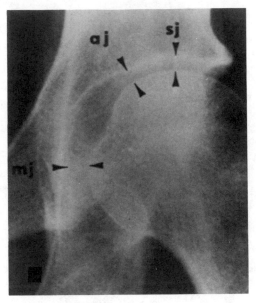

FIG 4E–2.
Joint measurements. (From Armbruster JG, et al: *Radiology* 1978; 128:1. Used by permission.)

Technique
Central ray: To center of pelvis perpendicular to plane of film.
Position: Anteroposterior.
Target-film distance: 40 inches.

Measurements (Fig 4E–2 and Table 4E–1)

SJ = Super or joint space, the distance from the femoral head cortex to the acetabular line at 90° from the horizontal.

AJ = Axial joint space, the distance from the femoral head to the acetabular line just lateral to the acetabular fossa.

MJ = Medial joint space, the distance from the femoral head cortex to the acetabular line along a horizontal line through the center of the femoral head.

*Ref: Armbruster JG, et al: *Radiology* 1978; 128:1.

MEASUREMENT OF THE WIDTH
OF THE HIP JOINT SPACE

TABLE 4E–1.

Medial, Superior, and Axial Joint Space (in Millimeters)*

		Medial	Average (Range) Superior	Axial
Total hips	≤40 yrs	8	4	4
		(4–13)	(3–6)	(3–7)
	>40 yrs	8	4	4
		(4–14)	(2–7)	(2–7)
Male hips	≤40 yrs	9	4	4
		(6–13)	(3–7)	(3–7)
	>40 yrs	9	4	4
		(4–14)	(2–7)	(2–7)
Female hips	≤40 yrs	8	4	4
		(4–10)	(3–7)	(3–7)
	>40 yrs	8	4	4
		(5–12)	(2–6)	(3–6)
Total male hips		9	4	4
		(4–14)	(2–7)	(2–7)
Total female hips		8	4	4
		(4–12)	(2–7)	(3–7)

*From Armbruster JG, et al: *Radiology* 1978; 128:1. Used by permission.

Source of Material
Analysis of over 300 normal anteroposterior hip radiographs.

ACETABULAR AND ARTICULAR CARTILAGE
MEASUREMENTS IN PERTHES' DISEASE BY MR*

Technique

1. 0.35 T superconductive magnet and a T1-weighted spin-echo sequence (700/30: repetition time [TR] msec/echo time [TE] msec).
2. 1.5 T magnet with a 600/20 pulse sequence.
3. Examinations performed with patients supine with the hips in neutral
   position. 10 mm thick coronal and axial sections obtained.

Measurements (Fig 4E−3)

Ref: Rush BH, et al: *Radiology* 1988; 167:473−476.

ACETABULAR AND ARTICULAR CARTILAGE MEASUREMENTS IN PERTHES' DISEASE BY MR

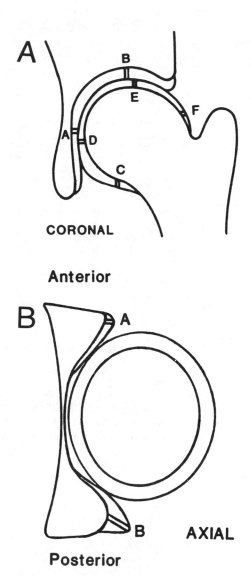

FIG 4E–3.

Measurement of articular and epiphyseal cartilage thickness. **A,** coronal view. A = medial acetabulum; B = superior acetabulum; C = inferior femoral head; D = medial femoral head; E = superior femoral head; F = lateral femoral head. **B,** axial view. A = anterior acetabular labrum; B = posterior acetabular labrum. (From Rush BH, et al: *Radiology* 1988; 167:473–476. Used by permission.)

The thickness of the femoral head cartilage was measured on the coronal image at four locations through the center of the femoral head. The superior and medial aspects of the acetabular cartilage were also measured.

ACETABULAR AND ARTICULAR CARTILAGE MEASUREMENTS IN PERTHES' DISEASE BY MR

The maximum thickness of the anterior and posterior aspects of the acetabular cartilage labrum was measured on the axial images.

The results of these measurements of both the normal and abnormal hips are given in Table 4E–2.

TABLE 4E–2.

Femoral Head Cartilage Thickness and Acetabular Cartilage Thickness in 20 Patients With Legg-Calvé-Perthes' Disease*†

Mean Thickness (mm)	Femoral Head Cartilage			
	Inferior	Medial	Superior	Lateral
Normal side	2.3 (18)	2.3 (18)	2.3 (17)	2.1 (18)
Abnormal side	5.2 (20)	5.9 (19)	4.2 (19)	5.0 (17)
Mean difference‡	3.2 (18)	3.4 (17)	1.8 (16)	2.8 (15)

Mean Thickness (mm)	Acetabular Cartilage			
	Medial	Superior	Anteroinferior	Posteroinferior
Normal side	2.4 (18)	2.9 (17)	2.2 (17)	4.0 (17)
Abnormal side	5.2 (19)	5.4 (20)	4.7 (18)	7.7 (19)
Mean difference‡	2.9 (17)	2.9 (17)	2.4 (17)	3.9 (17)

*From Rush BH, et al: *Radiology* 1988; 167:473–476. Used by permission.
†Measurements were made as shown in Figure 4E–3. Numbers in parentheses are numbers of measurements available.
‡Abnormal − normal.

The acetabulum-head index *(AHI)* and acetabulum-head quotient *(AHQ)* were used for evaluation of the degree of containment of the femoral head (Fig 4E–4). Measurements were made from the cartilaginous surfaces of the femoral head and acetabulum.

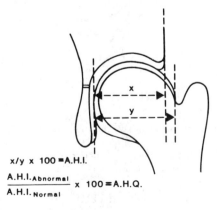

x/y x 100 = A.H.I.

$$\frac{A.H.I._{Abnormal}}{A.H.I._{Normal}} \times 100 = A.H.Q.$$

FIG 4E–4.
Assessment of containment of femoral head within the acetabulum. (From Rush BH, et al: *Radiology* 1988; 167:473–476. Used by permission.)

ACETABULAR AND ARTICULAR CARTILAGE MEASUREMENTS IN PERTHES' DISEASE BY MR

The AHI is a measure of the percent of the femoral head, with its cartilaginous rim, that is covered by superior acetabular cartilage. The results of these measurements are given in Table 4E−3.

TABLE 4E−3.

Degree of Containment of Femoral Head*†

| | AHI | | |
Case	Abnormal Side	Normal Side	AHQ
1	60.7	86.4	70.3
2	60.0	78.3	76.6
3	60.9	76.2	79.9
4	65.4	81.8	80.0
5	65.4	80.8	80.9
6	69.6	81.8	85.1
7	74.1	81.8	90.6
8	73.3	80.4‡	91.2
9	74.1	80.0	92.6
10	75.0	76.2	98.4
11	80.8	80.44‡	100.0
12	67.6	86.7	78.0
13	76.4	80.0	95.5
14	74.7	84.6	88.3
15	75.0	81.8	92.0
16	77.5	81.9	94.6
17	74.1	90.1	82.2
18	83.3	75.0	111.0
19	73.8	78.7	93.8
20	72.3	78.2	92.4

*From Rush BH, et al: *Radiology* 1988; 167:473−476. Used by permission.
†Degree of containment was determined as shown in Figure 4E−4.
‡Mean normal AHI used.

Source of Material

Data derived from 20 patients with Perthes' disease, ranging in age from 5 to 10 years, including 6 girls and 14 boys.

MEASUREMENT OF PROTRUSIO ACETABULI*

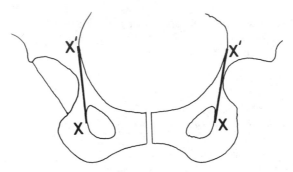

FIG 4E–5.
Adapted from Hubbard MJS: *AJR* 1969; 106:506.)

Technique
    Central ray: Perpendicular to plane of film centered over midpelvis.
    Position: Anteroposterior.
    Target-film distance: Immaterial.

Measurements (Fig 4E–5)
The outline of the dome of the acetabulum meets Köhler's line $X'X$. This line is drawn from the pelvic border of the ilium to the medial border of the body of the ischium.
    If the outline of the acetabular dome passes medial to line $X'X$, a protrusion exists.
    This method is applicable to serial roentgenograms of an individual patient but is not suitable for comparing patients.

Source of Material
The data are from 242 patients with a diagnosis of degenerative arthritis of the hip.

*Ref: Hubbard MJS: *AJR* 1969; 106:506.

THE ACETABULAR ANGLE
OF THE GROWING HIP*

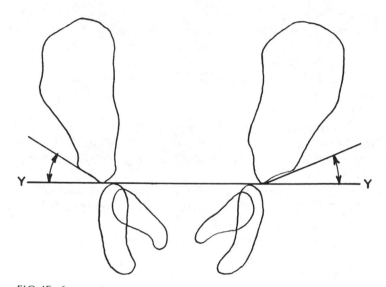

FIG 4E–6.

TABLE 4E–4.

Comparison of Acetabular Angles at Different Ages in All Categories*

	Mean Values (Degrees)			2-SD Range (Degrees)		
	Newborn	6 Mo	12 Mo	Newborn	6 Mo	12 Mo
White						
Male						
Right	25.8	19.4	19.1	34–17	26–12	26–12
Left	27.0	20.9	20.6	37–17	28–13	28–13
Female						
Right	28.3	22.1	20.5	38–18	30–14	28–13
Left	29.4	23.4	21.9	39–20	32–15	29–14
Black						
Male						
Right	24.8	21.4	20.5	34–15	31–12	29–12
Left	26.0	23.0	21.9	36–16	32–14	30–14
Female						
Right	27.7	23.9	22.5	38–18	32–16	30–15
Left	29.4	25.4	24.4	39–19	33–18	32–16

*Adapted from Caffey J, et al: *Pediatrics* 1956; 17:632.

*Ref: Caffey J, et al: *Pediatrics* 1956; 17:632.

THE ACETABULAR ANGLE
OF THE GROWING HIP*

Technique
Central ray: Perpendicular to plane of film centered to a point about 1 inch superior to the pubic symphysis.
Position: Anteroposterior.
Target-film distance: Immaterial.

Measurements (Fig 4E–6)
The acetabular angle is formed between a transverse line drawn through the right and left Y cartilages in the iliums (the Y-Y line) and an oblique line connecting the medial and lateral ends of the bony edge behind and above the acetabular face.

There are small differences in the left and right acetabular angles in all categories of patients (Table 4E–4.) There is also a distinct difference in size of the angles on both sides in females and males.

Congenital dislocation of the hip is all but unknown in blacks.

Source of Material
The radiologic findings were derived from 627 newborn infants, of whom 551 were later reexamined at 6 months and 527 at 12 months. This study did not include premature infants, children with Down's syndrome, children whose hips dislocated under observation, or children whose racial origins could not be determined accurately.

*Ref: Caffey J, et al: Pediatrics 1956; 17:632.

THE ILIAC ANGLE AND THE ILIAC INDEX OF THE GROWING HIP*

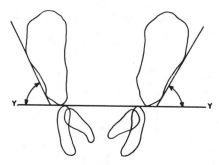

FIG 4E−7.

TABLE 4E−5.*†

Category	Mean	SD	2-SD Range	Actual Range
Acetabular angles in degrees				
Younger with Down's syndrome	16	4.5	25−7	29−9
Younger normals	28	4.7	37−18	44−12
Older with Down's syndrome	11	4.2	19−3	19−6
Older normals	22	4.2	8−14	34−8
Iliac angles in degrees				
Younger with Down's syndrome	44	6.5	56−30	58−35
Younger normals	55	5.5	66−44	67−43
Older with Down's syndrome	41	7.0	55−29	50−26
Older normals	58	7.0	72−43	74−44
Iliac indices				
Younger with Down's syndrome	60	9.9	80−49	87−48
Younger normals	81	8.0	97−65	97−68
Older with Down's syndrome	50	9.6	67−29	67−33
Older normals	79	9.0	96−60	101−62

*From Caffey J, Ross S: *AJR* 1958; 80:458. Used by permission.
†*Younger* means younger than 3 months; *older* means 3−12 months of age.

*Ref: Caffey J, Ross S: *AJR* 1958; 80:458.

THE ILIAC ANGLE AND THE ILIAC
INDEX OF THE GROWING HIP*†

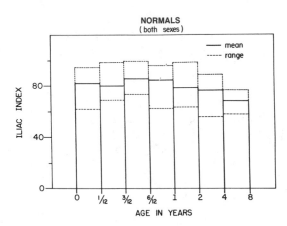

FIG 4E–8.
Variation of the normal iliac index with age. (Adapted from Astley R: *Br J Radiol* 1963; 36:2.)

Technique
   Central ray: Perpendicular to plane of film centered to a point about 1 inch superior to the pubic symphysis.
   Position: Anteroposterior.
   Target-film distance: Immaterial.

Measurements (Figs 4E–7 and 4E–8; Table 4E–5)
   The iliac angle is formed between a line drawn through the lower edges of the Y cartilages (the Y-Y line) and the oblique lines drawn through two points, the most lateral point of the iliac body below and the most lateral point on the iliac wing above.
   The iliac index is a combination of the iliac angle and the acetabular angle and may prove more useful than either single measurement. The iliac index is the sum of both acetabular angles and both iliac angles divided by 2. These measurements are useful in the diagnosis of Down's syndrome, where low values are obtained.
   Astley states that if the iliac index is less than 60 Down's syndrome is very possible. If it is more than 78, the child is probably normal. If it lies in between, only a qualified report can be given. If the index is between 60 and 68, Down's syndrome is probable, but a note must be added that 10% of normals occur in this range. If the index is between 68 and 78, the child probably does

Ref: Caffey J, Ross S: *AJR* 1958; 80:458.
†*Ref:* Astley R: *Br J Radiol* 1963; 36:2.

THE ILIAC ANGLE AND THE ILIAC
INDEX OF THE GROWING HIP

not have Down's syndrome, but a notation must be added that 6% of those with Down's syndrome do occur in this range.

Source of Material

Caffey and Ross's data are based on a study of 48 infants with Down's syndrome who varied in age from 2 days to 12 months and on a previous study of 1,500 unselected newborn infants in whom the pelvis and hips were examined roentgenographically.

Astley's study is based on 106 normal children from birth to 8 years and on 34 children in whom there was a clinical question of Down's syndrome.

CRITERIA FOR DETECTION OF ABNORMALITY
OF THE GROWING HIP[*]

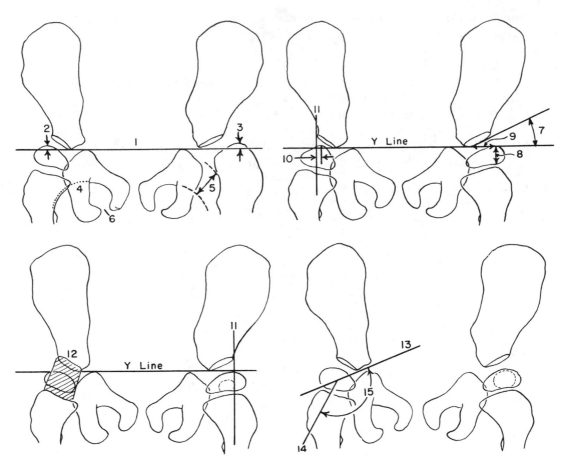

FIG 4E–9.
(Adapted from Meschan I: *Roentgen Signs in Clinical Diagnosis*. Philadelphia, WB Saunders Co, 1956.)

[*]Ref: Kohler A, Zimmer EA: *Borderlands of the Normal and Early Pathologic in Skeletal Roentgenology* (English translation by Case ST). Philadelphia, Grune & Stratton, 1956, pp 491–494.

CRITERIA FOR DETECTION OF ABNORMALITY
OF THE GROWING HIP*

Technique
Central ray: Passes through a point 1 inch below the center of the inguinal ligament, perpendicular to the plane of the film.
Position: Anteroposterior. The patient is placed flat on his back with the toe of the foot pointing somewhat to the median plane.
Target-film distance: Immaterial.

Measurements (Figs 4E–9 to 4E–11)

1 = Y symphyseal line, drawn horizontally through the cotyloid notches of the acetabula.
2 and 3 = Distances from the apex of the femoral head to the Y symphyseal line (1). Normally, these distances are equal.
4 = Shenton's line. Follows the upper arched contour of the obturator foramen, thus marking the lower margin of the pubic bone, and is continued as a regularly curved line into the lower border of the femoral neck.
5 = Break in continuity of Shenton's line, indicating dislocation or fracture.
6 = Fusion of the ischiopubic synchondrosis—may be delayed with dislocation.
7 = The angle of the acetabulum, the angle formed between a line from the cotyloid notch on the Y symphyseal line to the superior acetabular lip on that side. If this angle is more than 34° in the newborn or more than 25° in a child a year old, it may be said that a "steep acetabular roof" is present. (See also the section on the acetabular angle, page 297.)
8 = The diaphyseal interval, the distance between the diaphysis of the femur (which is conical in the period before ossification of the femoral head) and the Y symphyseal line. This distance should not be less than 6 cm.
9 = If in the newborn the distance of the pivotal point (point of intersection of line 8 and the Y symphyseal line) from the tip of the acetabular angle is more than 16 mm, the presence of a luxation must be suspected.
10 = This is the horizontal distance between the vertical line of Ombrédanne (see 11) and line 8. This distance is normally less than one half of the epiphyseal width (not illustrated).
11 = The vertical line of Ombrédanne, which intersects the upper jutting edge of the acetabular roof and is perpendicular to the Y symphyseal

CRITERIA FOR DETECTION OF ABNORMALITY
OF THE GROWING HIP*

line. The center of ossification of the normal femoral head lies below
the horizontal line and medial to the vertical line; in cases of
luxation, this center will be above and lateral, respectively.

12 = The parallelogram of Köpitz. A very near approach to a right angle is
normal; the head of the femur will be found very close to the center.
In cases of luxation of the hip, a rhomboid will be observed, and the
head of the femur will have an eccentric position.

13 = The guide line of the Y symphysis down from the center of the
acetabulum to the center of the head.

14 = The axis of the neck of the femur.

15 = The angle between 13 and 14, normally 120°–125°.

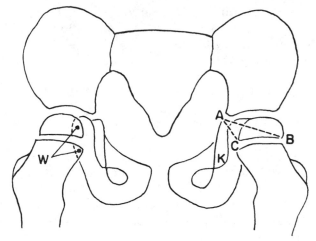

FIG 4E–10.
(Adapted from Meschan I: *Roentgen Signs in Clinical Diagnosis.* Philadelphia, WB Saunders Co, 1956.)

WW = Waldenström's overlap, a crescentic shadow formed by the
overlapping of the medial quadrant of the femoral head on the
posterior lip of the acetabulum. In normal hips the overlap
shadows are of equal size. If an inflammatory process is present or
an acetabular acclivity exists, the femoral head on that side will be
pushed laterally, diminishing the width of the overlap shadow.

K = Köhler's teardrop, the end-on view of the lower anterior acetabular
floor. The teardrops should be symmetrical bilaterally. See also
page 302.

ABC = Triangle formed by lines drawn from the cotyloid notch to both
margins of the femoral epiphyseal line. The sides of the triangle
should coincide with the triangle of the opposite hip. Inequality of
the two triangles is an early indication of anatomic imbalance and
hip-joint pathology.

MEASUREMENT OF THE BETA ANGLE
OF THE ACETABULUM FOR THE DETECTION
OF CONGENITAL HIP DYSPLASIA*

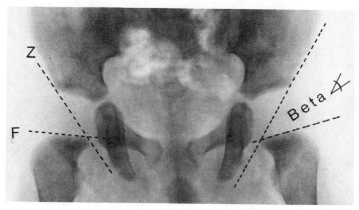

FIG 4E–12.
Measurement of the beta angle. (From Zsernaviczky J, Türk G: *Fortschr Geb Roentgenstr* 1975; 123:131. Used by permission.)

Technique
Central ray: Perpendicular to plane of film.
Position: Anteroposterior supine.
Target-film distance: Immaterial.

Measurements (Fig 4E–12)
The angle lies between a line drawn along the proximal end of the femur *(F)*, a line joining the edge of the femoral metaphysis and the edge of the acetabulum *(Z)*. The normal range is 50°–56°. Values above 56° indicate a definitely abnormal state in a child's hip joint.

Source of Material
Based on a study of 1,174 infantile hips.

Ref: Zsernaviczky J, Türk G: *Fortschr Geb Roentgenstr* 1975; 123:131.

DETECTION OF CONGENITAL DISLOCATION OF THE HIP BEFORE APPEARANCE OF CAPITAL FEMORAL EPIPHYSIS*

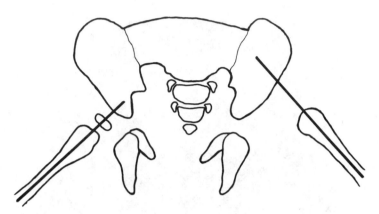

FIG 4E–13.

Technique
   Central ray: Projected over midpelvis perpendicular to plane of film.
   Position: Anteroposterior supine. The femora are abducted forcibly to at least 45° with appreciable inward rotation of the femora.
   Target-film distance: Immaterial.

Measurements (Fig 4E–13)
   The manipulation displaces the head medially, with the result that it is forced either into or out of the socket, depending on the presence or absence of dislocation, so that the head never assumes an intermediate position. If the hip is normal, the line of the femoral shaft will be directed toward the upper edge of the bony acetabular wall, but in the presence of congenital dislocation of the hip, it will point to the anterior superior iliac spine. Abduction should be 45° or more; otherwise, the roentgenograms may be misleading. A fair degree of inward rotation is also necessary because of the marked antetorsion of the femoral necks in newborns.

Source of Material
   This method is based on a study of 15,373 newborns, in which 14 cases of congenital dislocation of the hip were found (0.1%).

Ref: Andren L, Von Rosen S: *Acta Radiol* 1958; 49:89.

CRITERIA FOR DETECTION OF SLIPPED CAPITAL FEMORAL EPIPHYSIS*

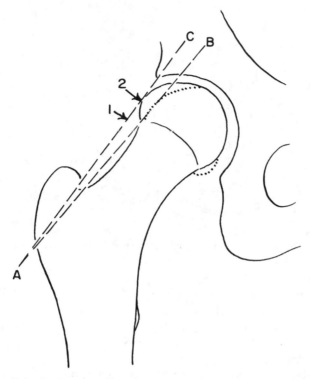

FIG 4E–11.
(Adapted from Martin HE: *Radiology* 1951; 56:842.)

AB = Line intersecting a superior lateral segment of the femoral head.

AC = Line tangential to the arc of the femoral head. When slipping occurs (*dotted line*), the head descends and the neck rides upward. Line *AC* therefore disappears, to overlie line *AB*, which is now a tangential line on the femoral head rather than an intersecting line.

1 and 2 = *Arrows* indicating the usual concavoconvexity at the superior epiphyseal junction.

Source of Material

These measurements were derived from the work of many investigators. The reader will find an extensive bibliography to these sources in the book by Köhler and Zimmer and in the article by Martin.

Ref: Martin HE: *Radiology* 1951; 56:842.

MEASUREMENT OF ACETABULAR DEPTH*

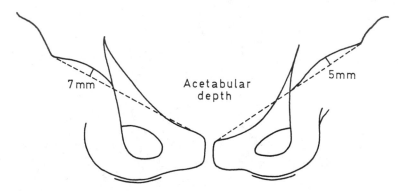

FIG 4E–14.
Measurement of acetabular depth. (Adapted from Murray RO: *Br J Radiol* 1965; 38:809.)

Technique
   Central ray: Perpendicular to plane of film.
   Position: Anteroposterior supine.
   Target-film distance: 120 cm.

Measurements (Fig 4E–14)
   A line is drawn between the edge of the articular surface of the acetabulum and the upper corner of the symphysis pubis on the same side.
   The average depth of the acetabulum in females was 12 mm, ranging from a maximum of 18 mm to a minimum of 9 mm. In males, the average was 13 mm, ranging from a maximum of 18 mm to a minimum of 7 mm. The mean figure was 12 mm. Murray believes that an acetabular depth of less than 9 mm is considered an imperfectly formed acetabulum, which may lead to osteoarthritis of the hip.

Source of Material
Based on a study of 25 males and 25 females, making a total of 100 hips.

*Ref: Murray RO: *Br J Radiol* 1965; 38:809.

EARLY DETECTION OF PERTHES' DISEASE:
THE TEARDROP DISTANCE*

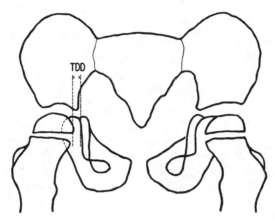

FIG 4E–15.

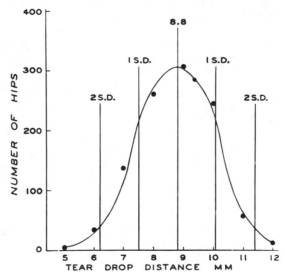

FIG 4E–16.
(From Eyring EJ, et al: *AJR* 1965; 93:382. Used by permission.)

*Ref: Eyring EJ, et al: *AJR* 1965; 93:382.

EARLY DETECTION OF PERTHES' DISEASE: THE TEARDROP DISTANCE

Technique
   Central ray: Perpendicular to plane of film centered over midpelvis.
   Position: Anteroposterior. Positioning does not alter the measurement,
   provided the femur is not rotated internally or externally more than 30°,
   flexed more than 30°, or abducted more than 15°.
   Target-film distance: 40 inches.

Measurements (Figs 4E–15 and 4E–16)
Measurement is made from the lateral margin of the pelvic teardrop to the medial border of the proximal femoral metaphysis. Measurements are independent of the age of the subject. The teardrop distance *(TDD)*, when greater than 11 mm, or more than 2 mm greater than that of the opposite hip, is a sensitive indicator of hip joint disease.

Source of Material
The data are based on a study of 1,070 normal hips of persons from 1 to 11 years and on 49 hips affected by Perthes' disease.

The Lower Extremity

MEASUREMENT OF THE DEGREE OF ANTEVERSION OF THE FEMORAL NECK

Direct Method of Budin and Chandler*

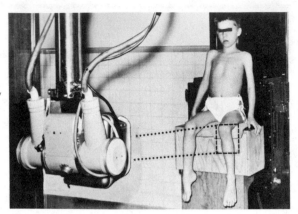

FIG 4F–1.
Position of patient in relation to the x-ray tube, showing approximate size of field. (From Budin E, Chandler E: *Radiology* 1957; 69:209. Used by permission.)

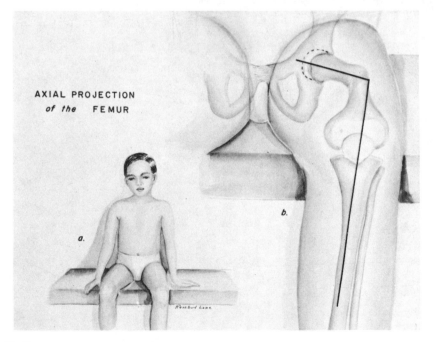

FIG 4F–2.
Axial view of femur, showing axis of the neck and tibial reference line. (From Budin E, Chandler E: *Radiology* 1957; 69:209.

*Ref: Budin E, Chandler E: *Radiology* 1957; 69:209.

MEASUREMENT OF THE DEGREE OF ANTEVERSION OF THE FEMORAL NECK

Direct Method of Budin and Chandler

Technique

1. *Central ray:* Projected along the axis of the femur, with the patient being rotated as is necessary. The beam is centered on the femoral neck (Fig 4F–1).
2. *Position:* The patient sits with knees flexed to 90° on a wooden box that has been placed on the footrest of the vertical x-ray table. In limiting the field size, it is important to include the upper third of the tibia on the film as a reference line (Figs 4F–2 and 4F–4) and yet narrow the field so that the gonads are completely shielded from the primary beam of radiation. This can be checked with boys by using a light-beam localizer; for girls, a field 2 inches wide is adequate. The use of a lead shield to cover the gonads will provide further protection. Repetition of examination should be avoided.
3. *Target-film distance:* 48 inches.
4. *Technical factors:* 100 ma, 6 seconds, 90–100 kvp. Because of the high ma value, this procedure probably should not be attempted on children more than 6 years of age unless they are unusually thin.

Measurements

This method consists of visualizing the femur in the true axial projection, with the coronal plane (or the bicondylar plane) defined by the axis of the flexed tibia, which is perpendicular to it. Only one plane is perpendicular to a line. It can be readily shown geometrically that the projection of the long axis of the tibia in any degree of flexion is always perpendicular to the bicondylar plane. Thus the actual angle that the femoral neck makes with the coronal plane is directly recorded on the film. This is illustrated in Figure 4F–3,A, where the horizontal line is perpendicular to the axis of the tibia and the angle of anteversion is the angle formed with this horizontal line by the axis of the femoral head and neck. A constant check on the adequacy of the positioning of the patient is the visualization of the cross-section of the upper femoral shaft on the film when it is taken properly.

Source of Material

The figures for normal degrees of anteversion (Table 4F–1) are averages adapted from reports of four different investigators and include measurements on 259 children and 54 anatomic specimens.

MEASUREMENT OF THE DEGREE OF ANTEVERSION OF THE FEMORAL NECK

TABLE 4F–1.

Normal Degrees of Anteversion, Showing Progression With Age*

Age	Anteversion (in Degrees)
Birth to 1 yr	30–50
2 yr	30
3–5 yr	25
6–12 yr	20
12–15 yr	17
16–20 yr	11
20 yr	8

*From Billing L: *Acta Radiol* 1954; Suppl 110. Averages adapted from several investigators.

Direct Method of Budin and Chandler

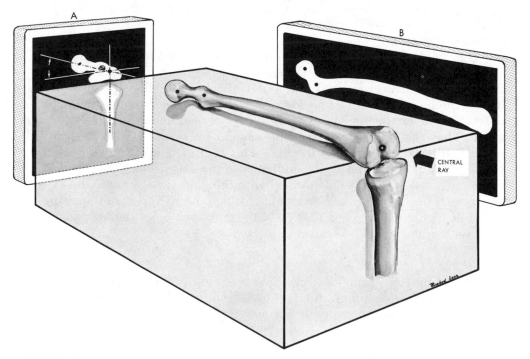

FIG 4F–3.
Femur and tibia in examining position in relation to central ray. **A,** cassette in position for axial view as projected, with angle of anteversion indicated. **B,** cassette illustrating angle measured on lateral view of femur. (From Budin E, Chandler E: *Radiology* 1957; 69:209. Used by permission.)

MEASUREMENT OF THE DEGREE OF ANTEVERSION OF THE FEMORAL NECK

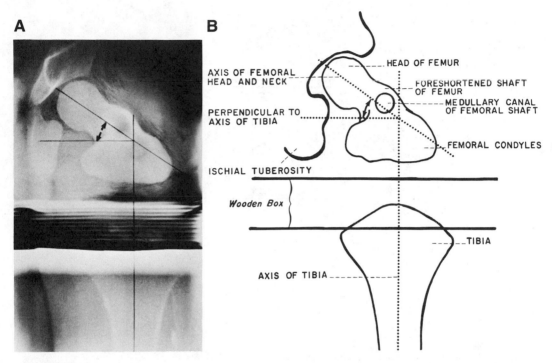

FIG 4F–4.
A, roentgenogram of left femur in axial projection, showing measurement of anteversion. **B,** diagram of anatomic parts seen in film. (From Budin E, Chandler E: *Radiology* 1957; 69:209. Used by permission.)

316

MEASUREMENT OF FEMORAL ANTEVERSION BY CT*

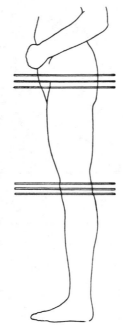

FIG 4F–5.
Diagram of locales from which sections were reviewed. (From Weiner DS, et al: *Orthopedics* 1978; 1:299. Used by permission.)

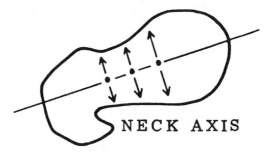

FIG 4F–6.
Drawing reflecting construction of cervical axis. (From Weiner DS, et al: *Orthopedics* 1978; 1:299. Used by permission.)

Ref: Weiner DS, et al: *Orthopedics* 1978; 1:299.

MEASUREMENT OF FEMORAL ANTEVERSION
BY CT

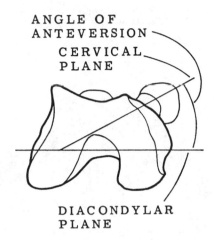

ANGLE OF ANTEVERSION

CERVICAL PLANE

DIACONDYLAR PLANE

FIG 4F–7.
Drawing of anteversion angle and diacondylar plane. (From Weiner DS, et al: *Orthopedics* 1978; 1:299. Used by permission.

Technique

1. The studies were performed on a Picker TR-120 prototype scanner. Slice thickness and other parameters not stated.
2. Several slices were taken through the femoral neck and femoral condyles.
3. No special device is required, just good immobilization.

Measurements (Figs 4F–5 to 4F–8)

1. Determine the axis of the femoral neck by connecting three points equidistant between the superior and inferior cortical surfaces.
2. Determine the axis of the distal femoral condyles by connecting two points at the widest flare of the condyles (diacondylar plane).
3. Photographs of the tomographic sections with marked axes are superimposed and the angle measured by a plastic goniometer.

The authors did not use the "table-top" method or condylar volume centers because of the variable shape of the condyles.

MEASUREMENT OF FEMORAL ANTEVERSION BY CT

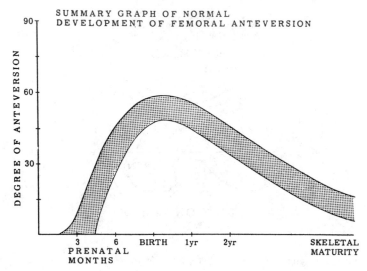

FIG 4F–8.
The ranges of normal anteversion. (From Weiner DS, et al: *Orthopedics* 1978; 1:299. Used by permission.)

Source of Material
Based on a study of cadaver specimens and 24 healthy subjects.

THE MUSCLE CYLINDER RATIO IN INFANCY*

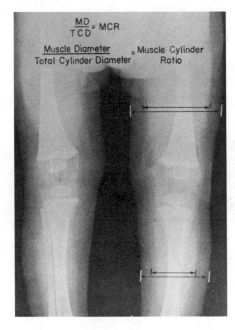

FIG 4F–9.
Determination of the muscle cylinder ratio. (From Litt RE, Altman DH: *AJR* 1967; 100:80. Used by permission.

Technique
    Central ray: Perpendicular to plane of film centered over extremity.
    Position: Anteroposterior supine.
    Target-film distance: Immaterial.

Measurements (Fig 4F–9)
    The muscle cylinder ratio (MCR) represents the ratio of muscle diameter (MD) to total cylinder diameter (TCD). In the normal infant, this ratio is between 0.64 and 0.72, i.e., the diameter of the muscle mass in the extremity constitutes approximately two thirds of the diameter of the limb. If this ratio is below 0.64 or above 0.72, the physician should be alerted to a group of disorders affecting soft tissues. See Litt and Altman* for this list of diseases.

Source of Material
Data based on a study of 300 patients.

Ref: Litt RE, Altman DH: *AJR* 1967; 100:80.

AXIAL RELATIONSHIPS OF THE KNEE JOINT*

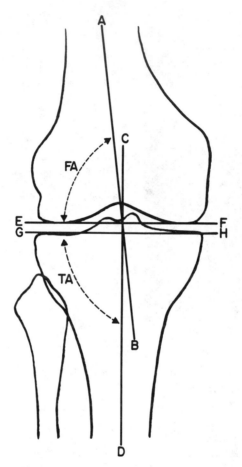

FIG 4F−10.

TABLE 4F−2.*

	FA	TA
Male	75°−85°	85°−100°
Female	75°−85°	87°−98°
Average	81°	93°

*From Keats TE, et al: *Radiology* 1966; 87:904. Used by permission.

*Ref: Keats TE, et al: *Radiology* 1966; 87:904.

AXIAL RELATIONSHIPS OF THE KNEE JOINT

Technique
   Central ray: Passes through a point about ½ inch below the tip of the patella, so that it will pass directly through the knee joint space, perpendicular to the plane of the film.
   Position: Anteroposterior.
   Target-film distance: Immaterial.

Measurements (Fig 4F–10 and Table 4F–2)

AB = Line drawn along the midaxis of the femoral shaft.
CD = Line drawn along the midaxis of the tibial shaft.
 EF = Line tangent to the articular surfaces of the condyles.
GH = Line tangent to the lateral and medial extremities of the tibial
        plateau.
FA = Femoral angle at intersection of AB and EF.
TA = Tibial angle at intersection of CD and GH.

Source of Material
   The data were based on a study of 50 normal adult subjects, equally divided between males and females ranging in age from 18 to 66 years.

SAGITTAL PLANE RELATION OF FEMORAL CONDYLES TO THE LONG AXIS OF THE FEMUR*

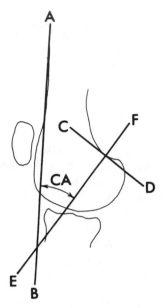

FIG 4F–11.
(Adapted from Lindahl O, Movin A: *Acta Radiol Diagn* 1970; 10:108. Used by permission.)

Technique
   Central ray: Projected through the knee joint space, perpendicular to the plane of the film.
   Position: True lateral.
   Target-film distance: Immaterial (Lindahl used 100 cm).

Measurements (Fig 4F–11)

AB = Line drawn along the anterior cortical demarcation of shaft of the femur.
CD = Plane for the floor of the intercondylar fossa (the intercondylar plane).
EF = Perpendicular to line CD intersecting line AB.
CA = Angle formed by roof of intercondylar fossa and long axis of femur.

   Mean value, 34.0° ± 0.5°; range, 26° to 44°. Right and left sides in same patient showed differences of 0.2° ± 0.2°.

Source of Material
Two hundred normal knee joints of 100 patients without knee complaints.

*Ref: Lindahl O, Movin A: *Acta Radiol Diagn* 1970; 10:108.

PATELLA POSITION IN THE NORMAL KNEE JOINT*

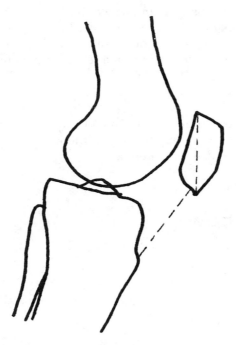

FIG 4F–12.
Measurement of patella and patellar tendon. (Adapted from Insall J, Salvati E: *Radiology* 1971; 101:101. Used by permission.)

Technique
Central ray: Perpendicular to plane of film central over joint.
Position: Lateral with knee semiflexed.
Target-film distance: Immaterial.

Measurements (Fig 4F–12)
The length of the patellar tendon was measured on its deep or posterior surface from its origin on the lower pole of the patella to its insertion into the tibial tubercle. The point of insertion is usually represented by a clearly defined notch that can be utilized as a point of reference if the tendon cannot be adequately visualized. The greatest diagonal length of the patella was measured.

It was found that these two measurements are approximately equal and that normal variation does not exceed 20%.

Source of Material
Data based on study of 114 knees without patellar disease.

*Ref: Insall J, Salvati E: *Radiology* 1971; 101:101.

MEASUREMENT FOR ASSESSING THE HEIGHT OF THE PATELLA*

This technique may be used in place of the preceding entry in those cases in which there is lack of definition of the posterior surface of the patellar tendon and loss of sharpness of the notch on the tibia, or in cases in which the lower limit of the tendon does not coincide with the notch of the tibial tubercle.

Technique
   Central ray: Perpendicular to plane of film.
   Position: Lateral with 30% flexion of the knee.
   Target-film distance: Immaterial.

Measurement (Fig 4F—13)

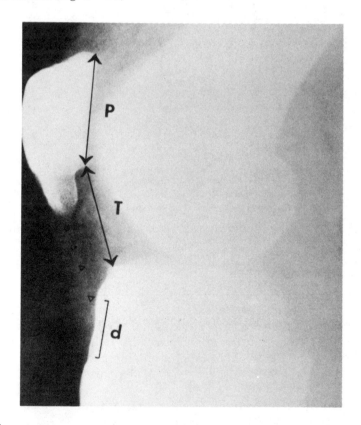

FIG 4F—13.
Low kv exposure radiograph illustrating an example of measurement of the distance (P) between the upper and lower limits of the articular surface of the patella, and the shortest distance (T) between this same lower limit and the tibial plateau. (From de Carvalho A, Andersen AH, Topp S, et al: *Int Orthop* 1985; 9:195—197. Used by permission.)

Ref: de Carvalho A, et al: *Int Orthop* 1985; 9:195—197.

MEASUREMENT FOR ASSESSING THE HEIGHT OF THE PATELLA

The ratio of T/P is calculated and the ranges for patella infera, normal, and patella alta are shown in Table 4F–3.

TABLE 4F–3.

Limits of Confidence of the T/P Ratio*

	Lower Limits (Patella Infera)					Upper Limits (Patella Alta)				
Levels of significance										
Two-sided	0.01	0.02	0.05	0.10	0.20	0.20	0.10	0.05	0.02	0.01
One-sided	0.005	0.01	0.025	0.05	0.10	0.10	0.05	0.025	0.01	0.005
T/P ratio	0.56	0.59	0.64	0.68	0.72	1.06	1.11	1.15	1.20	1.23

*From de Carvalho A, Andersen AH, Topp S, et al: *Int Orthop* 1985; 9:195–197. Used by permission.

Source of Material

Data derived from a study of 150 subjects without knee complaints, ages 20 to 60 years.

MEASUREMENTS OF RELATIONSHIPS OF THE PATELLOFEMORAL JOINT*

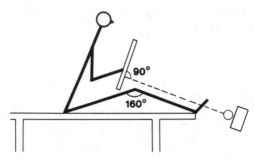

FIG 4F–14.
Roentgen technique. (From Laurin CA, et al: *Clin Orthop* 1979; 144:16. Used by permission.)

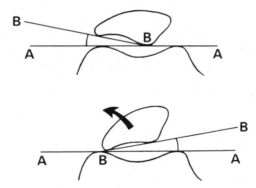

FIG 4F–15.
The lateral patellofemoral angle. (From Laurin CA, et al: *Clin Orthop* 1979; 144:16. Used by permission.)

Ref: Laurin CA, et al: *Clin Orthop* 1979; 144:16.

MEASUREMENTS OF RELATIONSHIPS OF THE PATELLOFEMORAL JOINT

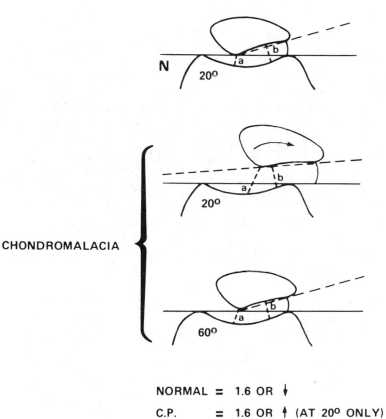

NORMAL = 1.6 OR ↓

C.P. = 1.6 OR ↑ (AT 20° ONLY)

FIG 4F–16.
The patellofemoral index. (From Laurin CA, et al: *Clin Orthop* 1979; 144:16. Used by permission.)

Technique (Figs 4F–14 to 4F–16)

Central ray: Directed parallel to the anterior border of the tibia and the patellofemoral space perpendicular to film.

Position: Patient seated with knees in 20° of flexion. The feet are plantar flexed.

Target-film distance: Immaterial.

MEASUREMENTS OF RELATIONSHIPS OF THE PATELLOFEMORAL JOINT

Measurements

1. The lateral patellofemoral angle (Fig 4F–15). The drawing is that of a left knee, and the left side of the drawing is the lateral side of the knee. Line *AA* joins the summits of the femoral condyles. Line *BB* joins the limits of the lateral patellar facet. The angle lies above line *AA* and, when normal, is always open laterally. In instances of patellar tilt with subluxation *(below)*, the lateral patellofemoral angle is open medially or the lines are parallel.
2. The patellofemoral index (Fig 4F–16). The index corresponds to the ratio of the thickness of the medial patellofemoral interspace *(a)* over the lateral patellofemoral interspaces *(b)*. In normal individuals, this ratio is 1.6, because the medial patellofemoral interspace is equal to or slightly greater than the lateral patellofemoral interspace. In patients with chondromalacia patellae, there is tilt of the patella with an increase in the medial interspace, and the patellofemoral index will be more than 1.6.

Source of Material

Normal measurements determined from 100 normal patients and 100 patients with chondromalacia patellae and 30 patients with patellar subluxation.

MEASUREMENT OF THE METAPHYSEAL-DIAPHYSEAL ANGLE FOR THE DIFFERENTIATION OF PHYSIOLOGIC BOWING OF THE KNEES AND TIBIA VARA*

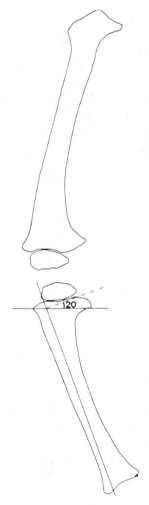

FIG 4F–17.
Tibia vara, the metaphyseal angle. (From Levine AM, Drennan JC: *J Bone Joint Surg* 1982; 64A:1158. Used by permission.)

Ref: Levine AM, Drennan JC: *J Bone Joint Surg* 1982; 64A:1158.

MEASUREMENT OF THE METAPHYSEAL-DIAPHYSEAL ANGLE FOR THE DIFFERENTIATION OF PHYSIOLOGIC BOWING OF THE KNEES AND TIBIA VARA

Technique
   Central ray: Centered over knees.
   Position: Anteroposterior standing.
   Target-film distance: Immaterial.

Measurement (Fig 4F—17 and Table 4F—4)
A line is drawn perpendicular to the longitudinal axis of the tibia, and another is drawn through the two beaks of the metaphysis to determine the transverse axis of the tibial metaphysis. The metaphyseal-diaphyseal angle is bisected by those two lines.

TABLE 4F—4.

Results

	Metaphyseal-Diaphyseal Angle (Degrees)	
	Average	Range
Physiologic bowing (age)		
11—20 mo	5.1 ± 2.8	0—11
21—30 mo	3.7 ± 3.1	0—10
Tibia vara (age)		
11—20 mo	16.4 ± 4.3	8—22
21—30 mo	13.7 ± 4.3	7—22

The author's data show that in 29 of 30 affected extremities with an initial metaphyseal-diaphyseal angle of more than 11.0 degrees, radiographic changes of tibia vara developed. However, only 3 of 58 extremities with a metaphyseal-diaphyseal angle of 11.0 degrees or less later had any of the diagnostic changes. This measurement allows accurate early diagnosis of bow-leg deformity.

Source of Material
Data based on 52 limbs of children with physiologic bowing and 32 limbs of children with tibia vara (Blount's disease).

MEASUREMENT OF THE TIBIAL PLATEAU ANGLE FOR DETERMINATION OF DEPRESSION DUE TO FRACTURE*

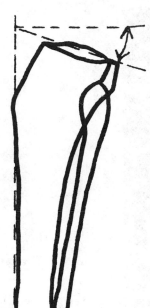

FIG 4F—18.
Method of measuring plateau angle. (Adapted from Moore TM, et al: *J Bone Joint Surg* 1974; 56A:155. Used by permission.)

Technique
Central ray: Perpendicular to plane of film centered over joint.
Position: Lateral.
Target-film distance: Immaterial.

Measurements (Fig 4F—18)
The angle of the tibial plateau is defined by a line drawn tangential to the tibial crest, a second line tangential to the proximal tibial articular surfaces, and a third line perpendicular to the tibial crest line. The interval found between the second and third lines defines the angle.

The normal angles range from 7° to 22° with a mean of 14° and a standard deviation of ± 3.6°. This angle is useful in determining the degree of depression of the tibial plateau due to fracture.

Source of Material
Data based on a study of 50 true lateral roentgenograms of normal knees.

*Ref: Moore TM, et al: *J Bone Joint Surg* 1974; 56A:155.

MEASUREMENT OF TIBIAL TORSION BY CT*

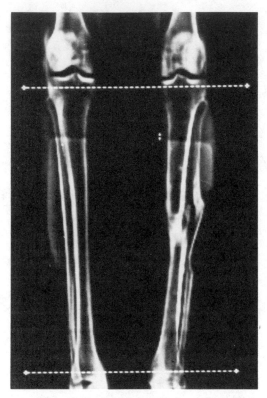

FIG 4F–19.
AP digital two-dimensional image (topogram) for determination of the proximal and distal planes of reference reduces the number of scans required. (From Jend HH, et al: *Acta Radiol Diagn* 1981; 22:271. Used by permission.)

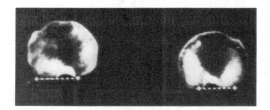

FIG 4F–20.
Axial CT image of the proximal tibiae just above the head of the fibula. The *tangent* to the dorsal border forms the proximal line of reference. (From Jend HH, et al: *Acta Radiol Diagn* 1981; 22:271. Used by permission.)

Ref: Jend HH, et al: *Acta Radiologic Diagn* 1981; 22:271.

MEASUREMENT OF TIBIAL TORSION BY CT

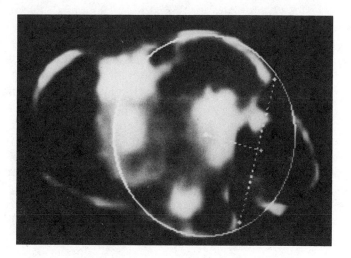

FIG 4F–21.
Axial scan of the left distal tibia just above the talocrural joint space. The distal line of reference is formed by the *pilon centerpoint,* i.e., the midpoint of the circle that fits into the tibial pilon, includes the fibular notch of the tibia but excludes the medial malleolus, and the midpoint of a line over the fibular notch. (From Jend HH, et al: *Acta Radiol Diagn* 1981; 22:271. Used by permission.)

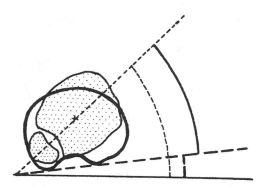

FIG 4F–22.
Proximal line of reference *(small dashes)* and distal line of reference *(large dashes)* form an angle with the horizontal line. Subtraction of the proximal from the distal angle results in the angle of tibial torsion *(solid arc).* (From Jend HH, et al: *Acta Radiol Diagn* 1981; 22:271. Used by permission.)

MEASUREMENT OF TIBIAL TORSION BY CT

Technique

1. Delta-Scan FS (Technicare) or Somatom 2 (Siemens). Scanning parameters not stated.
2. Patient was placed in supine position and two-dimensional localization image obtained. Transverse sections were taken through the proximal tibia and the distal tibia near the talocrural joint.
3. No special devices required, but the stretched legs are immobilized.

Measurement (Figs 4F—19 to 4F—23)

A tangent to the dorsal border of the proximal tibia forms the proximal line of reference.

The distal lines of reference are formed by joining the center of a circle outlining the distal tibia and fibular notch (excluding the medial malleolus bulge) to the midpoint of the fibular notch in the tibia. All lines, circles, and angles are formed on the computer image, but can be performed manually.

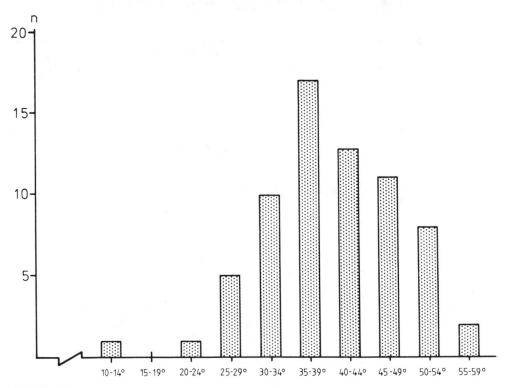

FIG 4F—23.
Distribution of angles of tibial torsion in mean value 40° ± 9°. (From Jend HH, et al: *Acta Radiol Diagn* 1981; 22:271. Used by permission.)

MEASUREMENT OF TIBIAL TORSION BY CT

Source of Material

Seventy healthy limbs in 61 patients of both sexes. Ages were not stated; patients were all adults.

MEASUREMENT OF THE AXIAL ANGLES
OF THE ANKLE*

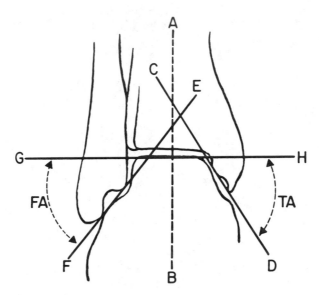

FIG 4F—24.

TABLE 4F—5.*

	Males	Females	Average
FA	45°–63°	43°–62°	52°
TA	45°–61°	49°–65°	53°

*From Keats TE, et al: *Radiology* 1966; 87:904. Used by permission.

Technique

    Central ray: Perpendicular to plane of film projected through the center of the talotibial joint.

    Position: Anteroposterior, with great toe pointing slightly medially.

    Target-film distance: Immaterial.

Measurements (Fig 4F—24 and Table 4F—5)

AB = The axis of the shaft of the tibia. This line is perpendicular to the horizontal plane of the ankle joint and is continuous with the vertical axis of the talus.

*Ref: Keats TE, et al: *Radiology* 1966; 87:904.

MEASUREMENT OF THE AXIAL ANGLES
OF THE ANKLE

CD = Line tangent to the articular surface of the medial malleolus.

EF = Line tangent to the articular surface of the lateral malleolus.

GH = Line tangent to the articular surface of the talus.

FA = Fibular angle at the intersection of EF and GH.

TA = Tibial angle at the intersection of CD and GH.

Source of Material

The data were based on a study of 50 normal adult subjects, equally divided between males and females ranging in age from 18 to 85 years.

MEASUREMENT OF THE WIDTH OF
THE ANKLE JOINT*

Technique
  Central ray: Perpendicular to plane of film centered over the ankle joint.
  Position: Anteroposterior, with patient sitting or supine, and lateral.
  Target-film distance: 120 cm.

Measurements (Fig 4F–25)
  The six measurements were averaged. Figure 4F–26 shows the average joint space in each measuring point.

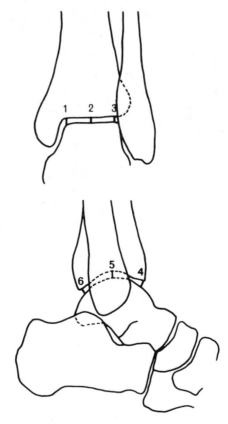

FIG 4F–25.
Measuring points of the ankle. (From Jonsson K, et al: *Acta Radiol Diagn* 1984; 25:147–149. Used by permission.)

Ref: Jonsson K, et al: *Acta Radiol Diagn* 1984; 25:147–149.

MEASUREMENT OF THE WIDTH OF
THE ANKLE JOINT

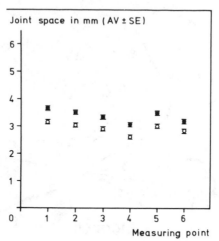

FIG 4F–26.
Average joint space in each measuring point. Men = *closed circles;* women = *open circles.* (From Jonsson K, et al: *Acta Radiol Diagn* 1984; 25:147–149. Used by permission.)

Figure 4F–27 shows the average joint space related to age.

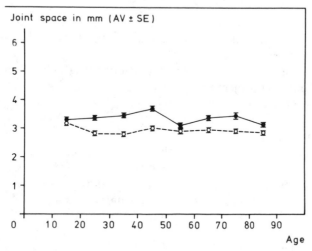

FIG 4F–27.
Average joint space related to age. Men = *closed circles;* women = *open circles.* (From Jonsson K, et al: *Acta Radiol Diagn* 1984; 25:147–149. Used by permission.)

The average joint space in men was 3.4 mm ± 0.4 mm and in women 2.9 mm ± 0.4 mm. The joint space is wider in the medial part in the AP view.

Source of Material
Data are based on a study of 160 normal adults, 80 men and 80 women.

AXIAL RELATIONSHIPS OF THE NORMAL CALCANEUS*

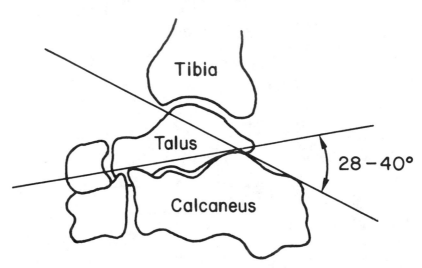

FIG 4F–28.
Boehler's angle.

Technique
Central ray: The ankle is placed against the film so that the lateral mal-
leolus is in the central ray.
Position: Lateral. The foot is perpendicular to the film, and the two mal-
leoli should be projected directly over one another.
Target-film distance: Immaterial.

Measurements
Boehler's angle (Fig 4F–28) for the normal calcaneus is formed between a
line tangent to the upper contour of the tuberosity of the calcaneus and a line
uniting the highest point of the anterior process with the highest point of the
posterior articular surface. This angle normally averages 30°–35°. Less than
28° is definitely abnormal and represents poor position.

Source of Material
The normal range of this measurement has been derived from radiographs
of approximately 1,900 patients who were treated for fracture of the os calcis.
In each case, both the normal and injured os calcis were radiographed.

*Ref: Boehler L: J Bone Joint Surg 1931; 13:75.

AXIAL RELATIONSHIPS OF THE FOOT AND CRITERIA FOR DETERMINATION OF CONGENITAL ABNORMALITIES

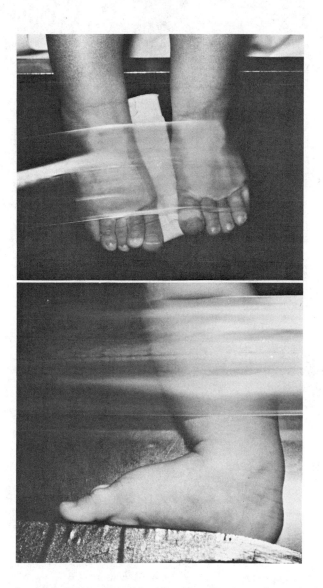

FIG 4F–29.
Proper positioning of a child's foot for AP and lateral radiographs. A wooden wedge is used on the lateral film to dorsiflex the foot as much as possible and to show the presence or absence of equinas. The position of the bones is not affected by holding the foot in the restrictive plastic strap to procure the anteroposterior view. (From Keim HA: *Clin Orthop* 1970; 70:133. Used by permission.)

AXIAL RELATIONSHIPS OF THE FOOT AND CRITERIA FOR DETERMINATION OF CONGENITAL ABNORMALITIES

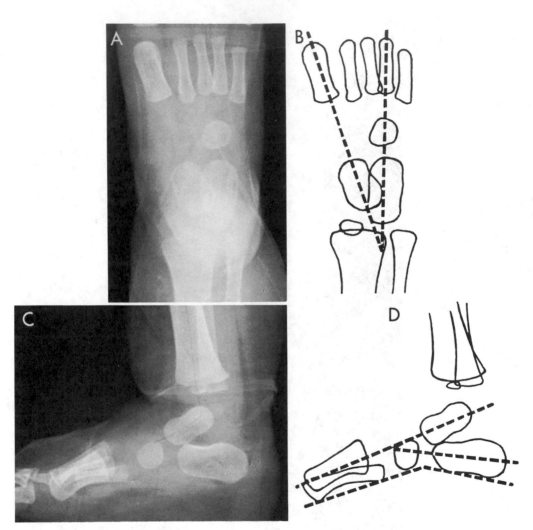

FIG 4F–30.
Normal foot. **A** and **B,** AP projection. The angle between the talus and calcaneus varies with age. In infants and young children, the angle is between 30° and 50° (weight bearing). In children older than 5 years, the talocalcaneal angle varies from 15° to 30° (weight bearing). The line through the midtalus points to the head of the first metatarsal. The line through the midcalcaneus points to the head of the fourth metatarsal. The midtalar and midcalcaneal lines generally coincide with midshaft lines of the first and fourth metatarsals, respectively. Lines of metatarsal shafts are very nearly parallel. **C** and **D,** lateral projection. The midtalar line and the line through the shaft of the first metatarsal coincide in children over 5 years of age on weight bearing, but in infants and young children the talus is positioned more vertically, and the midtalar line passes inferiorly to the shaft of the first metatarsal. An obtuse angle is formed by the line through the inferior cortex of the fifth metatarsal, ranging from 150° to 175° (weight bearing). The midtalar line and midcalcaneal line form an acute angle that varies normally from 25° to 50° (weight bearing). (**A** and **B** from Templeton AW: *AJR* 1965; 93:374. Drawings from Davis LA, Hatt WS: *Radiology* 1955; 64:818. Used by permission.)

AXIAL RELATIONSHIPS OF THE FOOT AND CRITERIA FOR DETERMINATION OF CONGENITAL ABNORMALITIES

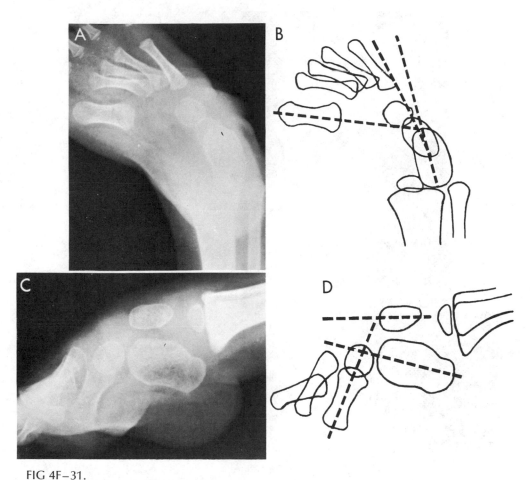

FIG 4F–31.

Clubfoot. **A** and **B,** AP projection. The talocalcaneal angle approaches 0° or is even reversed. Midtalar line points lateral to normal position. Midcalcaneal line points lateral to normal position. The midtalar line and the line through the shaft of the first metatarsal now form an angle. There is a loss of parallelism of metatarsals, with convergence posteriorly. **C** and **D,** lateral projection. The midtalar line and the line through the shaft of the first metatarsal form an obtuse angle. Midtalar and midcalcaneal lines approach parallelism. (From Davis LA, Hatt WS: *Radiology* 1955; 64:818. Used by permission.)

AXIAL RELATIONSHIPS OF THE FOOT AND CRITERIA FOR DETERMINATION OF CONGENITAL ABNORMALITIES

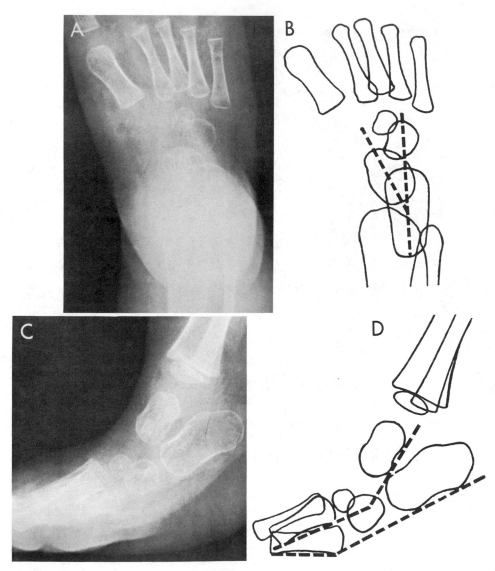

FIG 4F–32.
"Rocker" deformity (overcorrected clubfoot). **A** and **B,** AP projection. The angle between the calcaneus and talus is less than average. The forefoot may or may not be normal. **C** and **D,** lateral projection. Reverse angle between inferior cortex of calcaneus and fifth metatarsal. Reverse angle between inferior cortex of talus and first metatarsal in severe cases. (From Davis LA, Hatt WS: *Radiology* 1955; 64:81. Used by permission.)

AXIAL RELATIONSHIPS OF THE FOOT AND CRITERIA FOR DETERMINATION OF CONGENITAL ABNORMALITIES

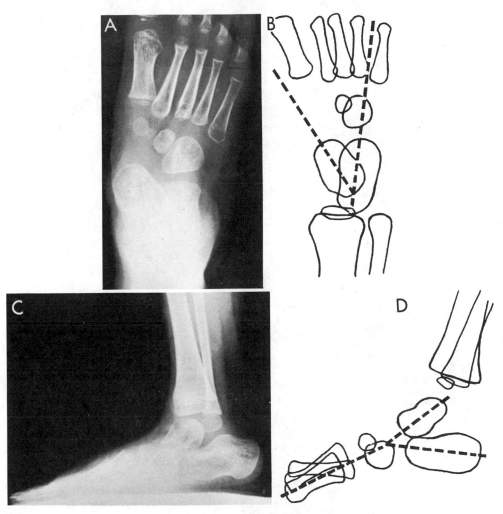

FIG 4F–33.

Flatfoot. **A** and **B,** AP projection. Increased talocalcaneal angle. **C** and **D,** lateral projection. The line of the first metatarsal makes an angle instead of coinciding with the midtalar line. Frequently there is an increased talocalcaneal angle. (From Davis LA, Hatt WS: *Radiology* 1955; 64:81. Used by permission.)

AXIAL RELATIONSHIPS OF THE FOOT AND CRITERIA FOR DETERMINATION OF CONGENITAL ABNORMALITIES

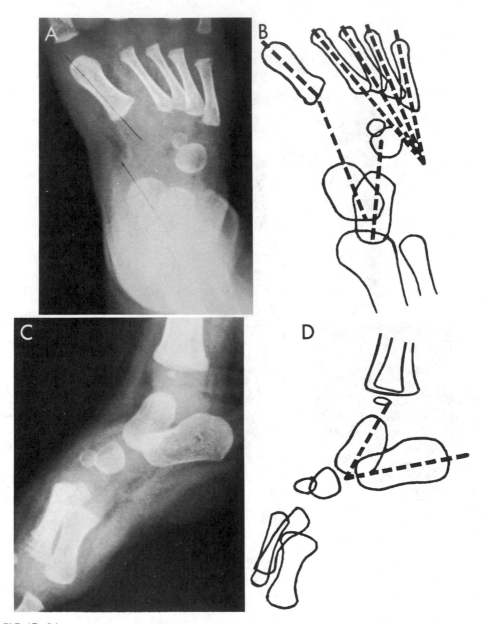

FIG 4F—34.
Metatarsus varus. **A** and **B,** AP projection. There is an increased angle between the midtalar line and the line of the shaft of the first metatarsal. The lines of the metatarsals converge posteriorly. The midcalcaneal line runs lateral to the normal position. **C** and **D,** lateral projection. The angle between the midcalcaneal and midtalar lines may increase. (From Davis LA, Hatt WS: *Radiology* 1955; 64:81. Used by permission.)

AXIAL RELATIONSHIPS OF THE FOOT AND CRITERIA FOR DETERMINATION OF CONGENITAL ABNORMALITIES*

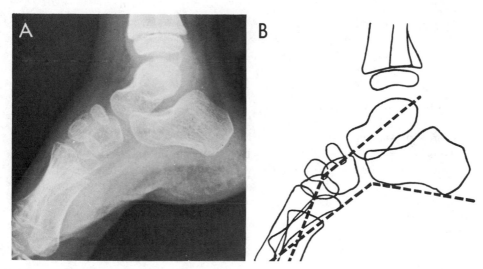

FIG 4F–35.
Pes cavus. The AP projection is unchanged from the normal. **A** and **B,** lateral projection. Increased angle between the line through the inferior cortex of the calcaneus and inferior cortex of the fifth metatarsal. There is now an angle between the midtalar line and the line through the shaft of the first metatarsal. (From Davis LA, Hatt WS: *Radiology* 1955; 64:81. Used by permission.)

Technique
    Central ray: Perpendicular to plane of film, over midportion of foot in both projections.
    Position: Anteroposterior and lateral. Technique must be carefully standardized. *Slight variations in rotation in either projection can markedly alter the relationship of the bones, as shown on the film.* For the anteroposterior view, the knees must be held together and must fall in a plane that is perpendicular to the film (Fig 4F–29,A). The tendency of the technologist to "correct" the abnormality by placing the foot normally on the cassette must be discouraged. For the lateral projection (Fig 4F–29, B), the technique for a lateral ankle view is the correct one. Templeton and coworkers exert pressure against the foot with a plastic board in both projections to simulate weight bearing.
    Target-film distance: Immaterial.

Ref: Davis LA, Hatt WS: *Radiology* 1955; 64:81. Used by permission.

AXIAL RELATIONSHIPS OF THE FOOT AND CRITERIA FOR DETERMINATION OF CONGENITAL ABNORMALITIES

Measurements

Figure 4F–30: Normal foot. Recorded angles with weight bearing.

Figure 4F–31: Clubfoot.

Figure 4F–32: "Rocker" deformity.

Figure 4F–33: Flatfoot.

Figure 4F–34: Metatarsus varus.

Figure 4F–35: Pes cavus.

Source of Material

Davis and Hatt's diagrams are not based on any statistically valid sample. They are arranged as a guide for the radiologist in describing certain abnormalities. No particular numbers are assigned to the angles, and the context should be interpreted in a manner similar to that for any other descriptive radiologic finding.

The angles of the normal foot reported by Templeton et al. are based on AP and lateral weight-bearing roentgenograms of 160 normal children, ages 12 days to 12 years.

AXIAL RELATIONSHIPS OF THE FOOT AND CRITERIA FOR DETERMINATION OF CONGENITAL ABNORMALITIES*

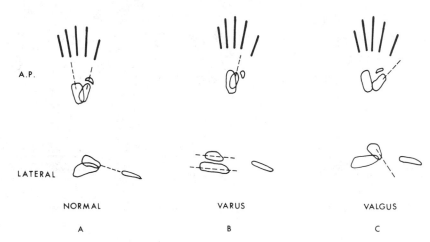

FIG 4F—36.

Diagrammatic representation of hindfoot and forefoot relationships. **A,** normal hindfoot. The talar axial line intersects or points slightly medial to the first metatarsal base. The navicular is situated directly opposite the head of the talus. The calcaneus points toward the fourth metatarsal base, making a definable angle with the talus. On the lateral projection, the anterior portion of the talus is slightly plantarflexed, the calcaneus slightly dorsiflexed. The talar axial line points down the shaft of the first metatarsal. **B,** hindfoot varus. The talocalcaneal angle is decreased, with these two bones more nearly parallel to each other or actually superimposed. The navicular is medially displaced, and the axial talar line points lateral to the first metatarsal base. On the lateral projection, the calcaneus and talus are both more nearly horizontal and parallel to each other. **C,** hindfoot valgus. The talocalcaneal angle is increased, with navicular and other midfoot bones displaced lateral to the talus. The talar axial line will pass medial to the first metatarsal base. On the lateral projection, the talus is more nearly vertical than normal. (From Ozonoff MB: *Pediatric Orthopedic Radiology*. Philadelphia, WB Saunders Co, 1979, pp 288—289. Used by permission.)

*Ref: Ozonoff MB: *Pediatric Orthopedic Radiology*. Philadelphia, WB Saunders Co, 1979, pp 288—289.

AXIAL RELATIONSHIPS OF THE FOOT AND CRITERIA FOR DETERMINATION OF CONGENITAL ABNORMALITIES

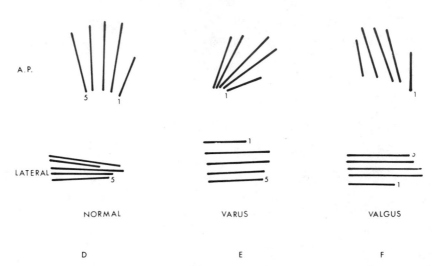

FIG 4F–37.

D, normal forefoot. The metatarsals converge proximally with overlap at the bases. On the lateral projection, the fifth metatarsal is most plantar, with the other metatarsals being superimposed. **E,** forefoot varus. The forefoot is narrowed, with increased convergence at the bases and more than normal superimposition. On the lateral projection, a ladder-like arrangement is seen with the first metatarsal highest. **F,** forefoot valgus. The forefoot is broadened with the metatarsals more nearly parallel than normal and with decreased overlap at the bases. On the lateral projection, a ladder-like arrangement is rarely seen, because the degree of eversion is rarely enough to show this finding. If it is present, however, the first metatarsal will be most plantar. (From Ozonoff MB: *Pediatric Orthopedic Radiology*. Philadelphia, WB Saunders Co, 1979, pp 288–289. Used by permission.)

MEASUREMENT OF THE FEET OF NORMAL INFANTS AND CHILDREN*

Technique
Central ray: Perpendicular to plane of film.
Position: Standing. For the AP projection, the knee was flexed and the beam directed at the head of the talus. For the true lateral and maximum dorsiflexion lateral radiographs, the ankle was held in neutral or maximally dorsiflexed, the beam directed at the talus.
Target-film distance: Immaterial.

Measurements (Fig 4F–38, A through K)

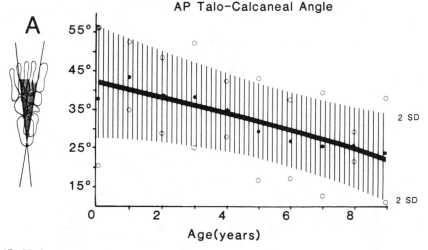

FIG 4F–38,A.
A–K, the mean and standard deviations for each of the ten angles and the calculated talocalcaneal index were plotted for each of the ten age groups. *Solid lines* show the mean changes with age; *shaded areas,* the normal ranges; *solid circles,* the mean measurements for each age group; *open circles,* two standard deviations for each age group. (From Vanderwilde R, et al: *J Bone Joint Surg* 1988; 70A: 407–414.)

Ref: Vanderwilde R, et al: *J Bone Joint Surg* 1988; 70A:407–414.

MEASUREMENT OF THE FEET OF NORMAL
INFANTS AND CHILDREN

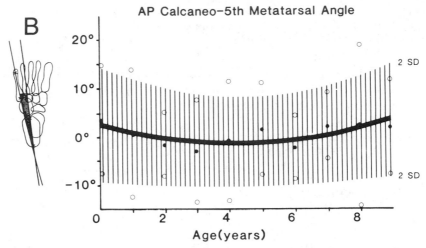

FIG 4F–38,B.

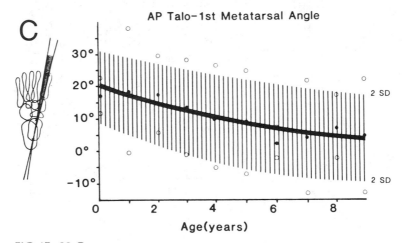

FIG 4F–38,C.

MEASUREMENT OF THE FEET OF NORMAL INFANTS AND CHILDREN

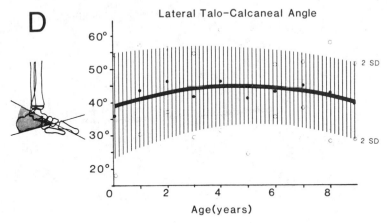

FIG 4F−38,D.

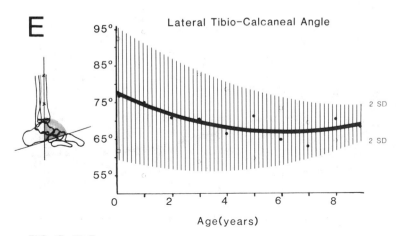

FIG 4F−38,E.

MEASUREMENT OF THE FEET OF NORMAL
INFANTS AND CHILDREN

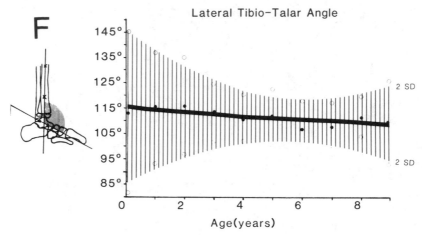

FIG 4F–38,F.

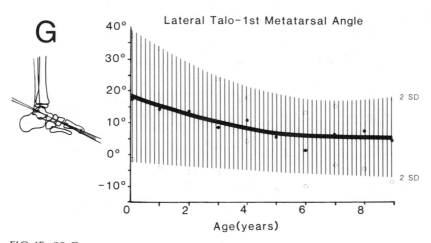

FIG 4F–38,G.

MEASUREMENT OF THE FEET OF NORMAL INFANTS AND CHILDREN

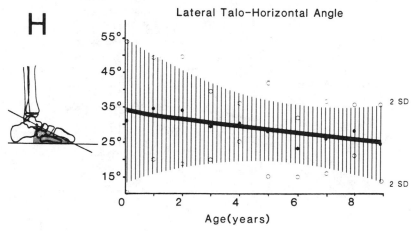

FIG 4F–38,H.

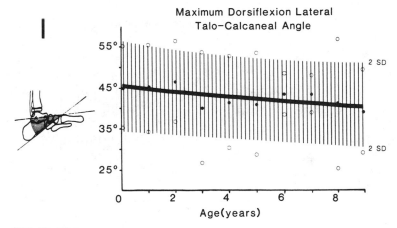

FIG 4F–38,I.

MEASUREMENT OF THE FEET OF NORMAL
INFANTS AND CHILDREN

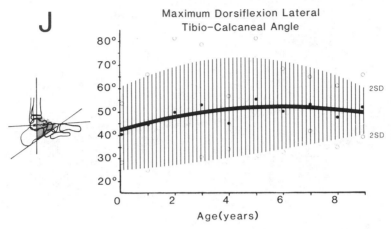

FIG 4F–38,J.

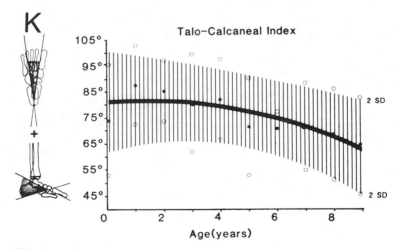

FIG 4F–38,K.

Source of Material

Data based on radiographs of 74 normal infants and children ranging in age from 6 to 127 months, including 39 boys and 35 girls.

MEASUREMENT OF THE HEEL PAD AS AN AID
TO DIAGNOSIS OF ACROMEGALY*

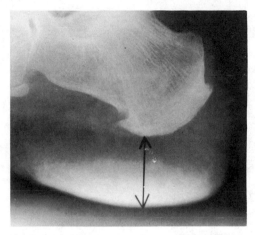

FIG 4F–39.
(From Steinbach HL, Russell W, *Radiology* 1964; 82:418. Used by permission.)

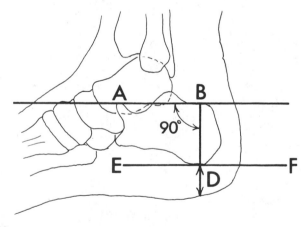

FIG 4F–40.
(From Kho KM, Wright AD, Doyle FH: *Br J Radiol* 1970; 43:119. Used by permission.)

*Ref: Steinbach HL, Russell W: *Radiology* 1964; 82:418.

MEASUREMENT OF THE HEEL PAD AS AN AID
TO DIAGNOSIS OF ACROMEGALY

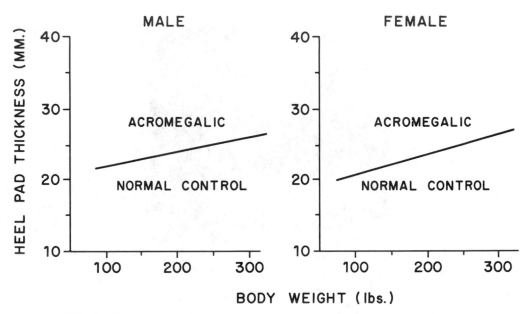

FIG 4F—41.
(From Kho KM, Wright AD, Doyle FH: *Br J Radiol* 1970; 43:119. Used by permission.)

Technique
   Central ray: Perpendicular to plane of film centered over the calcaneus.
   Position: Lateral.
   Target-film distance: 40 inches.

Measurements (Figs 4F—39 and 4F—40; Table 4F—6)
   The heel pad is measured at the shortest distance between the calcaneus and the plantar surface of the skin. Kho and colleagues* recommend the method shown in Figure 4F—40.
   Line *AB* joins the anterior and posterior angles on the superior surface of the calcaneus. Parallel to this line draw line *EF* parallel to the lowest point on the calcaneus. A line perpendicular to this point to the skin surface gives the heel pad thickness *(D)*.
   Heel pad thickness is related to body weight (Fig 4F—41). Puckette and Seymour† found a higher mean value in blacks than in whites and noted that age and sex did not appear to influence heel pad thickness.

*Ref: Kho KM, Wright AD, Doyle FH: *Br J Radiol* 1970; 43:119.
†Ref: Puckette SE, Seymour EQ: *Radiology* 1967; 88:982.

MEASUREMENT OF THE HEEL PAD AS AN AID
TO DIAGNOSIS OF ACROMEGALY

TABLE 4F–6.

Heel Pad Thickness in Controls[*]

		Upper Limit	
Mean	SD	Male	Female
18.6 mm	2.6 mm	25 mm	23 mm

[*]From Kho KM, Wright AD, Doyle FH: *BR J Radiol* 1970; 43:119. Used by permission.

Source of Material

Steinbach and Russell studied 29 patients with unequivocal clinical and laboratory evidence of acromegaly. The control group included 103 normal subjects.

Kho and colleagues studied 79 patients with untreated acromegaly and 52 normal control subjects.

Note: Several articles have appeared on heel pad thickness. Most of the articles are listed as references in Kho et al.

Two other measurements used less frequently as an aid in the diagnosis of acromegaly are:

1. The Sesamoid index,[‡] which is the product of the two longest perpendicular diameters of the medial sesamoid bone at the metacarpophalangeal joint of the first digit. Median index is 20; range is 12 to 29.
2. Skin thickness.[§] This measurement requires the use of a block of wood to flatten the skin surface. Normal measurements are compared with those found in several types of endocrine disease.

Comment: The value of heel-pad thickness in the diagnosis of acromegaly is controversial because of the wide variation among normal persons.[†]

[‡]*Ref*: Kleinberg DL, Young IS, Kupperman HS: *Ann Intern Med* 1966; 64:1075.
[§]*Ref*: Sheppard RH, Meema HE: *Ann Intern Med* 1967; 66:531.
[†]*Ref*: Puckette SE, Seymour EQ: *Radiology* 1967; 88:982.

LENGTH PATTERN OF METATARSAL BONES*

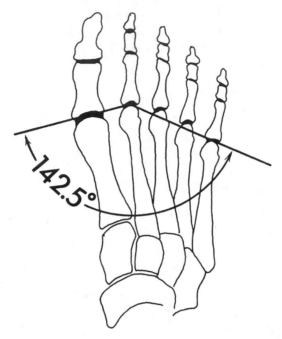

FIG 4F–42.
(Adapted from Gamble FO, Yale I: *Clinical Foot Roentgenology.* Baltimore, Williams & Wilkins Co, 1966, p 158. Used by permission.)

Technique
Central ray: Perpendicular to plane of film, over midportion of foot.
Position: Anteroposterior.
Target-film distance: Immaterial.

Measurements (Fig 4F–42)
Total joint line angle 142.5° mean. First metatarsal is shorter than second. Second metatarsal is longest. Third metatarsal is shorter than second. Fourth metatarsal is shorter than third. Fifth metatarsal is shorter than fourth.

Source of Material
Gamble and Yale used 279 foot roentgenograms.

Ref: Gamble FO, Yale I: *Clinical Foot Roentgenology.* Baltimore, Williams & Wilkins Co, 1966, p 158.

CHAPTER 5

The Respiratory System and Thymus

FAT THICKNESS OF THE CHEST
WALL IN INFANTS*

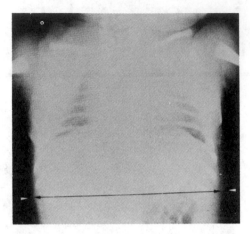

FIG 5–1.
Measurement of subcutaneous fat. (From Kuhns LR, et al: *Radiology* 1974;111:665. Used by permission.)

TABLE 5–1.

Control Double Fat Thickness
and Gestational Age*

Gestation (Weeks)	No. of Infants	Fat Thickness (mm)		
		−2SD	Mean	+2SD
<30	20	0	0	0
30–31+	9	0	1.9	2.9†
32–33+	17	2.3	3.2	4.1
34–35+	21	2.3	3.7	5.1
36–37+	23	2.7	4.1	5.5
38–39+	19	2.6	5.1	7.7
40–41+	38	3.1	5.8	8.6

*From Kuhns LR, et al: *Radiology* 1974;111:665. Used by permission.
†Range rather than ±2 standard deviations given since only 9 control newborn infants at this age qualified for the study.

Technique
   Central ray: Perpendicular to plane of film centered over midchest.
   Position: Anteroposterior supine.
   Target-film distance: 40 inches.

Ref: Kuhns LR, et al: *Radiology* 1974; 111;665.

FAT THICKNESS OF THE CHEST WALL IN INFANTS

Measurements (Fig 5–1 and Table 5–1)

A line is drawn between the ends of the tenth and eleventh ribs on the chest film, and this line is extended through the fat layer on each side. Skin and fat thickness are measured to the closest tenth of a millimeter. Since slight rotation has been found to decrease fat thickness on one side and increase it on the other, the sum of the two fat thicknesses is calculated for each infant. Gestational age can be estimated from dental and shoulder maturation as seen in chest films. (See section on skeletal maturation, pages 00 and 00.) Greater than normal subcutaneous fat in a newborn may give a clue that his mother is a latent diabetic.

Source of Material

Control studies were made on 147 white newborn infants, with estimated gestational ages from 24 to 42 weeks, who had respiratory problems.

THE LEVEL OF BIFURCATION OF TRACHEA IN ADULT AND CHILD*

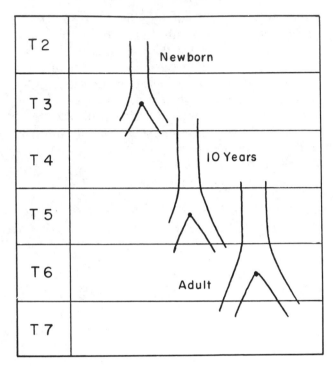

FIG 5–2.
Vertebral levels of trachea bifurcation.

Technique
Central ray: To fourth thoracic vertebra.
Position: Posteroanterior.
Target-film distance: 72 inches.

Measurements (Fig 5–2)
Newborn, third thoracic vertebra; 10-year-old, fifth thoracic vertebra; adult, sixth thoracic vertebra.

Source of Material
Caffey quotes the work of Mehnert.† The number of cases studied by Mehnert is not known.

*Ref: Caffey J: *Pediatric X-ray Diagnosis*, ed 3. Chicago, Year Book Medical Publishers, Inc, 1956.

†Ref: Mehnert E: Über topographische Alterveränderungen des Atmungsapparates. Jena, 1901.

MEASUREMENT OF TRACHEA DIAMETER IN THE NEWBORN INFANT*

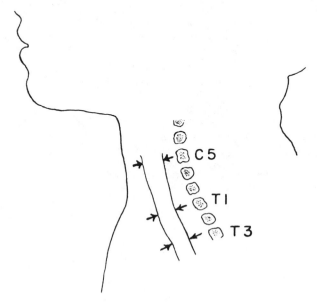

FIG 5-3.

Technique
    Central ray: Anteroposterior to fourth thoracic vertebra.
                    Left lateral: To fourth thoracic vertebra on midcoronal plane.
    Position: Anteroposterior, left lateral.
    Target-film distance: 36 inches.
    Films taken in maximum inspiration.

Ref: Donaldson SW, Tompsett AC: *AJR* 1952; 67:785.

MEASUREMENT OF TRACHEA DIAMETER
IN THE NEWBORN INFANT

Measurements (Fig 5–3 and Table 5–2)

TABLE 5–2.

	C5	T1	T3
Anteroposterior diameter of trachea			
Average diameter (mm)	4.5	3.9	3.5
Lateral diameter of trachea*			
Minimum diameter (mm)	2	1	1
Maximum diameter (mm)	7	6	5

*Donaldson and Tompsett found that this diameter was quite variable. Also, they considered a 3-mm anteroposterior diameter in the upper thorax to be the lower limit of normal.

Source of Material
Studies of 350 normal infants were made within 24 hours after birth.

MEASUREMENT OF TRACHEAL DIMENSIONS IN CHILDREN AND ADOLESCENTS BY CT*

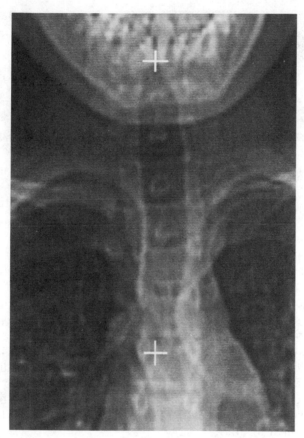

FIG 5–4.
Part of an anteroposterior slit radiograph (scout view) in a 14-year-old girl. The computer readily gave the distance between the vocal cords and the carina, identified by the *crosses*. (From Griscom NT: *Radiology* 1982;145:361. Used by permission.)

*Ref: Griscom NT: *Radiology* 1982; 145:361.

MEASUREMENT OF TRACHEAL DIMENSIONS
IN CHILDREN AND ADOLESCENTS BY CT

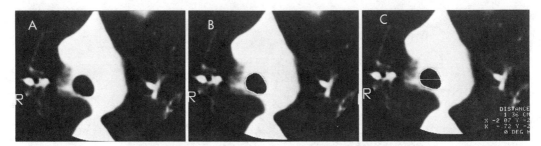

FIG 5−5.
A, magnified 10-mm section through the trachea and the arch of the aorta in an 18-year-old girl. The window is 1,000 CT units, and the center of the window is at −500. **B,** the same section after tracing through the pixels with a CT number of 500 ± 37, preparatory to determination of the luminal cross-sectional area by the computer. **C,** the same section showing measurement of the coronal diameter. Most tracheal cross sections in children and adolescents are more nearly round than this one, which is flattened by the aortic arch. (From Griscom NT: *Radiology* 1982;145:361. Used by permission.)

Technique

1. GE 8800 CT/T scanner with scan times of 9.6 seconds (occasionally 4.8 seconds or 5.7 seconds). Contiguous 10-mm sections from above the pulmonary apices to below the tracheal bifurcation.
2. Patients were scanned in the supine position. Children aged 6 years and older were studied with near full inspiration. Children aged 4 to 6 years were told to stop breathing during the scan, and those under 4 years were obtained during sedation and quiet respiration.
3. Scout views were obtained (AP usually) to localize sections and measure tracheal length.

Measurements (Figs 5−4 and 5−5)

Each section was analyzed for coronal and sagittal diameters and cross-sectional areas, using the electronic cursor on images enlarged × 3.

Windows of 1,000 HU were set with the center at -500 HU. The "blink" system was adjusted at 74 units, so that pixels with a CT number between −463 and −537 blinked once each second. Diameters and cross-sectional areas were measured, using the blinking pixels as the tracheal margin.

Mean values for each subject were calculated, excluding those slices showing the subglottic narrowing and the supracoronal lateral flaring of the trachea (Figs 5−6 to 5−8).

MEASUREMENT OF TRACHEAL DIMENSIONS
IN CHILDREN AND ADOLESCENTS BY CT

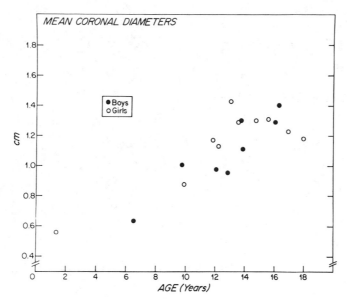

FIG 5–6.
Mean coronal diameters, plotted against age, showing each of the first 18 cases. *Solid circles* = boys; *open circles* = girls. (From Griscom NT: *Radiology* 1982;145:361. Used by permission.)

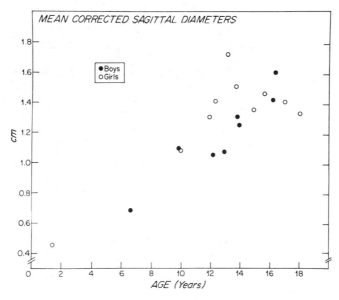

FIG 5–7.
Mean corrected sagittal diameters vs. age. (From Griscom NT: *Radiology* 1982;145:361. Used by permission.)

MEASUREMENT OF TRACHEAL DIMENSIONS
IN CHILDREN AND ADOLESCENTS BY CT

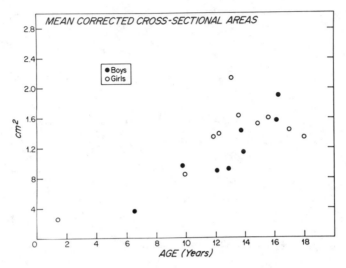

FIG 5–8.

Mean corrected cross-sectional areas vs. age. (From Griscom NT: *Radiology* 1982;145:361. Used by permission.)

Source of Material

Fifteen patients aged 1 to 19 years being scanned for possible pulmonary metastases. None of the subjects had prior thoracotomy, current or prior mediastinal or cervical mass, or pulmonary metastases more than 2 cm in diameter. Three of the patients were scanned twice at intervals.

DIMENSIONS OF THE NORMAL TRACHEA*

Technique
   Central ray: Perpendicular to plane of film.
   Position: Posteroanterior and lateral with maximum inspiration.
   Target-film distance: 10 feet (3.05 m). Magnification factor 1.08.

Measurements (Fig 5–9)

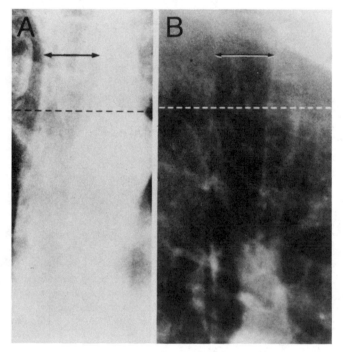

FIG 5–9.
Level of measurement *(solid line)* of coronal **(A)** and sagittal **(B)** tracheal diameters, 2 cm above projected top of aortic arch *(broken line)*. (From Breatnach E, et al: *AJR* 1984;142:903–906. Used by permission.)

The internal diameter of the tracheal air column was measured at a level 2 cm above the projected top of the aortic arch on both PA and lateral films. Measurements were made of the air column alone, excluding the tracheal wall.

The dimensions of the trachea related to age are given in Table 5–3.

Ref: Breatnach E, et al: *AJR* 1984; 142:903–906.

TABLE 5–3.

Mean Coronal and Sagittal Tracheal Diameters in Normal Subjects by Gender and Age*†

Age Group (Yrs)	Male			Female		
	No. of Subjects	Tracheal Diameter (mm): Mean ± SD		No. of Subjects	Tracheal Diameter (mm): Mean ± SD	
		Coronal	Sagittal		Coronal	Sagittal
10–19	26	15.5±2.8	15.4±3.1	22	14.4±1.6	14.5±1.3
20–29	81	18.7±2.0	19.3±2.0	98	15.7±1.6	15.6±1.7
30–39	72	19.2±2.1	19.7±2.4	64	16.0±1.8	16.3±2.3
40–49	69	19.5±2.3	20.3±2.2	45	16.6±2.0	16.8±2.2
50–59	80	19.2±2.3	20.4±2.6	65	16.5±1.6	17.0±2.0
60–69	71	19.5±2.2	20.7±2.5	48	16.8±2.0	17.2±2.3
70–79	31	19.7±2.2	20.8±1.8	36	16.4±2.4	16.5±2.3

*From Breatnach E, et al: AJR 1984;142:903–906. Used by permission.
†Coronal and sagittal tracheal diameters were defined as the internal diameters of the tracheal air column as measured at a level 2 cm above the projected top of the aortic arch on posteroanterior and lateral radiographs, respectively.

DIMENSIONS OF THE NORMAL TRACHEA

Source of Material

Data are based on studies of chest films of 808 patients with no clinical or radiological evidence of respiratory disease. There were 430 men and 378 women ranging in age from 10 to 79 years.

ANGLE OF TRACHEAL BIFURCATION*

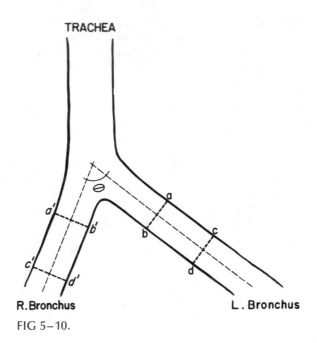

R. Bronchus   L. Bronchus

FIG 5–10.

Technique

Central ray: To the fourth thoracic vertebra.

Position: Posteroanterior.

Target-film distance: 40 inches for patients under age 1 year; 72 inches for all other patients.

Measurements (Fig 5–10)

Draw a straight line in the middle of each bronchus parallel to the walls of the bronchus.

Bifurcation angle θ is given in Figures 5–11 and 5–12. Mean and 95% confidence limits are shown.

Ref: Alavi SM, Keats TE, O'Brien WM: AJR 1970; 108:546.

ANGLE OF TRACHEAL BIFURCATION

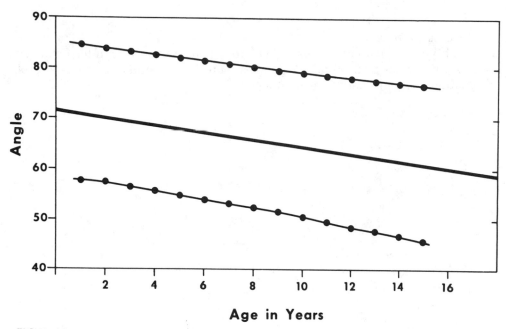

FIG 5–11.
Ninety-five percent confidence band for people under 16 years of age. Regression equation based on male and female data.

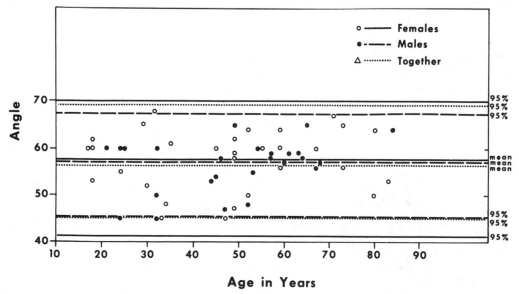

FIG 5–12.
Ninety-five percent confidence band for people over 16 years of age.

ANGLE OF TRACHEAL BIFURCATION

Source of Material

Eighty-seven patients whose chest roentgenograms were interpreted as normal. Forty-one males and 46 females were in the study. Twenty-nine of the patients were under 16 years of age.

MEASUREMENT OF THE RIGHT PARATRACHEAL STRIPE IN CHILDREN AND ADULTS*

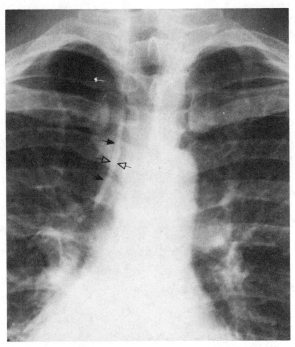

FIG 5–13.
The right paratracheal stripe. The *open arrows* outline the stripe at a level 2 cm above the superior extent of the azygous arch. *Arrows* 1 cm above and 1 cm below indicate the range within which the width of the stripe was measured. (From Savoca CJ, et al: *Radiology* 1977;122:295. Used by permission.)

Technique
   Central ray: Projected through the midchest.
   Position: Posteroanterior.
   Target-film distance: 72 inches.

Measurements (Fig 5–13)
   The right paratracheal stripe in normal children measures 0.5 to 3 mm, and any stripe 4 mm or wider is reliable evidence of disease affecting the trachea, mediastinum, or pleura.
   The right paratracheal stripe in a normal adult measures 1 to 4 mm. A measurement of 5 mm or more is reliable evidence of disease.

Ref: Children: Savoca CJ, et al: *Pediatr Radiol* 1978; 6:203. Adults: Savoca CJ, et al: *Radiology* 1977; 122:295.

MEASUREMENT OF THE RIGHT PARATRACHEAL STRIPE IN CHILDREN AND ADULTS

Source of Material

Data for children were derived from 50 children aged 5 months to 15 years. Adult data were derived from end-inspiration chest films of 1,259 normal subjects.

MEASUREMENT OF THE POSTERIOR TRACHEAL BAND*

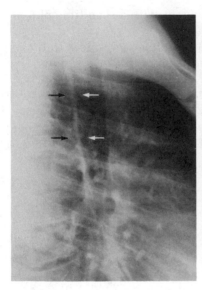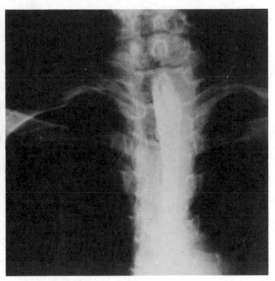

FIG 5–14.
The normal posterior tracheal band. (From Bachman AL, Teixidor HS: *Br J Radiol* 1975; 48:352. Used by permission.)

Technique
Central ray: Perpendicular to plane of film centered over midchest.
Position: Lateral upright.
Target-film distance: 72 inches.

Measurements (Fig 5–14)
The posterior tracheal band is uniform in width, measuring up to 3 mm (rarely to 4 mm) in thickness. Width greater than 4.5 mm is considered pathologic in a follow-up study by Putman et al.†

Source of Material
Based on a study of 200 normal individuals in whom 182 posterior tracheal bands could be visualized.

*Ref: Bachman AL, Teixidor HS: *Br J Radiol* 1975; 48:352.
†Ref: Putman, et al: *Radiology* 1976; 121:533.

MEASUREMENT OF NORMAL MEDIASTINAL LYMPH NODES BY CT*

Technique

1. CT scans performed using a GE 8800 scanner with a scan time of 5.6 seconds.
2. Contiguous 1.0 cm thick sections from the pulmonary apices to the lung bases are obtained in the supine position at full inspiration. Scans are obtained after bolus injection of 50–75 cc of Conray 60%.

Measurement

The number and size of lymph nodes were recorded at defined sites using the node mapping scheme of the American Thoracic Society (Fig 5–15 and Table 5–4).

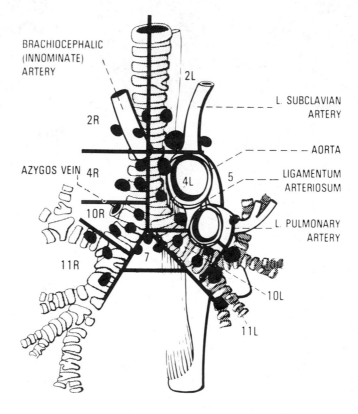

FIG 5–15.
American Thoracic Society lymph-node mapping scheme. Locations of regions 6, 8R, and 8L are not illustrated because they lie in front of or behind other regions in drawing. Definitions of all regions are listed in Table 5–4. (From Tisi GM, et al: *Am Rev Resp Dis* 1983; 127:659–664. Used by permission.)

*Ref: Glazer GM, et al: *AJR* 1985; 144:261–265.

MEASUREMENT OF NORMAL MEDIASTINAL LYMPH NODES BY CT

TABLE 5−4.

American Thoracic Society Definitions of Regional Nodal Stations*

X	Supraclavicular nodes.
2R	Right upper paratracheal nodes; nodes to the right of the midline of the trachea, between the intersection of the caudal margin of the innominate artery with the trachea and the apex of the lung.
2L	Left upper paratracheal nodes: nodes to the left of the midline of the trachea, between the top of the aortic arch and the apex of the lung.
4R	Right lower paratracheal nodes: nodes to the right of the midline of the trachea, between the cephalic border of the azygos vein and the intersection of the caudal margin of the brachiocephalic artery with the right side of the trachea.
4L	Left lower paratracheal nodes: nodes to the left of the midline of the trachea, between the top of the aortic arch and the level of the carina, medial to the ligamentum arteriosum.
5	Aortopulmonary nodes: subaortic and para-aortic nodes, lateral to the ligamentum arteriosum or the aorta or left pulmonary artery, proximal to the first branch of the left pulmonary artery.
6	Anterior mediastinal nodes: nodes anterior to the ascending aorta or the innominate artery.
7	Subcarinal nodes: nodes arising caudal to the carina of the trachea but not associated with the lower-lobe bronchi or arteries within the lung.
8	Paraesophageal nodes: nodes dorsal to the posterior wall of the trachea and to the right or left of the midline of the esophagus.
9	Right or left pulmonary ligament nodes: nodes within the right or left pulmonary ligament.
10R	Right tracheobronchial nodes: nodes to the right of the midline of the trachea, from the level of the cephalic border of the azygos vein to the origin of the right-upper-lobe bronchus.
10L	Left peribronchial nodes: nodes to the left of the midline of the trachea, between the carina and the left-upper-lobe bronchus, medial to the ligamentum arteriosum.
11	Intrapulmonary nodes: nodes removed in the right- or left-lung specimen, plus those distal to the main-stem bronchi or secondary carina.

*From Tisi GM, et al: *Am Rev Resp Dis* 1983; 127:659−664. Used by permission.

Nodes in locations X, 9, and 11 were not analyzed. The longest and shortest node diameters in the transverse plane were recorded. The number and size of normal mediastinal lymph nodes are shown in Table 5−5.

MEASUREMENT OF NORMAL MEDIASTINAL LYMPH NODES BY CT

TABLE 5−5.

Numbers and Sizes of Normal Mediastinal Lymph Nodes in 56 Patients*

Region	No. of Patients With Nodes Visible in Region	Nodes			
		No. (Mean ± SD)	Maximum No.	Shortest Diameter, mm (Mean ± SD)	Sum of Diameters, mm (Mean ± SD)
2R	53	2.1±1.3	6	3.5±1.3	8.0±3.1
2L	42	1.9±1.6	6	3.3±1.6	7.6±4.0
4R	56	3.2±2.0	10	5.0±2.0	11.1±3.9
4L	47	2.1±1.6	7	4.7±1.9	10.8±4.2
5	33	1.2±1.1	3	4.7±2.1	11.8±5.0
6	48	4.8±3.5	12	4.1±1.7	10.3±4.2
7	53	1.7±1.1	6	6.2±2.2	14.3±4.6
8R	32	1.0±1.1	4	4.4±2.6	10.1±6.1
8L	25	0.8±1.2	6	3.8±1.7	8.9±3.9
10R	56	2.8±1.3	7	5.9±2.1	13.6±4.0
10L	39	1.0±0.8	3	4.0±1.2	9.4±2.3

*From Glazer GM, et al: *AJR* 1985; 144:261−265. Used by permission.

Source of Material

Data are based on CT studies of 56 adult patients with no evidence of neoplasia. The group included 31 men, 21 to 75 years of age, and 25 women, 18 to 82 years of age.

MEASUREMENT OF THE HILA*

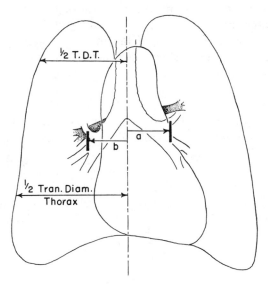

FIG 5–16.

Technique
Central ray: To fourth thoracic vertebral body.
Position: Posteroanterior chest.
Target-film distance: 72 inches.

Measurements (Fig 5–16)
Mean width for right and left hila: 5.56 ± 0.12 cm. Minimum width, 3.5 cm; maximum width, 7.0 cm.

Sum of transverse diameters of right and left hili = 11.0 ± 0.03 cm.

In at least 84% of the cases the difference between the right and left hilus did not exceed 1.0 cm.

Lateral border of the hilus is the margin farthest from the midline (midline to b and to a in Figure 5–16) but not including the first branchings of each pulmonary artery. Rigler and his co-workers* found that in 100 patients with proved bronchogenic carcinoma the mean sum of the hili diameters was 13 cm. If either hilus is more than 7.0 cm or if the sum of the diameters is 13 cm, the chance of abnormality is about 90%.

However, in a study of 541 cases of proved bronchogenic carcinoma, Lodwick, Keats, and Dorst† found that only 31.9% of the cases had a total trans-

*Ref: Rigler LG, O'Laughlin BJ, Tucker RC: *Radiology* 1952; 59:683.
†Ref: Lodwick G, Keats, TE, Dorst J: *Radiology* 1958; 71:370.

verse diameter greater than 13 cm; only 36.8% of the cases had a unilateral measurement greater than 7.0 cm; 13.5% had a total transverse diameter of less than the mean normal diameter of 11 cm.

In the very early bronchogenic cancer cases, hilar measurements were abnormal in only 19.4% of the cases.

Source of Material

Chest roentgenograms of 100 consecutive patients over 40 years of age, made as hospital routine on admission, were studied.

MEASUREMENT OF THE HILAR HEIGHT RATIO FOR DETECTION OF HILAR DISPLACEMENT*

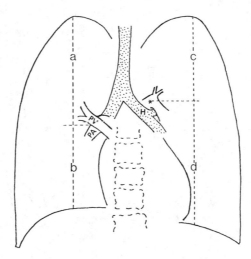

FIG 5–17.

Calculation of the hilar height ratio. (From Homer MJ: *Radiology* 1978; 129:11. Used by permission.)

Technique

Central ray: Perpendicular to plane of film centered over midchest.

Position: Posteroanterior, inspiratory phase.

Target-film distance: 72 inches.

Measurements (Fig 5–17)

A line parallel to the thoracic spine is drawn from the highest point of the pulmonary apex to the diaphragm. An intersecting line is drawn from the midpoint of the hilus, perpendicular to the vertical line. The lateral angle, designated by the midpoint of the right hilus, is joined by the right upper lobe pulmonary vein *(PV)* crossing the right basal pulmonary artery *(PA)*. The left hyparterial bronchus *(H)* must be identified in order to determine the midpoint of the left hilus (*). The right hilar height ratio = a/b; left hilar height ratio = c/d.

In normal patients, the right hilus is positioned in the lower half of the hemithorax, while the left hilus is positioned in the upper half of its hemithorax. The normal right hilar height ratio, therefore, should be greater than 1 and the left hilar height ratio less than 1. When these values are abnormal, pulmonary volume changes or intrapulmonary and subphrenic abnormal processes are present.

Source of Material

Data were obtained from films of 90 normal patients. There was no significant difference between males and females.

*Ref: Homer MJ: *Radiology* 1978; 129:11.

MEASUREMENTS FOR RADIOLOGIC
EVALUATION OF FUNNEL CHEST*

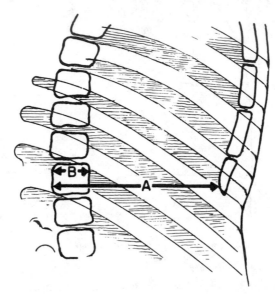

FIG 5–18.
(Adapted from Backer O, et al: *Acta Radiol* 1961; 55:249.)

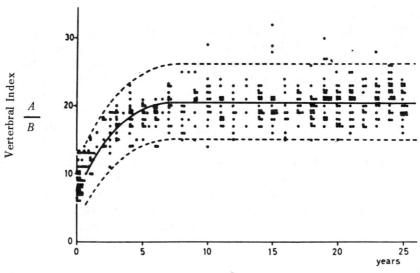

FIG 5–19.
(From Backer O, et al: *Acta Radiol* 1961; 55:249. Used by permission.)

*Ref: Backer O, et al: *Acta Radiologica* 1961; 55:249.

MEASUREMENTS FOR RADIOLOGIC
EVALUATION OF FUNNEL CHEST

Technique
   Central ray: Perpendicular to plane of film centered over midchest.
   Position: True lateral.
   Target-film distance: Immaterial.

Measurements (Figs 5–18 and 5–19)
The vertebral index indicates the percentage ratio between the minimum sagittal diameter of the chest, measured from the posterior surface of the vertebral body to the nearest point on the body of the sternum *(A)*, and the sagittal diameter of the vertebral body at the same level *(B)*. Figure 5–19 shows the vertebral index in normal persons. The *solid line* represents the mean curve. The 95% range lies between the broken lines. This method is applicable in assessment of the late results of operation, which heretofore has been based on subjective estimation.

Source of Material
The data are based on a normal series of 445 subjects, 197 males and 248 females, about equally distributed in 5-year age groups from 0 to 25 years.

MEASUREMENT OF THE STRAIGHT-BACK SYNDROME*

Absence of the normal thoracic kyphosis is a recently accepted cause of "pseudo heart disease." Roentgenographically, the heart is usually normal in size and configuration, but in some patients it is "pancake" in appearance, and in other patients it is displaced to the left with prominence of the pulmonary arteries.

Technique
> *Central ray:* PA chest: to fourth thoracic vertebral body.
> > Lateral chest: centered over midchest.
> *Position:* Posteroanterior and true lateral.
> *Target-film distance:* Posteroanterior: 72 inches.
> > Lateral: 72 inches.

Measurements (Table 5−6)

TABLE 5−6.

	No.	AP Chest Diam (cm)	AP/Transthoracic Ratio (%)
Straight-back syndrome patients			
Males	12	10.6	35.8
Females	12	9.8	37.3
Normal patients			
Males	50	14.2	47.0
Females	50	12.0	45.7

Source of Material
Twenty-four men and women in whom loss of thoracic kyphosis was the only somatic fault.

*Ref: Twigg HL, et al: *Radiology* 1967; 88:274.

MEASUREMENT OF RETROSTERNAL
SOFT TISSUE*

TABLE 5–7.

Width of the Retrosternal Soft Tissue*

Sex	Age Range (yr)	Mean Age (yr)	Distance from Manubrio-sternal Joint (cm)†	No. of Cases	Mean (mm)	SD (mm)	SE (mm)
Normal subjects							
Males	20–39	28.4	2	43	2.35	1.00	0.15
			4	43	2.35	1.34	0.20
			6	41	2.68	1.52	0.24
	42–59	49.2	2	33	2.64	1.11	0.19
			4	33	2.64	0.99	0.17
			6	31	3.03	1.30	0.23
	61–72	64.3	2	12	3.42	1.38	0.40
			4	13	3.46	1.61	0.45
			6	13	4.46	1.61	0.45
Females	20–40	29.7	2	33	2.12	1.16	0.20
			4	33	2.33	1.36	0.23
			6	33	2.88	1.34	0.23
	41–59	49.9	2	23	2.26	1.48	0.31
			4	22	2.59	1.56	0.33
			6	23	3.17	1.77	0.37
	63–78	69.2	2	8	2.38	1.19	0.42
			4	8	2.25	0.71	0.25
			6	8	3.25	1.49	0.53
All measurements analyzed together		41.5		453	2.67	1.38	0.065
Subjects with obstructive emphysema							
Males	22–78	57.7	2	8	1.75	0.89	0.31
			4	8	1.63	0.92	0.32
			6	8	1.63	1.30	0.46

*From Jemelin C, Candardjis G: *Radiology* 1973; 109:7. Used by permission.
†Indicates the point at which the measurement was taken.

Technique
Central ray: Perpendicular to plane of film centered over midchest.
Position: True lateral upright.
Target-film distance: 180 cm.

Ref: Jemelin C, Candardjis G: *Radiology* 1973; 109:7.

MEASUREMENT OF RETROSTERNAL
SOFT TISSUE

Measurements (Table 5–7)

Measurements made 2, 4, and 6 cm below the sternal margin of the manubriosternal sternal joint. These measurements are useful in detecting abnormalities of the retrosternal soft tissues.

Source of Material

Data based on a study of 380 chest films of normal patients, male and female, ranging in age from 20 to 78 years.

MEASUREMENT OF THE NORMAL THYMUS BY CT*

Technique

1. CT scans were performed on a GE 8800 scanner using a scan time of 5.6 sec and a 2.5 sec interscan delay.
2. Contiguous 1-cm thick slices were obtained at full inspiration. Contrast infusion was administered by bolus.

Measurements (Fig 5–20)

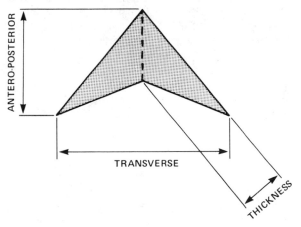

FIG 5–20.
(From Francis IR, et al: *AJR* 1985; 145:249–254.)

The craniocaudal extent, maximum AP and transverse dimensions, and thickness were measured as shown in Figure 5–20.

The normal measurements are given in Table 5–8.

Ref: Francis IR, et al: *AJR* 1985;145:249–254.

MEASUREMENT OF THE NORMAL
THYMUS BY CT

TABLE 5–8.

Thymic Measurements in Patients With Normal Glands*

Age Group (yr)	No. of Patients	Mean Dimension in cm (SD)			
		Thickness	Anteroposterior	Craniocaudal	Transverse
0–10	23	1.50(0.46)	2.52(0.82)	3.53(0.99)	3.13(0.85)
10–20	31	1.05(0.36)	2.56(0.88)	4.99(1.25)	3.05(1.17)
20–30	13	0.89(0.16)	2.38(0.72)	5.38(1.80)	2.87(0.86)
30–40	8	0.99(0.34)	2.48(0.86)	5.00(1.12)	3.38(1.37)
40–50	3	0.93(0.58)	2.23(0.93)	6.67(2.08)	3.17(0.76)
50–60	4	0.58(0.33)	0.58(0.33)	2.00(1.15)	1.43(0.48)

*From Francis IR, et al: *AJR* 1985; 145:249–254. Used by permission.

Source of Material

Data based on CT examination of 309 normal patients ranging in age from 6 weeks to 81 years.

CHAPTER 6

The Cardiovascular System

MEASUREMENT OF THE HEART IN CHILDREN

Cardiothoracic Index

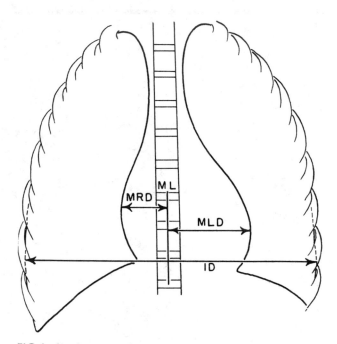

FIG 6–1.

TABLE 6–1.

First Year of Life*

Age Range (wk)	No. of Cases	Mean Cardiothoracic Index	Range (Within 1 SD)
0–3	52	0.55	0.60–0.50
4–7	36	0.58	0.64–0.52
8–15	71	0.57	0.62–0.51
16–23	42	0.57	0.62–0.51
24–31	27	0.56	0.61–0.50
32–39	35	0.56	0.61–0.51
40–47	19	0.54	0.60–0.49
48–55	22	0.53	0.57–0.49

*Data from Bakwin H, Bakwin RM: *Am J Dis Child* 1935; 49:861.

TABLE 6-2.

First 6 Years of Life[†]

Age (YR)	No. of Cases	Mean Cardio-thoracic Index	Actual Total Range
0-1	357	0.49	0.65-0.39
1-2	211	0.49	0.60-0.39
2-3	183	0.45	0.50-0.39
3-4	152	0.45	0.52-0.40
4-5	87	0.45	0.52-0.40
5-6	33	0.45	0.50-0.40

†Data from Maresh MM, Washburn AH: *Am J Dis Child* 1938; 56:33.

TABLE 6-3.

7 to 12 Years[‡]

Age in (YR)	No. of Cases	Total Transverse Diameter of Heart (CM)	Internal Diameter of Thorax (CM)	Normal Range
Boys				
7	35	9.2	19.7	0.49-0.43
8	32	9.4	20.5	0.49-0.42
9	35	9.5	21.1	0.49-0.41
10	21	9.8	21.5	0.49-0.43
11	21	9.9	22.0	0.49-0.43
12	19	10.1	23.0	0.46-0.40
Girls				
7	36	9.1	19.3	0.50-0.44
8	32	9.3	20.0	0.50-0.44
9	28	9.5	20.6	0.49-0.43
10	22	9.7	20.9	0.49-0.43
11	24	9.9	22.0	0.49-0.41
12	21	10.4	22.9	0.49-0.41

‡Data from Lincoln EM, Spillman R: *Am J Dis Child* 1928; 35:791.

MEASUREMENT OF THE HEART IN CHILDREN*†‡

Cardiothoracic Index

Technique
  Central ray: Perpendicular to plane of film centered over midpoint of chest.
  Positions:

1. Bakwin and Bakwin: anteroposterior erect. No timing according to phase of respiration.
2. Maresh and Washburn: infants, posteroanterior supine; from age 3 or 3½ years, posteroanterior erect.
3. Lincoln and Spillman: posteroanterior erect. Moderately deep inspiration.

Target-film distances:

1. Bakwin and Bakwin: 2 meters.
2. Maresh and Washburn: infants, 1.5 meters (5 feet); from 3 or 3½ years, 2.1 meters (7 feet).
3. Lincoln and Spillman: 6 feet.

Measurements (Fig 6–1; Tables 6–1 to 6–3)

MRD = Maximum transverse diameter of the right side of the heart, which is a line drawn from the midline of the spine to the most distant point on the right cardiac margin.
MLD = Maximum transverse diameter on the left side of the heart.
  ID = Internal diameter of the thorax drawn parallel to the transverse cardiac diameters through the tip of the dome of the right side of the diaphragm. It extends from the right to the left pleural surface.

The total transverse cardiac diameter is the sum of *MRD* and *MLD*. The cardiothoracic index is obtained by dividing the sum of *MRD* and *MLD* by *ID*. Originally, the heart was considered pathologically enlarged when the ratio exceeded 0.50. Experience has demonstrated that there is a considerable range for the normal values of the cardiothoracic index, the range being widest during the first year of life.

Ref: Bakwin H, Bakwin RM: *Am J Dis Child* 1935; 49:861.
†*Ref:* Maresh MM, Washburn AH: *AM J Dis Child* 1938; 56:33.
‡*Ref:* Lincoln EM, Spillman R: *Am J Dis Child* 1928; 35:791.

MEASUREMENT OF THE HEART IN CHILDREN

Source of Material

Bakwin and Bakwin: Data based on study of 165 infant boys and 146 infant girls born in Bellevue Hospital. Only infants of white antecedents were studied.

Maresh and Washburn: Data based on study of 38 normal boys and 29 normal girls examined by the Child Research Council every 3 months since birth. One thousand twenty-six roentgenograms were measured.

Lincoln and Spillman: Study made over a period of 7 school years and based on yearly roentgenograms of 246 normal school children.

Transverse Cardiac Diameter (Ages Between 4 and 16 Years)

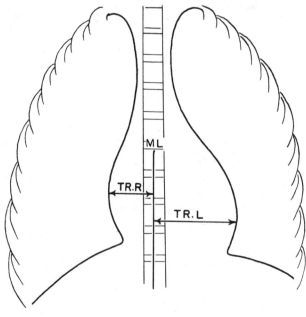

FIG 6–2.

MEASUREMENT OF THE HEART IN CHILDREN

TABLE 6—4.

Percent Deviation From Average*

% Minus					Average %	% Plus				
25	20	15	10	5		5	10	15	20	25
51	55	58	62	65	**69**	72	76	79	83	86
52	56	59	63	66	**70**	73	77	80	84	87
52	56	59	63	67	**71**	75	79	83	86	90
53	57	61	64	68	**72**	76	80	83	87	91
54	58	62	65	69	**73**	77	81	84	88	92
55	59	63	66	70	**74**	78	82	85	89	93
57	60	64	68	71	**75**	70	82	86	90	94
58	61	64	68	72	**76**	80	84	88	91	95
59	62	65	69	73	**77**	81	85	89	92	96
59	62	66	70	74	**78**	82	86	90	94	98
60	63	67	71	75	**79**	83	87	91	95	99
61	64	68	72	76	**80**	84	88	92	96	100
62	65	69	73	77	**81**	85	89	93	97	101
63	66	70	74	78	**82**	86	90	94	98	102
63	66	71	75	78	**83**	87	91	95	100	104
64	67	71	76	80	**84**	88	92	97	101	105
65	68	72	76	81	**85**	89	94	98	102	106
66	69	73	77	82	**86**	90	95	99	103	107
67	70	74	78	83	**87**	91	96	100	104	108
67	70	75	79	84	**88**	92	97	101	106	110
68	72	76	80	85	**89**	93	98	102	107	111
69	72	76	81	86	**90**	94	99	104	108	112
70	73	77	82	86	**91**	96	100	105	109	113
71	74	78	83	87	**92**	97	101	106	110	114
71	74	79	84	88	**93**	98	102	107	112	117
72	75	80	85	89	**94**	99	103	108	113	118
72	76	81	85	90	**95**	100	105	109	114	119
73	77	82	86	91	**96**	101	106	110	115	120
74	78	82	87	92	**97**	102	107	112	116	120
74	78	83	88	93	**98**	103	108	113	118	123

MEASUREMENT OF THE HEART IN CHILDREN

% Minus					Average %	% Plus				
25	20	15	10	5		5	10	15	20	25
75	79	84	89	94	**99**	104	109	114	119	124
75	80	85	90	95	**100**	105	110	115	120	125
76	81	86	91	96	**101**	106	111	116	121	126
77	82	87	92	97	**102**	107	112	117	122	127
78	82	88	93	98	**103**	108	113	118	124	129
79	83	88	94	99	**104**	109	114	120	125	130
80	84	89	95	100	**105**	110	116	121	126	131
81	85	90	95	101	**106**	111	117	122	127	132
82	86	91	96	102	**107**	112	118	123	128	133
82	86	92	97	103	**108**	113	119	124	130	135
83	87	93	98	104	**109**	114	120	125	131	136
84	88	94	99	105	**110**	116	121	127	132	137
85	89	94	100	105	**111**	117	122	128	133	138
85	90	95	101	106	**112**	118	123	129	134	139
85	90	96	102	107	**113**	119	124	130	136	141
86	91	97	103	108	**114**	120	125	131	137	142
87	92	98	104	109	**115**	121	127	132	138	143
88	93	99	104	110	**116**	122	128	133	139	144
89	94	99	105	111	**117**	123	129	135	140	145
89	94	100	106	112	**118**	124	130	136	142	147
90	95	101	107	113	**119**	125	131	137	143	149
91	96	102	108	114	**120**	126	132	138	144	150
92	97	103	109	115	**121**	127	133	139	145	151
93	98	104	110	116	**122**	128	134	140	146	152
93	98	105	111	117	**123**	129	135	141	148	153
94	99	105	112	118	**124**	130	136	143	149	155
95	100	106	113	119	**125**	131	138	144	150	156
96	101	107	113	120	**126**	132	139	145	151	157
97	102	108	114	121	**127**	133	140	146	152	158
97	102	109	115	122	**128**	134	141	147	154	160
98	103	110	116	123	**129**	135	142	148	155	161
99	104	111	117	124	**130**	137	143	150	156	162
100	105	111	118	124	**131**	138	144	151	157	163
101	106	112	119	125	**132**	139	145	152	158	164

*From Esguerra-Gomez GE: *Bol Clin Marly* 1949; 11: nos. 5–8. Used by permission.

TABLE 6–5.
Prediction of Transverse Cardiac Diameter in Children*†

Height		Weight lb	35		40		45												55	60	65	70	75	80	85	90
in	cm	kg	14	15	16	17	18	19	20	21	22	23	24	25	26	27	28	29	30	31	32	33	34	35	36	37	38	39	40	41
30	76		86	89																										
	77		86	89																										
31	78		85	88	91																									
	79		85	88	91																									
	80		84	87	90																									
32	81		84	87	90	92																								
	82		83	86	89	92																								
	83		83	86	89	91																								
33	84		82	85	88	91	93																							
	85		82	85	88	90	93																							
34	86		81	84	87	90	92																							
	87		81	84	86	89	92	94																						
	88		80	83	86	89	91	93																						
	89		80	83	85	88	91	93																						
35	90		79	82	85	88	90	92	95																					
	91		79	82	84	87	90	92	94																					
36	92		79	81	84	87	89	91	94																					
	93		78	81	83	86	89	91	93	96																				
37	94		78	80	83	86	88	90	93	95																				
	95		77	80	82	85	88	90	92	95																				

Group		c1	c2	c3	c4	c5	c6	c7	c8	c9	c10	c11	c12	c13	c14	c15	c16
38	96	77	80	82	85	87	89	92	94	96							
	97	76	79	82	84	87	89	91	94	96							
	98	76	79	81	84	86	89	91	93	95							
39	99	76	78	81	83	86	88	90	93	95							
	100	75	78	80	83	85	88	90	92	94							
40	101	75	77	80	83	85	88	90	92	94	97						
	102	74	77	80	82	84	87	89	91	93	96						
	103	74	77	79	82	84	86	89	91	93	95						
	104	74	76	79	81	84	86	88	91	92	94	97					
41	105	73	76	78	81	83	86	88	90	92	94	96	98				
42	106	73	76	78	80	83	85	87	89	91	93	96	98				
	107	73	75	78	80	82	85	87	89	91	93	95	98				
	108	72	75	77	80	82	84	86	88	91	92	95	97				
43	109	73	75	77	79	82	84	86	88	90	92	94	97				
	110	72	74	77	79	81	84	86	88	90	92	94	96				
44	111	71	74	76	79	81	83	85	87	89	91	94	96	99			
	112	71	74	76	79	81	83	85	87	89	91	93	95	99			
	113	71	73	76	78	80	83	85	87	89	91	93	95	98			
45	114	70	73	76	78	80	82	84	86	88	90	92	94	98			
	115	70	73	75	78	80	82	84	86	88	90	92	94	97			
46	116	70	73	75	77	79	81	83	85	87	89	91	93	95	97	99	
	117	70	72	75	77	79	81	83	85	87	89	91	93	95	97	99	100
	118	69	72	74	77	78	81	83	85	87	88	90	92	94	96	98	100
47	119	69	72	74	76	78	80	82	84	86	88	90	92	94	96	98	99
	120	69	71	74	76	78	80	82	84	86	88	90	92	94	96	97	99
	121		71	73	76	78	80	82	84	87	89	91	93	95	97	98	100
48	122		70	73	75	77	79	81	83	85	87	89	91	93	95	97	100
	123		70	73	75	77	79	81	83	85	87	89	91	94	96	98	100
49	124		70	72	74	76	78	80	82	84	86	88	90	92	94	97	99
	125		70	72	74	76	78	80	82	84	86	88	90	92	93	95	98

TABLE 6–5 (cont.).

Weight

Height in	Height cm	14	15	35 lb / 16	17	40 lb / 18	19	45 lb / 20	21	50 lb / 22	23	24	55 lb / 25	26	60 lb / 27	28	65 lb / 29	30	31	70 lb / 32	33	75 lb / 34	35	80 lb / 36	37	38	85 lb / 39	40	90 lb / 41
50	126			72	74	76	78	80	82	84	86	87	89	91	93	95	96	98	100	102									
	127				73	76	78	80	82	83	85	87	89	91	93	94	96	98	100	101									
	128					75	77	79	81	83	85	87	89	90	92	94	96	97	99	101									
	129					75	77	79	81	83	85	86	88	90	92	94	95	97	99	101	102								
51	130						77	79	81	82	84	86	88	90	92	93	95	96	98	100	102	102	104	105	107	108	110	111	112
	131						76	78	80	82	84	86	88	89	91	93	94	96	98	100	101	102	104	105	106	108	109	110	112
52	132						76	78	80	82	84	85	87	89	91	93	94	96	98	99	101	102	103	105	106	107	109	110	111
	133						76	78	80	82	83	85	87	89	90	92	94	95	97	99	101	101	103	104	106	107	109	110	111
53	134								79	82	83	85	87	88	90	92	93	95	97	98	100	101	103	104	105	107	108	109	111
	135								79	81	83	84	86	88	90	91	93	95	97	98	100	101	102	104	105	106	108	109	110
54	136									81	82	84	86	88	89	91	93	94	96	98	99	101	102	103	105	106	107	109	110
	137									80	82	84	86	87	89	91	92	94	96	97	99	100	102	103	104	106	107	108	109
	138										82	84	85	87	89	90	92	94	96	97	98	100	101	103	104	105	107	108	109
	139										82	83	85	87	88	90	92	93	95	97	98	99	101	102	104	105	106	107	108
55	140											83	85	86	88	90	91	93	95	96	98	99	101	102	103	105	106	107	108
	141												84	86	88	89	91	92	95	96	97	99	100	102	103	104	106	107	108
56	142												84	86	87	89	91	92	94	96	97	98	100	101	103	104	105	107	108
	143														87	88	90	92	94	95	97	98	100	101	102	104	105	106	107
57	144														87	88	90	92	93	95	96	98	99	101	102	103	105	106	107
	145															88	90	91	93	95	96	97	99	100	102	103	104	105	107
58	146															88	89	91	93	94	96	97	99	100	101	103	104	105	107
	147																89	91	92	94	95	97	98	100	101	102	104	105	106
	148																89	90	92	94	95	96	98	99	101	102	103	104	106
	149																	90	92	93	95	96	98	99	100	102	103	104	105
59	150																88	90	92	93	94	96	97	99	100	101	102	104	105
	151																		91	93	94	95	97	98	100	101	102	103	105
60	152																		91	92	94	95	97	98	99	101	102	103	105

*From Esguerra-Gomez GE: *Bol Clin Marly* 1949; 11: nos. 5–8. Used by permission.

†$D \text{ (in cm)} = 2\sqrt{\dfrac{\text{weight (Kg)}}{\text{height (m)}}}$

MEASUREMENT OF THE HEART IN CHILDREN

Transverse Cardiac Diameter

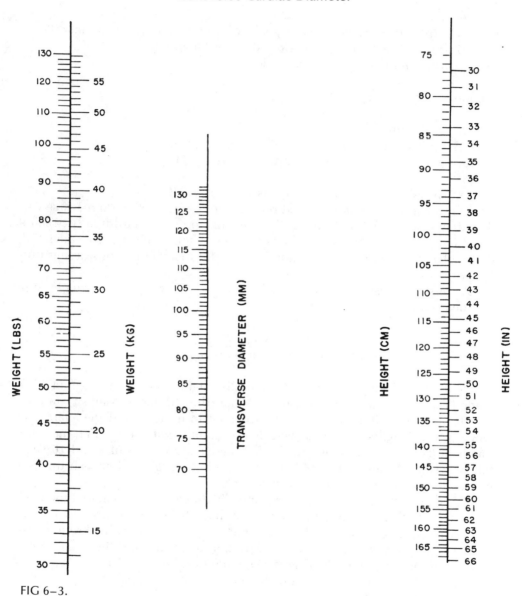

FIG 6–3.

Nomogram for prediction of transverse diameter in children. $D \text{ (cm)} = 2\sqrt{\dfrac{\text{weight (kg)}}{\text{height (m)}}}$. (Adapted from Esguerra-Gomez GE: *Radiology* 1951; 57:217.)

MEASUREMENT OF THE HEART IN CHILDREN*

Technique
Central ray: Perpendicular to plane of film centered over midchest.
Position: Erect, posteroanterior. Moderate inspiration.
Target-film distance: At least 6 feet.

Measurements (Fig 6–2)

ML = Midline.
TR.R = Maximum transverse cardiac diameter, right.
TR.L = Maximum transverse cardiac diameter, left.

Transverse cardiac diameter equals TR.R plus TR.L.

These measurements are based on measured length of the transverse cardiac diameter in relation to the anthropometric index. In children between 9 and 16 years of age, the mean values show an insignificant negative deviation that probably coincides with accumulation of fat in subcutaneous tissues during growth periods.

A constant to establish a predicted cardiac transverse diameter in children was determined. The constant is:

$$\frac{\text{Weight (kg)} \times 100,000}{\text{Height (cm)} \times (\text{transverse diameter})^2} = 2.47$$

With the aid of this constant, prediction tables and a nomogram were made (Tables 6–4 and 6–5; Fig 6–3). When the studies of Maresh* in relation to the prediction tables, the anthropometric indices, and the average of weights and heights were analyzed, it was found that the cardiac measurements of 81.2% of the examined children between the ages of 4 and 16 years fell between +10 and −10 percent of the prediction tables. Between the ages of 4 and 8 years, the percentage was 88.53%.

These records studied on the respective histograms establish that there exists a relationship between the transverse diameter of the heart and the anthropometric index not only in adults but in children as well. From 4 to 8 years of age, the histogram coincides with that of adults, and the slight minus deviation from 9 to 15 years of age is explained as the result of the subcutaneous accumulation of fat during growth periods.

Source of Material
The data are based on a study by Maresh, in which a group of 71 boys and 57 girls were examined radiologically several times a year over a period of more than 20 years. Of a total of 3,205 roentgenograms, only 3,190 gave the necessary data (transverse diameter of the heart, weight, and height). The data of Esguerra-Gomez are based exclusively on this group.

*Ref: Maresh MM: Pediatrics 1948; 2:382.

MEASUREMENT OF THE HEART
AND AORTA IN ADULTS

The Cardiothoracic Ratio*

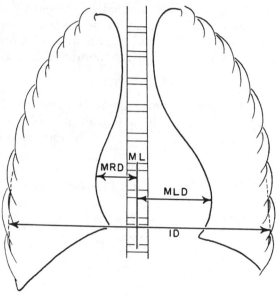

FIG 6–4.

Technique

    Central ray: Perpendicular to plane of film centered over midportion of chest.

    Position: Posteroanterior erect. Breathing suspended in midrespiration.

    Target-film distance: 6 feet.

Measurements (Fig 6–4)

MRD = Maximum transverse diameter of the right side of the heart, which is a line drawn from the midline of the spine to the most distant point on the right cardiac margin.

  ML = Midline of the spine.

MLD = Maximum transverse diameter on the left side of the heart.

   ID = Greatest internal diameter of the thorax, which is usually at the level of the apex or one space lower, measuring the inner borders of the ribs.

The transverse diameter *(TD)* of the heart = MRD + MLD.

$$\frac{\text{Maximum transverse diameter heart } (TD)}{\text{Maximum transverse diameter thorax } (ID)}$$

Ref: Danzer CS: *Am J Med Sci* 1919; 157:313.

MEASUREMENT OF THE HEART AND AORTA IN ADULTS

The normal heart is usually less than half the greatest diameter of the thorax. The normal cardiothoracic ratio varies between 39% and 50%, with an average of about 45%. Because of variations due to cardiac filling and phase of respiration, a margin of safety of 2% above the upper limit is claimed.

Source of Material
The method was tested on approximately 500 patients. In Danzer's opinion, the results of this test warrant its practicability and usefulness in the estimation of cardiac size, particularly in cases of moderate or early enlargement.

Cardiac Measurements in Systole and Diastole† (Table 6−6)

TABLE 6−6.

Differences in Heart Size	No. of Patients	Percent of Patients
0.0 to 0.3 cm.	169	52
0.4 to 0.9 cm.	113	41
1.0 to 1.7 cm.	22	7

1. Two chest films obtained on each of 359 patients.
2. Films taken during systole and diastole.
3. Summary of size changes in the widest transverse measurements of the heart.

Cardiac Measurement in the Anteroposterior Projection‡
A study of the cardiothoracic ratio in erect anteroposterior projection has shown an upper limit of cardiothoracic ratio of 55% and of heart diameter of 165 mm in males and 150 mm in females and has been shown to provide useful discrimination between normal and abnormal heart size.

†Ref: Gammill SL, et al: *Radiology* 1970; 94:115.
‡Ref: Kabala JE, Wilde P: *Br J Radiol* 1987; 60:981−986.

ANGIOCARDIOGRAPHIC CIRCULATION TIMES*

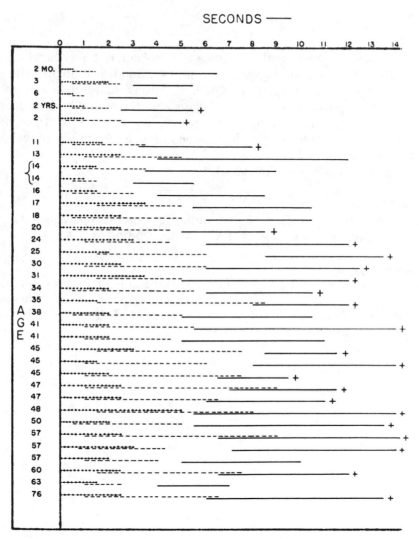

FIG 6–5.

Normal opacification periods of the superior vena cava, pulmonary artery and its main branches, and the aorta. Timing begins with the initial entry of the contrast medium into the intrathoracic veins. Note that, with few exceptions, there is no overlapping opacity of the pulmonary arteries and the aorta. *(Closed circles* = superior vena cava; *dashes* = pulmonary arteries; *solid line* = aorta; *plus sign* = unfilmed. (From Figley MM: *Radiology* 1954; 63:837. Used by permission.)

*Ref: Figley MM: *Radiology* 1954; 63:837.

ANGIOCARDIOGRAPHIC CIRCULATION TIMES

Technique
  Central ray: Perpendicular to plane of film centered over heart.
  Position: Children up to age 6 or 7 are examined recumbent, with no attempt to control respiration. Older children and adults are examined in a sitting position. Injection is begun with the initiation of a deep but not maximum inspiration, and the breath is held for 12 to 15 seconds during the entire filming cycle. Dosage is 1 cc for 2 pounds of weight up to a maximum of 50 cc.
  Target-film distance: Immaterial.

Measurements (Fig 6–5)
Circulation times are based on the author's visual estimate of the earliest and latest definite opacification of the structure studied.

Source of Material
The data are based on a study of angiocardiograms of 35 patients, most of whom were studied for intrathoracic masses and had no clinical evidence of cardiac disease or compression by the mass. Several of the patients had aneurysms or anomalous aortic branches.

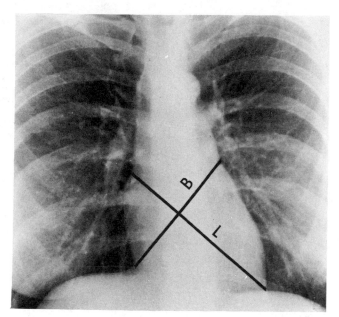

FIG 6–6.
(From Keats TE, Enge IP: *Radiology* 1965; 85:850. Used by permission.)

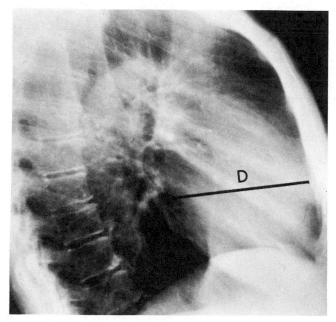

FIG 6–7.
(From Keats TE, Enge IP: *Radiology* 1965; 85:850. Used by permission.)

MEASUREMENT OF CARDIAC VOLUME*

TABLE 6–7.

Cardiac Volume in Children and Adolescents as Predicted by Body Weight*†

Body Weight (X) in Pounds	Cardiac Volume (Y) of Males (cc)			Cardiac Volume (Y) of Females (cc)		
		95% Confidence Limits			95% Confidence Limits	
	Mean	Upper Limit	Lower Limit	Mean	Upper Limit	Lower Limit
5	27	37	20	29	39	21
10	53	72	40	54	73	39
15	79	107	59	77	105	57
20	104	141	77	101	137	74
25	129	175	95	123	167	91
30	154	209	114	145	197	107
40	204	277	151	189	256	139
50	254	344	187	231	314	170
60	303	411	224	273	370	201
70	352	477	260	314	426	231
80	401	543	296	354	481	261
90	450	610	332	394	535	290
100	498	676	368	434	589	319
110	547	741	404	473	642	348
120	595	807	439	512	695	377
130	644	873	475	550	748	405
140	692	938	510	588	800	433
150	740	1004	545	626	852	461
160	788	1069	580	664	903	489
170	836	1134	616	702	954	516

*From Nghiem QX, Schreiber MH, Harris LC: *Circulation* 1967; 35:509. Used by permission.
†For males $Y = 5.620 \, X^{0.973}$ (linear correlation r = 0.982); for females $Y = 6.628 \, X^{0.907}$ (linear correlation r = 0.980).

*Ref: Nghiem QX, Schreiber MH, Harris LC: *Circulation* 1967; 35:509.

TABLE 6–8.

Comparison of Body Surface Area and Body Weight as Predictors of Cardiac Volume*†

Sample	No. of Subjects	Correlation Coefficient (r)	Regression Equation	95% Confidence Limits		% of Mean
				Upper Limit	Lower Limit	
Body surface area (Z)						
Limited data	261	0.981	Y = 284Z	413Z	155Z	±45
Males	132	0.980	Y = 295Z	434Z	156Z	±47
Females	129	0.987	Y = 273Z	388Z	159Z	±42
Body weight (X)						
Limited data	261	0.987	Y = 5.0X	6.6X	3.4X	±32
Males	132	0.990	Y = 5.2X	6.7X	3.7X	±29
Females	129	0.990	Y = 4.8X	6.4X	3.2X	±34
Total data	305	0.985	Y = 4.9X	6.6X	3.2X	±34
Males	158	0.985	Y = 5.1X	6.8X	3.5X	±32
Females	147	0.989	Y = 4.7X	6.3X	3.1X	±34

*From Nghiem QX, Schreiber MH, Harris LC: *Circulation* 1967; 35:509. Used by permission.
†The limited data included 261 subjects whose height and weight were known. Y = cardiac volume in cubic cm; X = body weight in pounds; Z = body surface area in square meters.

MEASUREMENT OF CARDIAC VOLUME

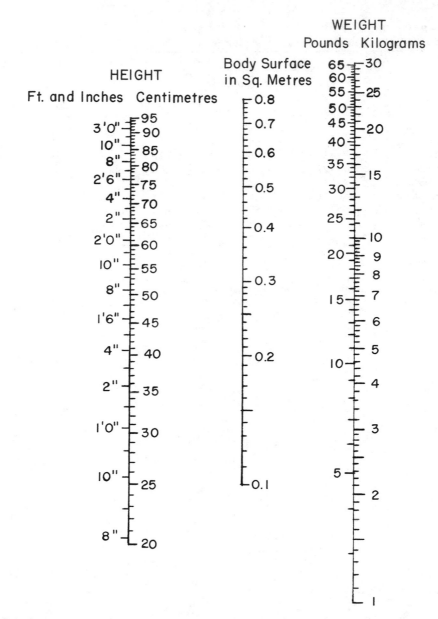

FIG 6–8.
Nomogram for the determination of body surface area of children. (Adapted from Documenta Geigy: *Scientific Tables,* ed 6. Basel, Switzerland, 1962.)

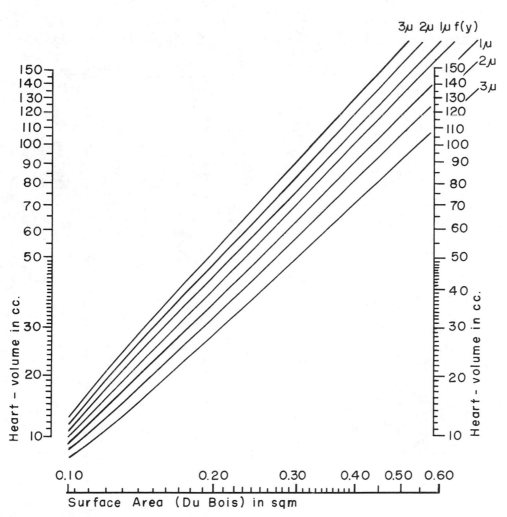

FIG 6–9.
Predicted normal heart volume compared with calculated heart volumes in infants. (From Lind J: *Acta Radiol* 1950; suppl 82. Used by permission.)

MEASUREMENT OF CARDIAC VOLUME

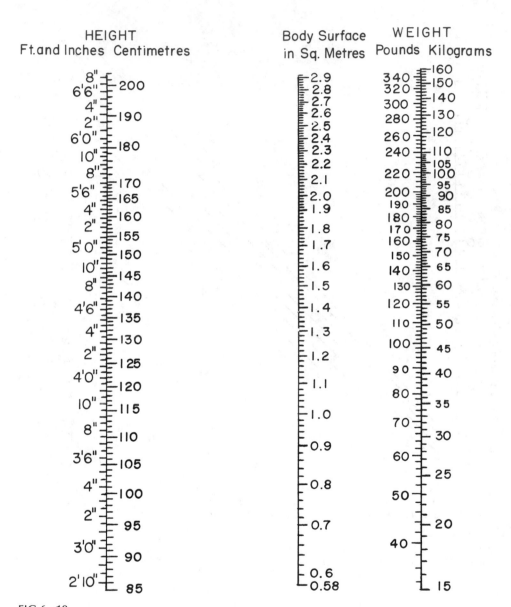

FIG 6–10.
Nomogram for the determination of body surface area of adults. (Adapted from Documenta Geigy: *Scientific Tables,* ed 6. Basel, Switzerland, 1962.)

MEASUREMENT OF CARDIAC VOLUME

TABLE 6−9.

Adults: Upper Limits of Normal*

	$\dfrac{\text{Heart Volumes}}{\text{Body Surface Area}} =$
Females	450−490 cc/m²
Males	500−540 cc/m²

*Data from Amundsen P: *Acta Radiol* 1959, suppl 181.

Technique

Central ray: Perpendicular to plane of film centered over midchest.

Position: Posteroanterior in adults and children and anteroposterior or posteroanterior in infants.

Target-film distance: 200 cm, 150 cm, or 100 cm.

Measurements (Figs 6−6 to 6−10; Tables 6−7 to 6−9)

L = Long diameter. This line extends from the junction of the superior vena cava and right atrium to the cardiac apex.

B = Broad diameter. This line extends from the junction of the right atrium and the diaphragm to a point on the left heart border at the junction of the pulmonary artery and left atrial appendage.

D = Depth; represents the greatest horizontal depth of the cardiac shadow.

Calculation of cardiac volume is based on the formula:

$$V = L \times B \times D \times K$$

The constant (K) will vary with the focal-film distances used: 200 cm, K = 0.42; 150 cm, K = 0.39; 100 cm, K = 0.38.

The calculated cardiac volume is correlated with body surface area.

Nomograms for the determination of body surface area for children and adults, derived from patient height and weight, are shown in Figures 6−8 and 6−10. The normal heart volumes for infants correlated with body surface area are shown in Figure 6−9.

For older children and adults, the variation of normal is sufficiently limited that, for practical purposes, it is adequate to divide the calculated volume by the body surface area and compare with normal standards on page 414.

Cardiac mensuration by volume determination is probably the most accurate method now available.

Source of Material

Nghiem et al. studied 305 subjects; 158 were males and 147 were females. Ages ranged from birth to 18 years, 9 months. Body surface area ranged from 0.18 to 1.87 m^2 and body weight from 6.2 to 167 lbs.

Lind's data on normal heart volumes in infants are based on a study of 293 children under 2 years of age, male and female. All were healthy.

The data on children from 4 to 7, 9 to 12, and 14 to 16 years are taken from Carlgren,* based on a study of 61 healthy children.

Amundsen's data are based on a study of 87 normal patients (29 males and 58 females).

*Ref: Carlgren LE *Acta Paediatr Scand* 1946; 33(suppl 6).

MEASUREMENT OF THE PEDIATRIC
AORTA BY CT*

Technique

1. Dynamic scanning was performed on a 9800 GE CT scanner.
2. Sixty percent iodinated contrast material was injected as a bolus with a dose of 3 cc/kg.
3. Scans were performed at 5 or 10 mm levels with the patient breathing quietly. Two-second scans were obtained.

Measurement (Fig 6–11)

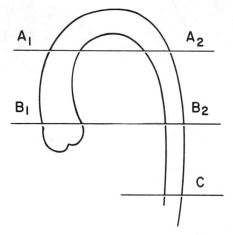

FIG 6–11.
Illustration of the thoracic aorta depicts the approximate levels of aortic measurement. (From Fitzgerald SW, et al: *Radiology* 1987; 165:667–669. Used by permission.)

Measurement of the aorta was obtained perpendicular to the long axis of the aorta at three levels with direct reading calipers. Level A was placed 1 cm caudal to the top of the aortic arch. Level B was 1 cm cranial to the aortic root. Level C was approximately 1 cm cranial to the dome of the right hemidiaphragm (Fig 6–12).

*Ref: Fitzgerald SW, et al: *Radiology* 1987; 165:667–669.

MEASUREMENT OF THE PEDIATRIC
AORTA BY CT

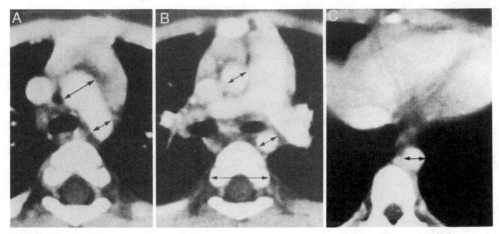

FIG 6–12.
Representative CT scans of a 2½-year-old boy obtained approximately **(A)** 1 cm caudal to the top of the aortic arch. **B,** 1 cm cranial to the aortic root. **C,** at the level of the dome of the right hemidiaphragm. The thoracic vertebral body width was measured coronally at level B. *Arrows* indicate sites of measurement. (From Fitzgerald SW, et al: *Radiology* 1987; 165:667–669. Used by permission.)

The distribution of aortic diameters as a function of age is shown in Figure 6–13.

MEASUREMENT OF THE PEDIATRIC
AORTA BY CT

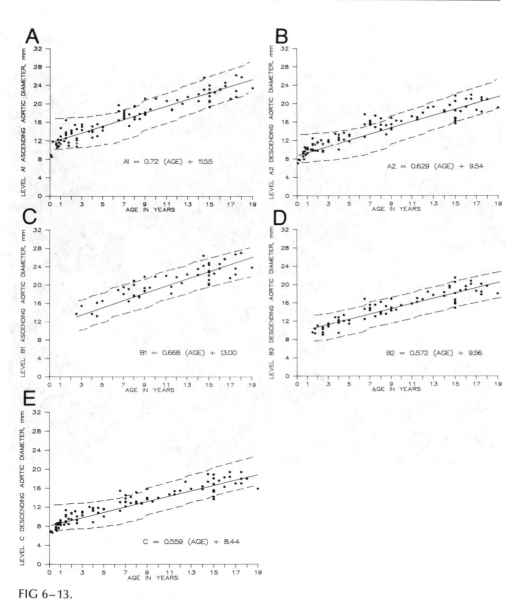

FIG 6–13.
Distributions of aortic diameters plotted versus age. The *solid lines* represent linear regression lines, and the *dashed lines* represent 95% confidence bands. **(a)** A_1 (ascending aortic diameter). **(b)** A_2 (descending). **(c)** B_1 (ascending). **(d)** B_2 (descending). **(e)** C (descending). (From Fitzgerald SW, et al: *Radiology* 1987; 165:667–669. Used by permission.)

Source of Material

Data are based on a CT study of 97 patients ranging in age from 2 weeks to 19 years.

MEASUREMENT OF CARDIAC
STRUCTURES BY CT*

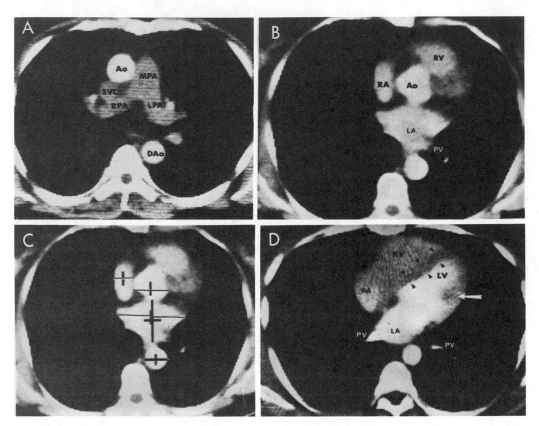

FIG 6–14.

After contrast administration in different patients 2 to 3 years after bypass graft surgery with normal hemodynamics and left ventriculogram within 24 hours after study. **A,** through pulmonary artery bifurcation *(MPA)*. **B,** plane of section passes through aortic root *(Ao)* and left atrium *(LA)* posteriorly. Low-density fat in pericardial space separates right atrium *(RA)* from aorta. On scans through aortic sinuses **(B)**, aorta has cloverleaf configuration. **C,** (same as **B**), location of measurements of right atrium, aortic root, left atrium, and descending aorta. **D,** through mitral valve. Artifact emanates from sternal wires. Opacified left atrium *(LA)* and left ventricular chamber *(LV)* with protruding papillary muscles *(arrow)* are well seen. Interventricular septum *(arrowheads)* separates right *(RV)* and left *(LV)* ventricles. RPA = right pulmonary artery; LPA = left pulmonary artery; SVC = superior vena cava; PV = pulmonary veins; RA = right atrium; RV = right ventricle; Ao = ascending aorta; DAo = descending aorta. (From Guthaner DF, et al: AJR 1979; 133:75. Used by permission.)

*Ref: Guthaner DF, et al: AJR 1979; 133:75.

MEASUREMENT OF CARDIAC
STRUCTURES BY CT

Technique

1. Varian CT scanner with 3-second scan time. Slice thickness: 10 mm.
2. Scanning was performed in the supine position during suspended moderate inspiration.
3. Studies were performed before and after bolus injection of 20 to 30 ml of Renografin-60 (Squibb).

Measurements (Fig 6–14 and Table 6–10)

Structures were measured as the diameter perpendicular to the long axis of a tubular organ (such as aorta or pulmonary artery) or the transverse diameter when seen in cross section.

The widest horizontal diameters of the atria were measured. The longest AP diameter of the left atrium was measured on a line perpendicular to the posterior wall of the aortic root at the level of the pulmonary veins. The right ventricle was measured from the atrioventricular groove at its most anterior extent to the indentation of the right ventricular septum.

Measurements were either by electronic calipers or from hard copies, using appropriate minification correction.

MEASUREMENT OF CARDIAC STRUCTURES BY CT

TABLE 6–10.

Cardiac CT Measurements in 15 Normal Patients*†

Structure		Scan Level			
	Arch	Pulmonary Artery Bifurcation	Aortic Root	Mitral Valve	Midventricle
Ascending aorta	3.3 ± 0.6 (N = 4)	3.2 ± 0.5 (N = 12)	3.7 ± 0.3 (N = 12)	. . .	. . .
Descending aorta	2.4 ± 0.3 (N = 8)	2.5 ± 0.4 (N = 12)	2.5 ± 0.3 (N = 12)	2.5 ± 0.4 (N = 12)	2.4 ± 0.3 (N = 10)
Arch	1.5 ± 1.2 (N = 6)	. . .	. . .	. . .	. . .
Right atrium	. . .	. . .	1.9 ± 0.8 (N = 12)	3.2 ± 1.2 (N = 12)	2.8 ± 0.4 (N = 6)
Left atrium	. . .	. . .	Transverse, 6.6 ± 1.0 (N = 12); AP, 3.8 ± 0.6 (N = 12)	Transverse, 6.9 ± 1.5 (N = 10); AP, 4.0 ± 0.9 (N = 10)	. . .
Superior vena cava	1.4 ± 0.4 (N = 8)	2.0 ± 0.4 (N = 10)	. . .	. . .	. . .
Main pulmonary artery	. . .	2.8 ± 0.3 (N = 10)	. . .	. . .	. . .
Left pulmonary artery	. . .	2.0 ± 0.2 (N = 6)	. . .	. . .	. . .
Right pulmonary artery	. . .	2.0 ± 0.4 (N = 8)	. . .	. . .	. . .
Right ventricular outflow tract	. . .	. . .	2.8 ± 1.1 (N = 10)	. . .	. . .
Right ventricle	. . .	. . .	. . .	5.8 ± 1.1 (N = 10)	5.8 ± 1.4 (N = 8)
Interventricular septum	. . .	. . .	. . .	. . .	0.8 ± 0.6 (N = 6)
Coronary sinus	. . .	. . .	. . .	. . .	0.9 ± 0.1 (N = 6)
Inferior vena cava	. . .	. . .	. . .	. . .	2.7 ± 0.6 (N = 5)

*From Guthaner DF, et al: *AJR* 1979; 133:75. Used by permission.
†Mean = ±1 SD; N = number of patients from whom measurements (cm) were taken at the indicated level.

MEASUREMENT OF CARDIAC STRUCTURES BY CT

Source of Material

Ten patients without heart disease and a normal cardiac examination and five patients with normal cardiac catheterization within 24 hours of CT scan, but with a history of aortocoronary bypass surgery 2 or more years earlier.

MEASUREMENT OF NORMAL LEFT
HEART DIMENSIONS BY MR*

Techniques

1. Electrocardiographically gated MRI examination was performed using a whole-body 0.6 T superconducting Technicare magnet with a spin-echo pulse sequence and an echo delay (TE) of 30 msec.
2. Images were oriented along the long and short axes of the left ventricle in planes similar to two-dimensional echocardiograms.
3. *Position:* Supine.

Measurements

Measurements of the left heart were made at end diastole and end systole in both long and short axis views. For each image plane, an initial series of contiguous images was obtained with either single or multislice technique for selection of appropriate levels for sets of single images at end systole and end diastole. The long axis images of the left ventricle were obtained in a plane through the aortic valve and the left ventricular apex (Fig 6–15).

Ref: Kaul S, et al: *AJR* 1986; 146:75–79.

MEASUREMENT OF NORMAL LEFT
HEART DIMENSIONS BY MR

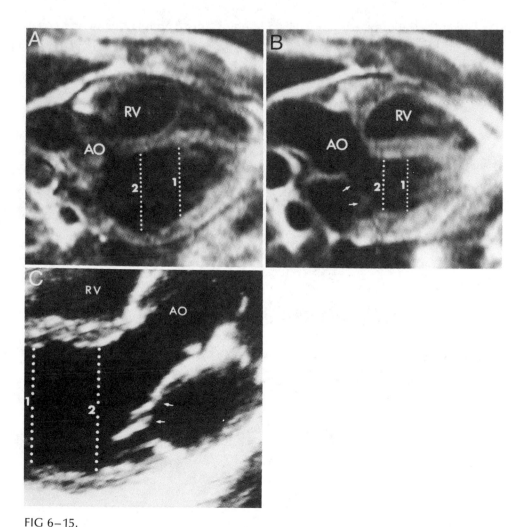

FIG 6–15.
Long-axis images of left ventricle in plane through aortic valve and apex, perpendicular to septum. **A,** MRI, diastole. **B,** MRI, systole. **C,** parasternal long-axis 2DE, diastole. *AO* = aortic sinuses; *RV* = right ventricle; *double arrows* = mitral valve plane. Left ventricular diameters were measured at mid-papillary muscle level *(1)* and chordal level *(2)*. (From Kaul S, et al: *AJR* 1986; 146:75–79. Used by permission.)

MEASUREMENT OF NORMAL LEFT
HEART DIMENSIONS BY MR

The left atrial dimension was best obtained from a contiguous image offset to the right (Fig 6–16).

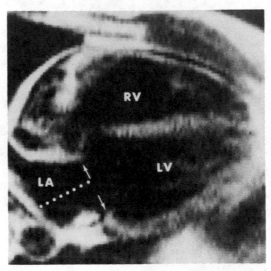

FIG 6–16.
Diastolic MRI through long axis of left ventricle at mitral valve and left atrial level. Anteroposterior mid-left-atrial diameter, from posterior left atrial wall to plane of mitral annulus, is indicated. *LA* = left atrium; *LV* = left ventricle; *RV* = right ventricle; *arrows* = mitral annulus. (From Kaul S, et al: *AJR* 1986; 146:75–79. Used by permission.)

The image plane was then rotated 90° to obtain short axis images of the heart at the chordal level (midway between the aortic valve and papillary muscle) and mid-papillary-muscle level, the level where the papillary muscle appears thickest (Fig 6–17).

MEASUREMENT OF NORMAL LEFT
HEART DIMENSIONS BY MR

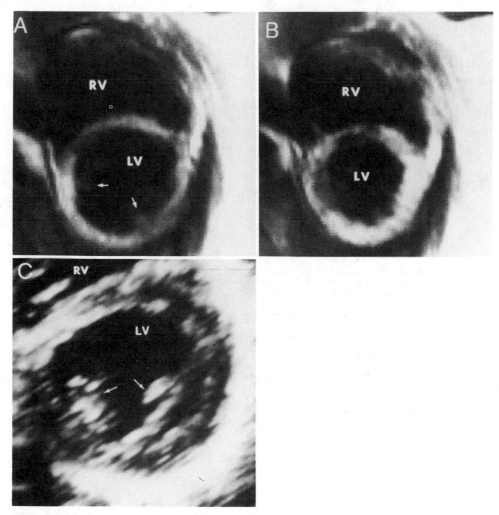

FIG 6–17.
Short-axis images of left ventricle at mid-papillary muscle level. **A,** MRI, diastole. **B,** MRI, systole. **C,** parasternal short-axis 2DE, diastole. *RV* = right ventricle; *LV* = left ventricle; *arrows* = papillary muscles. (From Kaul S, et al: *AJR* 1986; 146:75–79. Used by permission.)

MEASUREMENT OF NORMAL LEFT
HEART DIMENSIONS BY MR

The normal left ventricular dimensions are shown in Table 6–11.

TABLE 6–11.

Normal Left Ventricular Dimensions in 16 Subjects*†

Dimension: Location	Diastole	Systole
Left ventricular cavity diameter (mm)		
Chordal level	46.4 ± 5.5	33.6 ± 3.8
Papillary muscle level	43.4 ± 4.4	29.9 ± 4.8
Septum thickness (mm)		
Chordal level	10.3 ± 0.5	15.5 ± 1.4
Papillary muscle level	10.4 ± 1.8	15.6 ± 2.5
Posterior wall thickness (mm)		
Chordal level	10.2 ± 0.5	15.7 ± 1.0
Papillary muscle level	10.3 ± 1.2	15.4 ± 1.4
Left atrial diameter (mm)		
Anteroposterior	25.6 ± 4.2	. . .

*From Kaul S, et al: *AJR* 1986; 146:75–79. Used by permission.
†Left ventricular measurements were made at mid-papillary-muscle level and midway between the aortic valve and papillary muscle (chordal level). Measurements of the same structure from different planes are consolidated in this table.

Source of Material
Data based on MR studies of 16 normal asymptomatic subjects.

ECHOCARDIOGRAPHIC MEASUREMENTS IN NORMAL SUBJECTS FROM INFANCY TO OLD AGE*

Technique

1. All measurements were made from M-mode echocardiograms recorded on strip chart recorder.
2. Oldest children and adults were studied with a 2.25-MHz, 1.25-cm unfocused transducer. A 3.5-MHz, 1.25-cm transducer was used in younger children and a 5-MHz, 0.6-cm transducer in infants and very small children.
3. Subjects were studied in supine and left lateral decubitus positions.

Measurements (Figs 6–18 to 6–25; Tables 6–12 and 6–13)

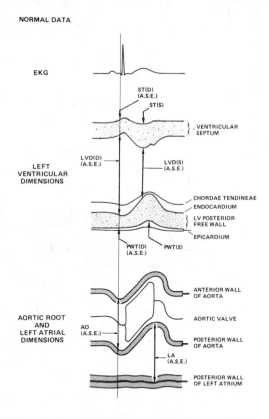

FIG 6–18.

Diagram of standards used to obtain various echocardiographic measurements, as recommended by the American Society of Echocardiography (A.S.E.). LVD(D) = left ventricular dimension at end-diastole; LVD(S) = left ventricular dimension at end-diastole; ST(D) = ventricular septal thickness at end-diastole; PWT(D) = left ventricular posterior wall thickness at end-diastole; PWT(S) = left ventricular posterior wall thickness at end-systole; AO = aortic root dimension at end-diastole; LA = maximal left atrial dimension; ST(S) = ventricular septal thickness at end-systole. (From Henry WL, et al: Circulation 1980; 62:1054. Used by permission of the American Heart Association.)

*Ref: Henry WL, et al: Circulation 1980; 62:1054.

ECHOCARDIOGRAPHIC MEASUREMENTS IN NORMAL SUBJECTS FROM INFANCY TO OLD AGE

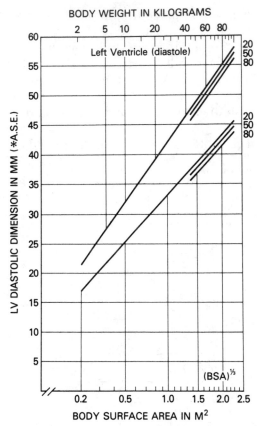

FIG 6–19.
Left ventricular *(LV)* dimension at end-diastole *(vertical axis)* plotted against body surface area *(BSA)* *(lower horizontal axis)* and body weight *(upper horizontal axis)*. This echocardiographic measurement was made according to standards recommended by the American Society of Echocardiography *(A.S.E.)* (From Henry WL, et al: *Circulation* 1980; 62:1054. Used by permission.)

ECHOCARDIOGRAPHIC MEASUREMENTS IN
NORMAL SUBJECTS FROM INFANCY TO OLD AGE

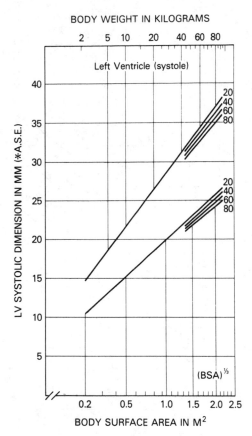

FIG 6–20.
Left ventricular *(LV)* dimension at end-systole *(vertical axis)* plotted against body surface area *(BSA)* and body weight *(horizontal axes).* (From Henry WL, et al: *Circulation* 1980; 62:1054. Used by permission.)

ECHOCARDIOGRAPHIC MEASUREMENTS IN NORMAL SUBJECTS FROM INFANCY TO OLD AGE

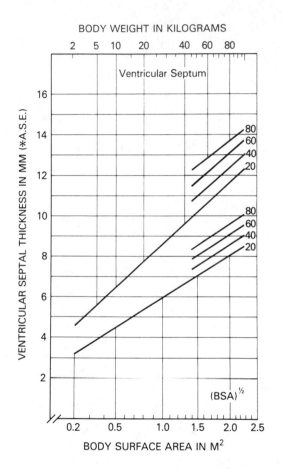

FIG 6–21.

Ventricular septal thickness plotted against body surface area *(BSA) (lower horizontal axis)* and body weight *(upper horizontal axis)*. This echocardiographic measurement was made according to standards recommended by the American Society of Echocardiography *(A.S.E)*. The two diverging *dark solid lines* that extend from a BSA of 0.2 m^2 to a BSA of 2.3 m^2 represent the 95% prediction intervals of measurements obtained in normal subjects from 30 days to 20 years of age. The 95% prediction intervals for adult subjects who are 40, 60, and 80 years of age are indicated by the *dark solid lines* that extend from a BSA of 1.4 m^2 to a BSA of 2.3 m^2. (From Henry WL, et al: *Circulation* 1980; 62:1054. Used by permission.)

ECHOCARDIOGRAPHIC MEASUREMENTS IN NORMAL SUBJECTS FROM INFANCY TO OLD AGE

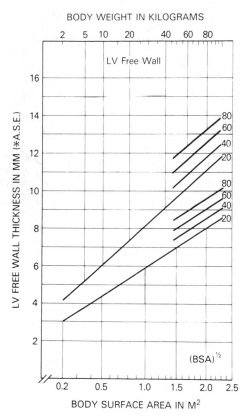

FIG 6–22.
Left ventricular *(LV)* free wall thickness *(vertical axis)* plotted against body surface area *(BSA)* and body weight *(horizontal axes)*. A.S.E. = American Society of Echocardiography. (From Henry WL, et al: *Circulation* 1980; 62:1054. Used by permission.)

ECHOCARDIOGRAPHIC MEASUREMENTS IN NORMAL SUBJECTS FROM INFANCY TO OLD AGE

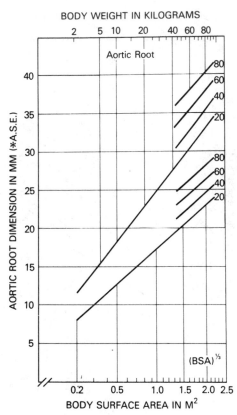

FIG 6–23.
Aortic root dimension *(vertical axis)* plotted against body surface area *(BSA)* and body weight *(horizontal axes)*. A.S.E. = American Society of Echocardiography. (From Henry WL, et al: *Circulation* 1980; 62:1054. Used by permission.)

ECHOCARDIOGRAPHIC MEASUREMENTS IN NORMAL SUBJECTS FROM INFANCY TO OLD AGE

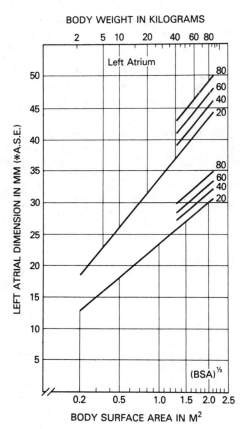

FIG 6–24.
Left atrial dimension *(vertical axis)* plotted against body surface area *(BSA)* and body weight *(horizontal axes)*. A.S.E. = American Society of Echocardiography. (From Henry WL, et al: *Circulation* 1980; 62:1054. Used by permission.)

ECHOCARDIOGRAPHIC MEASUREMENTS IN NORMAL SUBJECTS FROM INFANCY TO OLD AGE

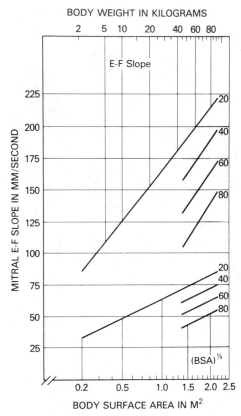

FIG 6–25.
Mitral EF slope *(vertical axis)* plotted against body surface area *(BSA)* and body weight *(horizontal axes).* The American Society of Echocardiography *(A.S.E.)* has not recommended standards for this measurement. (From Henry WL, et al: *Circulation* 1980; 62:1054. Used by permission.)

ECHOCARDIOGRAPHIC MEASUREMENTS IN NORMAL SUBJECTS FROM INFANCY TO OLD AGE

TABLE 6–12.

Equations for Predicting Normal Echocardiographic Measurements From Body Surface Area and Age*

Measurements	Equation
LV end-diastolic dimension†	$45.3 (BSA)^{1/3} - 0.03 (AGE) - 7.2 \pm 12\%$
LV end-systolic dimension†	$28.8 (BSA)^{1/3} - 0.03 (AGE) - 4.1 \pm 18\%$
Septal thickness†	$5.44 (BSA)^{1/2} + 0.03 (AGE) + 1.5 \pm 18\%$
LV free wall thickness†	$5.56 (BSA)^{1/2} + 0.03 (AGE) + 1.1 \pm 16\%$
Aortic root dimension†	$24.0 (BSA)^{1/3} + 0.1 (AGE) - 4.3 \pm 18\%$
Left atrial dimension†	$28.5 (BSA)^{1/3} + 0.08 (AGE) - 0.9 \pm 18\%$
Mitral EF slope	$161 (BSA)^{1/3} - 0.9 (AGE) - 36 \pm 45\%$

*From Henry WL, et al: *Circulation* 1980; 62:1054. Used by permission.
†Measurements made according to standards recommended by the American Society of Echocardiography. In these equations, body surface area (BSA) is expressed in square meters, age in years, dimensions and thicknesses in millimeters, and EF slope in millimeters per second.

TABLE 6–13.

Equations for Predicting Normal Echocardiographic Measurements From Body Weight and Age*†

Measurement	Equation
LV end-diastolic dimension†	$22.4 (WT)^{0.213} - 0.03 (AGE) - 7.2 \pm 12\%$
LV end-systolic dimension†	$14.2 (WT)^{0.213} - 0.03 (AGE) - 4.1 \pm 18\%$
Septal thickness†	$1.88 (WT)^{0.32} + 0.03 (AGE) + 1.5 \pm 18\%$
LV free wall thickness†	$1.92 (WT)^{0.32} + 0.03 (AGE) + 1.1 \pm 16\%$
Aortic root dimension†	$11.8 (WT)^{0.213} + 0.1 (AGE) - 4.3 \pm 18\%$
Left atrial dimension†	$14.1 (WT)^{0.213} + 0.08 (AGE) - 0.9 \pm 18\%$
Mitral EF slope	$79.4 (WT)^{0.213} - 0.9 (AGE) - 36 \pm 45\%$

*From Henry WL, et al: *Circulation* 1980; 62:1054. Used by permission.
†Measurements made according to standards recommended by the American Society of Echocardiography. In these equations, body weight (WT) is expressed in kilograms, age in years, dimensions and thicknesses in millimeters, and EF slope in millimeters per second.

Measurements were made according to the recommendations of the American Society of Echocardiology.

The thickness of the ventricular septum, posterior LV wall, and internal LV dimensions were measured with the ultrasound beam passing slightly caudal to the tip of the mitral valve. The internal dimension of LV at end-diastole was measured at the onset of QRS complex and end-systole when the septum was farthest from the anterior chest at the nadir of septal motion. Septal thickness was made at onset of QRS complex.

Aortic root and left atrial dimensions were recorded by angling the ultrasound beam from the mitral valve into the aortic root, adjusting orientation to demonstrate leaflets.

ECHOCARDIOGRAPHIC MEASUREMENTS IN NORMAL SUBJECTS FROM INFANCY TO OLD AGE

Source of Material

Two groups of normal subjects were studied and later pooled. One group of 92 subjects with no evidence of heart disease (most with normal 12 lead ECGs and normal blood pressures) ranged in age from 1 month to 23 years. The other group of 136 adults ranged in age from 20 years to 97 years, and none had evidence of hypertension or heart disease based on physical examination, ECG, chest x-ray, and echocardiogram.

MEASUREMENT OF THE AORTIC NIPPLE*

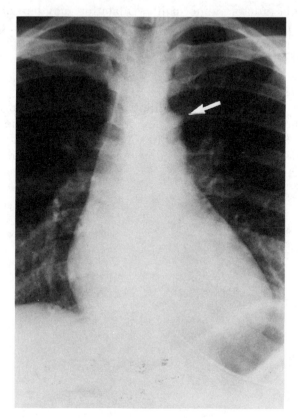

FIG 6–26.
Normal aortic nipple *(arrow).* (From Friedman AC, et al: *AJR* 1978; 131:599. Used by permission.)

Technique
Central ray: Perpendicular to plane of film centered to midchest.
Position: Posteroanterior erect.
Target-film distance: 72 inches.

Measurement (Fig 6–26)
The diameter of the aortic nipple is taken as the horizontal distance from the lateral wall of the aortic knob to the lateral wall of the nipple, through the midplane of the nipple.

The normal nipple ranges in size from 1 to 4 mm, taking the mean plus 2 SD as the upper limit of normal; dilatation of the vein beyond 4.5 mm is a

Ref: Friedman AC, et al: *AJR* 1978; 131:599.

useful sign of a circulatory abnormality. Dilatation may be due to absence of the inferior vena cava, hypoplasia of the left innominate vein, congestive failure, portal hypertension, Budd-Chiari syndrome, or superior or inferior vena caval obstruction.

Source of Material

Five hundred consecutive chest films of patients without known cardiovascular or pulmonary disease were reviewed. Children under the age of 10 were excluded. Seven of these demonstrated an aortic nipple. In addition, 9 aortic nipples previously encountered in normal patients were used in calculating the normal diameter.

MEASUREMENT OF THE INFUNDIBULUM
OF THE RIGHT VENTRICLE

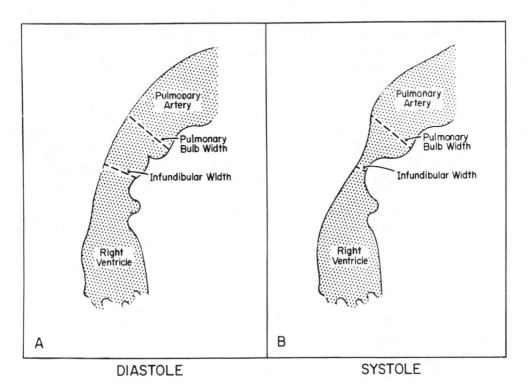

DIASTOLE   SYSTOLE

FIG 6–27.
(From Little TB, et al: *Circulation* 1963; 28:182. Used by permission.)

Infundibular/Bulb Ratio*

Normal range: 0.45–0.83. Average, 0.63 ± 0.08.

Infundibular Systolic/Diastolic Ratio†

In tetralogy of Fallot: 0.33–1.00. Average, 0.56.
In pulmonic valvular stenosis: 0.11–0.30. Average, 0.25.

*Ref: Little TB, et al: *Circulation* 1963; 28:182.
†Ref: Lester RG, et al: *AJR* 1965; 94:78.

MEASUREMENT OF THE INFUNDIBULUM
OF THE RIGHT VENTRICLE

Technique
    Central ray: Perpendicular to plane of film centered over midchest.
    Projection: True lateral angiocardiograms.
    Target-film distance: Immaterial.

Measurements (Fig 6–27)

1. The infundibular/bulb ratio. Several bulb measurements are averaged, and the ratio of the minimum systolic diameter to the average pulmonary diameter is obtained. Normal values are given on page 441. The critical ratio is 0.4. Figures below this level indicate significant systolic narrowing.
2. The infundibular systolic/diastolic ratio. Measurements are made of the infundibulum at its narrowest point in the systole and at the same point in the diastole. In all cases of tetralogy of Fallot, the ratio is greater than 0.33; in all cases of valvular stenosis, the ratio is less than 0.30. An infundibulum with significant obstruction, as measured by the infundibular/bulb ratio, and an infundibular systolic/diastolic ratio greater than 0.30 may not regress following valvulotomy.

Source of Material
    The data on the infundibular/bulb ratio are based on a study of 13 patients with pulmonary valvular stenosis and 30 control subjects.
    The infundibular systolic diameter/infundibular diastolic ratio is based on a study of 42 patients with tetralogy of Fallot and 19 patients with pulmonic valvular stenosis.

VENA CAVAL–LEFT VENTRICULAR
RELATIONSHIPS IN HEART DISEASE

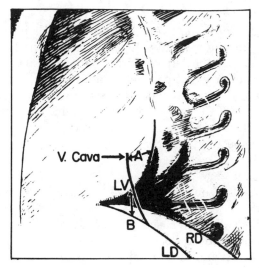

FIG 6–28.
LV = left ventricle; *V. Cava* = inferior vena cava; *RD* = right diaphragm; *LD* = left diaphragm. (From Hoffman RB, Rigler LG: *Radiology* 1965; 85:93.

Technique
Central ray: Perpendicular to plane of film centered over midchest.
Position: True lateral. Full inspiration.
Target-film distance: 6 feet.

Measurements (Fig 6–28)
With full inspiration and in true lateral projection, the shadow of the inferior vena cava in the retrocardiac space is not completely included in the cardiac silhouette. Eyler and associates[*] have shown that this relationship is useful in differentiating mitral stenosis from mitral insufficiency. With mitral insufficiency, the left ventricle projects behind the shadow of the inferior vena cava for a distance of 15 mm or more.

Keats and Rudhe[†] use this relationship in differentiating atrial secundum septal defects. In the atrial secundum septal defect, the inferior vena cava lies in part free in the retrocardiac space. In the ventricular septal defect, with large shunt, the vena cava is projected over the mass of the heart.

Hoffman and Rigler[‡] have defined two additional measurements for determining left ventricular enlargement. Measurement A in Figure 6–28 is de-

*Ref: Eyler WR, et al: *Radiology* 1959; 73:56.
†Ref: Keats TE, Rudhe U: *Radiology* 1964; 83:616.
‡Ref: Hoffman RB, Rigler LG: *Radiology* 1965; 85:93.

VENA CAVAL–LEFT VENTRICULAR
RELATIONSHIPS IN HEART DISEASE

fined as the distance that the left ventricle (LV) extends posteriorly to the posterior border of the inferior vena cava (v. cava) at a point 2 cm cephalad to the crossing of the cava and the left ventricle. This measurement is made on a plane extending posteriorly that parallels the horizontal plane of the vertebral bodies. Measurement B is the distance of this crossing caudad to the left leaf of the diaphragm. When A is more than 1.8 cm, one can postulate left ventricular enlargement with a considerable degree of certainty. When B is less than 0.75 cm, one can suspect left ventricular enlargement.

Source of Material

Eyler's data are based on a study of 214 cases of rheumatic heart disease, surgically explored.

Keats and Rudhe's data are based on a study of 32 patients with atrial secundum defects, ages 9 to 28 years; 36 patients with ventricular septal defects, ages 4 to 32 years, and 30 normal subjects, ages 4–36 years.

Hoffman and Rigler's data are based on a study of 270 subjects, including 122 normals, the remainder being patients with aortic and mitral valvular diseases and hypertension.

MEASUREMENT OF THE LEFT ATRIUM
ON THE FRONTAL FILM*

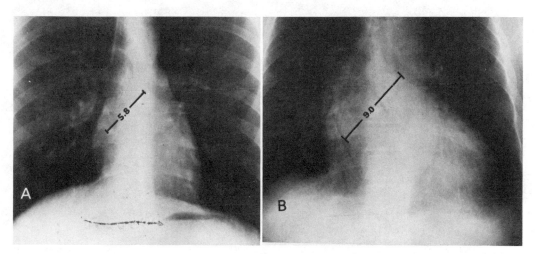

FIG 6–29.
Measurement of the left atrium. (From Higgins CB, et al: *AJR* 1978; 130:251. Used by permission.)

Technique
Central ray: Centered over midchest, perpendicular to film.
Position: Posteroanterior.
Target-film distance: 182.9 cm.

Measurements (Fig 6–29 and Table 6–14)
The left atrium is measured from the midpoint of the curvilinear margin of the double density to the midpoint of the inferior wall of the left bronchus.

TABLE 6–14.

Left Atrial Dimension for Normal and Abnormal Groups[*]

	Males			Females		
Group	Mean	SD	Range	Mean	SD	Range
Normal						
Decade 3	6.3	±0.6	5.1–7.4	5.9	±0.6	4.3–7.4
Decade 4	6.1	±0.6	5.0–7.4	6.1	±0.7	5.3–7.1
Decade 5	6.5	±0.9	5.6–7.6	5.8	±0.7	5.2–7.6
Decade 6	5.9	±0.9	5.5–6.6	6.1	±0.8	5.5–6.8
Abnormal	9.1	±1.5	6.6–12.4	8.2	±1.0	6.0–10.4

[*]From Higgins CB, et al: *AJR* 1978; 130:251. Used by permission.

Ref: Higgins CB, et al: *AJR* 1978; 130:251.

MEASUREMENT OF THE LEFT ATRIUM
ON THE FRONTAL FILM

The measurement is less than 7.0 cm in 98% of normal patients and greater than 7.0 cm in 90% of patients with left atrial enlargement. The measurement is less reliable in children.

Source of Material
One hundred forty-eight normal volunteers and 48 patients in whom there was echocardiographic left atrial enlargement. The study also included 30 pediatric patients with left atrial enlargement secondary to ventricular septal defect.

MEASUREMENT OF THE LEFT ATRIUM
IN THE LATERAL PROJECTION*

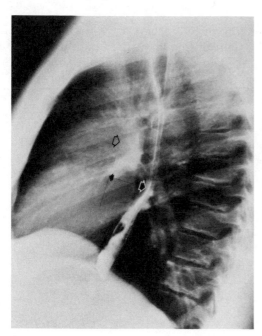

FIG 6–30.
Measurement of the left atrium in a normal patient. The right pulmonary artery *(open black arrow)* is seen as an oval density anterior to the major bronchi and slightly caudal to the left pulmonary artery *(curved arrow).* (From Westcott JL, Ferguson P: *Radiology* 1976; 118:265. Used by permission.)

TABLE 6–15.

Left Atrial Diameter (MM)*

	Female	Male
Normal	<36	<40
Borderline	36–38	40–42
Enlarged	>38	>42

*From Westcott JL, Ferguson P: *Radiology* 1976; 118:265. Used by permission.

Technique
   Central ray: Perpendicular to plane of film centered over midpoint of chest.
   Position: Upright lateral.
   Target-film distance: 6 feet.

Ref: Westcott JL, Ferguson P: *Radiology* 1976; 118:265.

MEASUREMENT OF THE LEFT ATRIUM IN THE LATERAL PROJECTION

Measurements (Fig 6–30)

To approximate the position of the anterior left atrial wall, a line is drawn downward from the anterior wall of the right pulmonary artery parallel to the long axis of the barium-filled esophagus. The maximum perpendicular distance from the line to the esophagus represents the left atrial diameter. Normal values are given in Table 6–15.

Source of Material

Data based on study of 82 adult patients.

ESOPHAGEAL DISPLACEMENT BY LEFT ATRIUM*

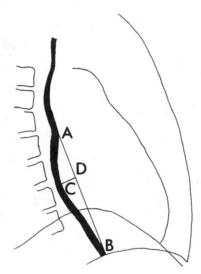

FIG 6–31.
(Adapted from Kaye J, et al: *Br J Radiol* 1955; 28:693.)

Technique

Central ray: Perpendicular to plane of film centered over midpoint of chest.

Position: Right anterior oblique with barium outlining the esophagus. Optimum degree of rotation determined during fluoroscopy. Full inspiration.

Target-film distance: 64 inches.

Measurements (Fig 6–31 and Table 6–16)

Line *AB* is drawn from the anterior aspect of the esophagus where it begins a backward sweep at the upper level of the left atrium to a point on the anterior aspect of the esophagus where it passes the left leaf at the diaphragm, or any more anterior portion above this point.

Line *CD* is the posterior displacement of the esophagus. Line *CD* is drawn perpendicular to line *AB* at the maximum displacement of the esophagus. The distance *CD* is measured in millimeters from line *AB* to the anterior wall of the esophagus.

---

*Ref: Kaye J, et al: *Br J Radiol* 1955; 28:693.

ESOPHAGEAL DISPLACEMENT BY LEFT ATRIUM

TABLE 6—16.

Posterior Displacement of the Esophagus in the Erect Anterior Oblique View[*]

	Mean Displacement	Standard Deviation	± 2 Standard Deviations
Normal	7.9 mm	3.0 mm	2–14 mm
Mitral value disease	19.6 mm	10.4 mm	0–40 mm

*From Kaye J, et al: *Br J Radiol* 1955; 28:693. Used with permission.

Source of Material

Fifty normal subjects and 50 patients with mitral valve disease. The diagnosis was based on clinical electrocardiographic and phonocardiographic findings. Age and sex incidence were similar in both groups.

MEASUREMENT OF THE NORMAL PULMONARY ARTERIES*

In Children

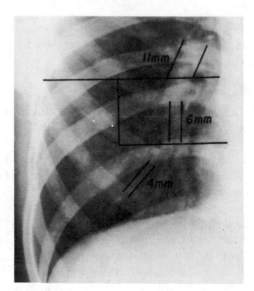

FIG 6–32.
(From Leinbach LB: *AJR* 1963; 89:995. Used by permission.)

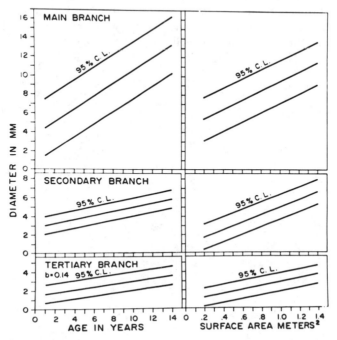

FIG 6–33.
(From Leinbach LB: *AJR* 1963; 89:995. Used by permission.)

*Ref: Leinbach LB: *AJR* 1963; 89:995.

MEASUREMENT OF THE NORMAL
PULMONARY ARTERIES

In Children

Technique
   Central ray: Perpendicular to plane of film centered over midchest.
   Position: Posteroanterior.
   Target-film distance: 6 feet.

Measurements (Fig 6–32)
   The right lower lung field is utilized. A horizontal line is drawn from the descending branch of the right pulmonary artery just below the right hilar shadow to the lateral chest wall. A perpendicular line is then drawn inferiorly from the midpoint of this line to meet a horizontal line drawn bisecting the distance from the upper line and the cardiophrenic reflection. In this way, a central square-shaped area and a peripheral L-shaped area are obtained. Three measurements are made: (1) the diameter of the right descending pulmonary artery is measured as it appears below the right hilus; (2) the diameter of the widest-caliber secondary arterial branch is measured in the central area; (3) the widest tertiary branch is then measured in the peripheral area. Normal measurements on function of age and surface area are shown in Figure 6–33. Normal values for surface area are found on page 414.

Source of Material
   The data are based on a study of 243 children ranging in age from infancy to 14 years. Each chest film used was interpreted as normal if the diaphragmatic level was the ninth posterior rib.

MEASUREMENT OF THE NORMAL PULMONARY ARTERIES

In Adults

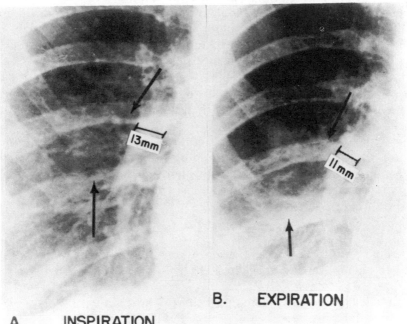

FIG 6–34.
(From Chang CH: *AJR* 1962; 87:929. Used by permission.)

TABLE 6–17.*

	Inspiration	Expiration	Range of Difference Between Inspiration and Expiration
Males	16 mm	15 mm	1–3 mm
Females	15 mm	14 mm	1–3 mm

*From Chang CH: *AJR* 1962; 87:929. Used by permission.

Technique
Central ray: Perpendicular to plane of film centered over midchest.
Position: Posteroanterior.
Target-film distance: 6 feet.

Measurements (Fig 6–34)
All films are obtained in deep inspiration and forceful expiration. The right descending pulmonary artery is measured on both inspiratory and expi-

MEASUREMENT OF THE NORMAL
PULMONARY ARTERIES

In Adults

ratory films at its widest point near the bifurcation of the artery from the lateral segment of the right middle lobe and above the branching of the middle basilar artery. This measurement point usually lies between the right eighth and ninth ribs posteriorly in deep inspiration. On expiration, it usually lies just below or over the right eighth rib posteriorly.

Normal values are shown in Table 6–17. Values greater than those shown are abnormal, and pulmonary hypertension is most likely present.* The expiratory measurement is always smaller than the inspiratory, and it is helpful in borderline cases.

These measurements are also useful in the diagnosis of pulmonary infarction.† With infarction, values ranging from 17 to 22 mm are noted on the right, and from 17 to 26 mm on the left, on inspiration. This dilatation usually appears within 24 hours of the onset of chest pain, and maximum dilatation occurs in 2 to 3 days.

Source of Material

The data on normal size are based on a study of 1,085 normal adults, including 432 males ranging in age from 18 to 70 years and 652 females ranging in age from 18 to 72 years.

Figures for pulmonary infarction are based on a study of 23 patients with pulmonary infarction.

*Ref: Chang CH: AJR 1962; 87:929.
†Ref: Chang CH, Davis WC: Clin Radiol 1965; 16:141.

RATIO OF PULMONARY ARTERY DIAMETER TO TRACHEA FOR ASSESSMENT OF PULMONARY VASCULARITY IN CHILDREN*

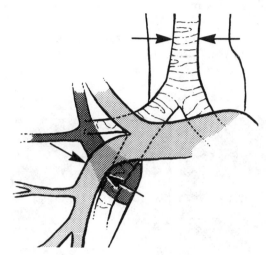

FIG 6–35.
Sites of measurement of right descending pulmonary artery and tracheal diameters. (From Coussement AM, Gooding CA: *Radiology* 1973; 109:649. Used by permission.)

Technique
    Central ray: Perpendicular to plane of film.
    Position: Posteroanterior or anteroposterior.
    Target-film distance: Immaterial.

Measurements (Fig 6–35)
The diameter of the right descending pulmonary artery was measured at the level where it parallels the right main bronchus and crosses the pulmonary vein, draining the right upper lobe. The diameter of the trachea was measured just above the impression of the aorta.

It was found that when a left-to-right shunt was present, the right descending pulmonary artery never had a diameter less than that of the trachea.

Source of Material
Data derived from chest films of 112 normal children and 102 children with left-to-right shunts. Ages ranged from 6 months to 14 years.

*Ref: Coussement AM, Gooding CA: *Radiology* 1973; 109:649.

MEASUREMENT OF CORONARY
ARTERY SIZE DURING LIFE*

Technique
 Central ray: Perpendicular to plane of film.
 Position: 30° RAO and 60° LAO.
 Target-film distance: Corrected for distortion by use of a calibrating object placed in same height above table as previously determined for the atrioventricular groove. Selective arteriograms performed by cine angiography.

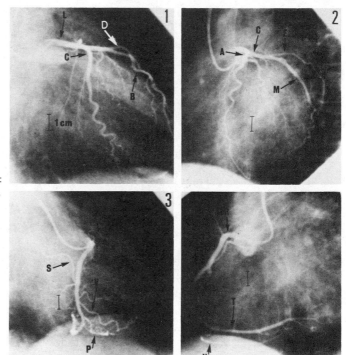

FIG 6–36.
(From MacAlpin RN, et al:
Radiology 1973; 108:567.
Used by permission.)

Ref: McAlpin RN, et al: *Radiology* 1973; 108:567.

MEASUREMENT OF CORONARY
ARTERY SIZE DURING LIFE

TABLE 6−18.

Major Coronary Artery Diameters[*]

	No.	Mean ± SD (Range), mm				
		LCA	LAD	CMFX	Proximal RCA	Distal RCA
Normal men	19	4.3±0.6 (3.4−5.5) n = 15‡	3.5±0.5 (2.9−4.7)	3.1±0.7 (1.7−4.1)	3.4±0.7 (2.3−4.5) n = 13§	2.9±0.7 (2.0−3.9) n = 13§
Normal women	7	3.5±0.7[a] (2.6−4.5) n = 6‡	2.9±0.4[a] (2.4−3.5)	2.6±0.6 (1.8−3.4)	3.0±0.5 (2.5−3.8)	2.5±0.6 (1.7−3.4)
All normals:	26	4.0±0.7 n = 21‡	3.4±0.5	3.0±0.7	3.2±0.6 n = 20§	2.7±0.7 n = 20§
"Floppy mitral valve" syndrome	8	3.9±0.4 (3.5−4.5)	3.2±0.5 (2.5−3.9)	2.9±0.5 (2.5−4.1)	3.5±0.6 (2.5−4.5)	2.9±0.6 (1.9−3.8)
Aortic stenosis	14	4.3±0.8 (3.0−5.2) n = 9‡	3.5±0.8 (2.4−5.0)	3.1±0.7 (1.9−4.4)	3.7±0.8[a] (2.8−5.5)	3.0±0.8 (1.8−4.5)
Aortic regurgitation	12	5.6±0.8[d] (4.1−6.5) n = 9‡	4.5±0.6[d] (3.2−5.7)	4.0±0.9[d] (2.1−5.3)	3.9±0.5[b] (3.2−4.9)	3.3±0.3[a] (2.8−3.9)
Mitral stenosis	11	4.3±0.4 (3.8−4.8) n = 7‡	3.4±0.7 (2.2−4.7)	3.2±0.8 (2.3−4.3)	3.5±0.8 (2.1−4.6) n = 10§	2.5±0.6 (1.5−3.4) n = 10§
Mitral regurgitation	9	4.6±0.5[a] (4.1−5.5) n = 7‡	3.8±0.5[a] (3.1−4.5)	3.2±0.5 (2.4−4.1)	3.8±0.8 (2.6−4.8)	3.2±0.7 (2.1−4.0)
Hypertrophic cardiomyopathy	8	4.4±0.7 (3.5−5.6) n = 6‡	4.2±1.0[a] (2.7−5.5)	3.0±0.4 (2.3−3.5)	4.1±0.6 (3.3−5.0)	3.5±0.5 (2.6−4.3) n = 7
Congestive cardiomyopathy	9	*	4.0±0.8[a] (3.0−5.5)	3.4±0.7 (2.3−5.5)	3.3±0.8 (2.7−3.8) n = 7§	2.7±0.2 (1.8−3.0) n = 7§

[*]From MacAlpin RN, et al: *Radiology* 1973; 108:567. Used by permission.

†In tests for significance of differences, normal women were compared with normal men, and patients with heart disease were compared with the total group of normals. a = $P < 0.05$; b = $P < 0.01$; c = $P < 0.001$; d = $P < 0.0001$. CMFX = left circumflex coronary artery; LAD = anterior descending coronary artery; LCA = left main coronary artery; RCA = right coronary artery.

‡Cases in which the LCA was too short to measure were excluded.

§Subjects with marked LCA preponderance were excluded.

MEASUREMENT OF CORONARY
ARTERY SIZE DURING LIFE

TABLE 6–19.

Coronary Artery Diameters[*][†]

	Mean ± SD (Range), mm				
	Distal LAD	Diagonal	Left Marginal	Right Ventricular Branch	Distal RCA Proximal RCA (Ratio)
Normal men	2.0±0.4 (1.6–3.1) n = 16	2.0±0.3 (1.3–2.3) n = 17	2.5±0.6 (1.6–3.3) n = 16	1.9±0.5 (1.2–2.7) n = 10§	0.86±0.11 (0.65–1.00) n = 13§
Normal women	1.8±0.2 (1.5–2.0) n = 5	2.0±0.3 (1.7–2.4) n = 4	1.9±0.2 (1.7–2.1) n = 4	1.2±0.6[a] (0.8–2.2) n = 5	0.82±0.09 (0.68–0.94) n = 7
All normals	1.9±0.3 n = 21	2.0±0.3 n = 21	2.4±0.5 n = 20	1.7±0.6 n = 15§	0.85±0.10 n = 20§
"Floppy mitral valve" syndrome	1.6±0.3 (1.3–2.1) n = 7	2.0±0.3 (1.6–2.5) n = 8	2.2±0.8 (1.5–3.2) n = 4	1.3±0.4 (1.0–1.8) n = 5	0.83±0.13 (0.66–1.00) n = 8
Aortic stenosis	2.2±0.4 (1.6–3.0) n = 13	2.4±0.7[b] (1.6–3.6) n = 7	2.6±0.6 (1.7–3.8) n = 7	1.5±0.5 (0.9–2.2) n = 8	0.81±0.07 (0.64–0.93) n = 14
Aortic regurgitation	2.6±0.5[c] (1.5–3.3) n = 12	2.5±0.4[b] (1.6–3.0) n = 10	2.9±0.7[a] (1.9–4.0) n = 6	1.9±0.2 (1.6–2.4) n = 8	0.85±0.07 (0.76–0.97) n = 12
Mitral stenosis	2.2±0.5 (1.8–3.1) n = 10	2.1±0.5 (1.3–2.6) n = 8	. . .	1.7±0.2 (1.2–2.1) n = 10	0.72±0.05[c] (0.64–0.81) n = 11
Mitral regurgitation	2.4±0.2[b] (2.2–2.9) n = 6	2.5±0.4[b] (1.9–3.0) n = 6	. . .	1.9±0.3 (1.3–2.1) n = 6	0.84±0.05 (0.76–0.90) n = 9
Hypertrophic cardiomyopathy	2.4±0.6[a] (1.7–3.2) n = 8	2.5±0.9[b] (1.5–3.9) n = 7	. . .	1.8±0.3 (1.5–2.1) n = 5	0.84±0.11 (0.66–0.95) n = 7
Congestive cardiomyopathy	2.4±0.4[b] (1.8–3.1) n = 8	2.4±0.3[b] (2.0–2.8) n = 7	. . .	. . .	0.82±0.10 (0.66–0.91) n = 7

[*]From MacAlpin RN, et al: *Radiology* 1973; 108:567. Used by permission.
[†]See Table 6–18 for abbreviations and annotations.

MEASUREMENT OF CORONARY ARTERY SIZE DURING LIFE

TABLE 6–20.

Coronary Cross-Sectional Area With Correction for Body Surface Area*†

	No.	Body Surface Area (BSA) (m²)	TCA (mm²)	TCA/BSA (mm²/m²)	LVCA (mm²)	LVCA/BSA (mm²/m²)
			Mean ± SD (Range)			
Normal men	19	1.96±0.15 (1.74–2.33)	25.7±4.8 (19–35)	13.3±2.9 (8.2–18.8)	22.7±4.8 (16–32)	11.8±2.8 (7.0–16.4)
Normal women	7	1.58±0.14[c] (1.37–1.76)	19.7±4.6[b] (15–29)	12.5±2.5 (10.0–16.5)	17.4±4.5[a] (13–27)	11.1±2.4 (8.0–5.2)
All normals	26	1.86±0.22	24.1±5.4	13.1±2.8	21.3±5.2	11.6±2.6
"Floppy mitral valve syndrome	8	1.74±0.17 (1.51–2.09)	24.7±5.6 (19–35)	14.1±2.2 (11.9–17.6)	21.7±3.6 (18–29)	12.4±1.2 (10.6–14.0)
Aortic stenosis	14	1.72±0.23 (1.33–2.10)	30.3±12.5[a] (16–52)	17.1±5.6[b] (10.7–31.1)	24.5±7.2 (13–38)	13.9±4.3[a] (6.5–19.8)
Aortic regurgitation	12	1.74±0.20 (1.46–2.10)	40.9±9.2[d] (26–56)	22.9±6.4[d] (13.9–34.3)	37.6±8.6[d] (24–53)	21.9±5.6[d] (11.2–31.0)
Mitral stenosis	11	1.75±0.26 (1.45–2.38)	27.3±9.2 (12–43)	15.5±4.1[a] (7.8–21.5)	22.6±7.5 (11–36)	12.8±3.4 (6.8–18.0)
Mitral regurgitation	9	1.65±0.18[a] (1.38–1.90)	31.9±7.5[b] (24–47)	19.3±3.7[d] (12.7–24.5)	28.5±6.6[b] (21–41)	17.3±3.5[d] (11.9–21.6)
Hypertrophic cardiomyopathy	8	1.70±0.21 (1.50–2.12)	35.0±10.5[c] (23–51)	20.5±5.4[d] (14.3–30.0)	31.2±9.8[b] (21–47) n = 7	18.6±5.4[c] (13.6–28.8) n = 7
Congestive cardiomyopathy	9	1.87±0.31 (1.37–2.45)	30.5±10.1[a] (17–46)	16.4±5.4[b] (10.4–27.0)	27.0±8.4[a] (16–43)	14.5±4.8[a] (9.0–25.0)

*From MacAlpin RN, et al: *Radiology* 1973; 108:567. Used by permission.
†BSA = body surface area; LVCA = left ventricular coronary area; TCA = total coronary area; a = P < 0.05, b = P < 0.01; c = P < 0.001; d = P < 0.0001.

Measurements (Fig 6–36)

The following measurements were made from LAO arteriograms; proximal right coronary artery (RCA) at a point not less than 0.5 cm or greater than 2.5 cm from its ostium; distal RCA (DRCA) at a point at the posterior atrioventricular groove after the last right ventricular branch has been given off but

MEASUREMENT OF CORONARY
ARTERY SIZE DURING LIFE

about 0.5 cm proximal descending to the origin of the PD and terminal left ventricular branches; the largest right ventricular branch of the right coronary artery (RCA) within the first 1 cm of that branch; proximal left circumflex coronary artery (CMFX) within the first 2 cm and proximal to its first marginal branch; the largest marginal branch of the CMFX within 1 cm of the origin of that branch; left coronary artery (LCA) within the last 0.5 cm before its bifurcation.

The following measurements of vessel lumen diameter were made from RAO arteriograms; proximal left anterior descending artery (LAD) within its first 1.5 cm proximal to the origin of its first septal and diagonal branches; the largest diagonal branch of the LAD (DIAG) within the first 1 cm of that branch; the distal LAD in the anterior interventricular groove about 1 cm distal to the origin of its last major diagonal branch; the PD within the first 1 cm of its course in the inferior interventricular groove. See Tables 6–18 to 6–20 for measurement data.

Source of Material

Arteriograms of 99 patients were included; the 53 men and 46 women ranged in age from 21 to 79 years. They included 27 normals; the remaining cases fell into the diagnoses indicated in the tables.

MEASUREMENT OF ACTUAL CORONARY ARTERY SIZE TO DETERMINE RELATIVE NARROWING*

TABLE 6–21.

Determination of the Diameter of Coronary Arteries*†

X (mm)	Y (mm)				
	3.0	3.5	4.0	4.5	5.0
0.5	0.4	0.3	0.3	0.3	0.2
1.0	0.8	0.7	0.6	0.5	0.5
1.5	1.2	1.0	0.9	0.8	0.7
2.0	1.6	1.3	1.2	1.0	0.9
2.5	2.0	1.7	1.5	1.3	1.2
3.0	2.3	2.0	1.8	1.6	1.4
3.5	2.7	2.3	2.1	1.8	1.6
4.0	3.1	2.7	2.3	2.0	1.9
4.5	3.5	3.0	2.6	2.3	2.1
5.0	3.9	3.3	2.9	2.6	2.3
5.5	4.3	3.7	3.2	2.9	2.6
6.0	4.7	4.0	3.5	3.1	2.8
6.5	5.1	4.3	3.8	3.4	3.0
7.0	5.5	4.7	4.1	3.6	3.3
7.5	5.8	5.0	4.4	3.9	3.5
8.0	6.2	5.4	4.7	4.2	3.7

*From Van Tassel R, et al: *AJR* 1972; 116:62. Used by permission.

†These values apply for a No. 7 French catheter (2.34 mm OD).

The size of the diameter of the image of the coronary artery, X, and the diameter of the image of the catheter, Y, are measured on the roentgenogram. If the true diameter of the catheter is 2.34 mm, then X and Y are used to locate the true diameter Z, of the coronary artery in the Table. Z = 2.34 (X/Y).

X = outside diameter of the image of the artery, as measured on the film (mm). Y = outside diameter of the image of the catheter, as measured on the film (mm). Z = true diameter of the artery at that point (mm).

TABLE 6–22.

Determination of the Diameter of Coronary Arteries*†

X (mm)	Y (mm)				
	3.0	3.5	4.0	4.5	5.0
0.5	0.4	0.4	0.3	0.3	0.3
1.0	0.9	0.8	0.7	0.6	0.5
1.5	1.3	1.1	1.0	0.9	0.8
2.0	1.8	1.5	1.3	1.2	1.1
2.5	2.2	1.9	1.6	1.5	1.3
3.0	2.6	2.3	2.0	1.8	1.6
3.5	3.1	2.6	2.3	2.1	1.8
4.0	3.5	3.0	2.6	2.4	2.1
4.5	4.0	3.4	3.0	2.6	2.4
5.0	4.4	3.8	3.3	2.9	2.6
5.5	4.8	4.1	3.6	3.2	2.9
6.0	5.3	4.5	4.0	3.5	3.2
6.5	5.7	4.9	4.3	3.8	3.4
7.0	6.2	5.3	4.6	4.1	3.7
7.5	6.6	5.7	4.9	4.4	4.0
8.0	7.0	6.0	5.3	4.7	4.2

*From Van Tassel R, et al: *AJR* 1972; 116:62. Used by permission.

†These values apply for a No. 8 French catheter (2.64 mm OD).

The size of the diameter of the image of the coronary artery, X and the diameter of the image of the catheter, Y, are measured on the roentgenogram. If the true diameter of the catheter is 2.64 mm, then X and Y are used to locate the true diameter Z, of the coronary artery in the Table. Z = 2.64 (X/Y).

X = outside diameter of the image of the artery, as measured on the film (mm). Y = outside diameter of the image of the catheter, as measured on the film (mm). Z = true diameter of the artery at that point (mm).

Technique

Central ray: Perpendicular to plane of film.

Position: Immaterial.

Target-film distance: Immaterial.

Measurements

The catheter size is used to compute the magnification factor. Tables 6–21 and 6–22 are used in the following manner: (1) select the row in the left-hand column corresponding to the size of the image of the coronary cath-

*Ref: Van Tassel R, et : *AJR* 1972; 116:62.

MEASUREMENT OF ACTUAL CORONARY ARTERY SIZE TO DETERMINE RELATIVE NARROWING

eter; (2) select the column corresponding to the size of the measured lumen of the coronary artery. The number at the intersection of the row and column is the actual size of the lumen of the coronary artery. An attempt should be made to take the measurement of the catheter in the plane in which the coronary artery is approximately parallel with the horizontal plane.

Source of Material

This entry relates to a technique of measurement, and statistical data are not provided. This technique may also be used to determine the exact size of other vascular structures, such as the aortic root and pulmonary arteries.

MEASUREMENT OF THE SIZE OF THE ARCH
OF THE AZYGOS VEIN[*]

In Children

TABLE 6–23.

Azygous Vein Width in Children*

Age	Birth to 6 Mo	6 to 24 Mo	2 to 7 Yr	8 to 14 Yr
Position	AP and PA supine and upright	PA upright	PA upright	PA upright
Mean ± 1 standard deviation	3.5 ± 1.3 mm	4.1 ± 1.0 mm	4.6 ± 1.2 mm	5.1 ± 1.6 mm

*From Wishart DL: *Radiology* 1972; 104:115. Used by permission.

Technique
Central ray: Perpendicular to plane of film centered over midchest.
Position: Supine and upright: AP and PA in infants aged birth to 6 months; others PA upright.
Target-film distance: 72 inches.

Measurements (Table 6–23 and Fig 6–37)
Measurements made from the outer margin of the vein and the inner margin of the tracheal wall at its greatest width.

Source of Material
Data based on routine chest wall radiographs in 429 children ranging in age from birth to 14 years.

Wishart states that respiratory activity, posture, and anatomic arrangement may cause changes in azygos vein width, making clinicoradiologic correlation uncertain.

*Ref: Wishart DL: *Radiology* 1972; 104:115.

MEASUREMENT OF THE SIZE OF THE ARCH OF THE AZYGOS VEIN*

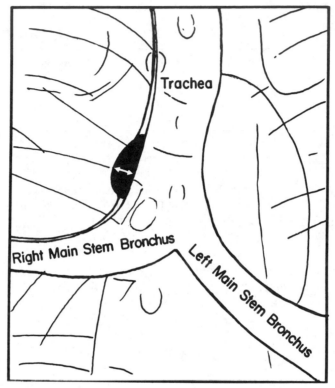

FIG 6–37.
(From Keats TE, Lipscomb G: *Radiology* 1968; 90:990. Used by permission.)

TABLE 6-24.

Normal Values*

Minimum	3 mm
Maximum	7 mm
Average	4.9 mm

*From Keats TE, Lipscomb G: *Radiology* 1968; 90:990.
Used by permission.

In Adults

Technique

Central ray: Perpendicular to plane of film centered over midchest.
Position: Posteroanterior, upright; inspiratory phase of respiration.
Target-film distance: 72 inches.

Ref: Keats TE, Lipscomb G: *Radiology* 1968; 90:990.

MEASUREMENT OF THE SIZE OF THE ARCH
OF THE AZYGOS VEIN

Measurements (Fig 6–37 and Tables 6–24)

The width of the azygos arches is measured perpendicularly to the trachea in the greatest transverse dimension of the arch. Measurement includes the wall of the trachea.

The normal ranges are exceeded in pregnancy, congestive heart failure, portal hypertension, and obstructions of the superior or inferior vena cava.

Source of Material

The data are based on a study of 200 normal adults, equally divided between males and females aged 20 to 60 years.

WIDTH OF THE AZYGOS VEIN RELATED
TO CENTRAL VENOUS PRESSURE*

Technique
  Central ray: Perpendicular to plane of film centered over midchest.
  Position: Anteroposterior. Patient supine on bed rolled flat. Maximum inspiration phase of respiration.
  Target-film distance: 40 inches.

Measurements (Fig 6–37 and Table 6–25)
  The azygos vein width is measured at its greatest diameter, perpendicular to the wall of the trachea. This measurement includes the mediastinal pleural reflection laterally and the tracheal wall medially.

TABLE 6–25.*

Width of Azygos Vein (mm)	Estimated CVP (to nearest cm)	95% Confidence Limits (to nearest cm)
4	3	0–10
6	5	0–12
8	8	1–15
10	11	4–18
12	14	7–21
14	17	10–24
16	19	12–26
18	22	15–29
20	25	18–32
22	28	21–35
24	31	24–38
26	33	26–40
28	36	29–43

*From Preger L, et al: *Radiology* 1969; 93:521. Used by permission.

Source of Material
  Fifty-four adult patients ranging in age from 23 to 77 years of age. In this group were patients with congestive heart failure, patients recovering from thoracic surgery, and recipients of renal transplants.

Ref: Preger L, et al: *Radiology* 1969; 93:521.

ANATOMIC LEVEL OF ORIGIN
OF AORTIC BRANCHES

In Newborns*

TABLE 6–26.

Location of Origin of Major Aortic Branches in Newborns*

Branches	Location With Reference to Vertebrae
Ductus	T3-T4
Celiac axis	Top T12 (Low T11 to Top L1)
Superior mesenteric	T12 L1 interspace (Mid T12 to Mid L1)
Renal	Top L1 (Low T12 to L1-2 interspace)
Inferior mesenteric	L3 (Mid L2 to Mid L3)
Aortic bifurcation	Top L4 (Mid L3 to Top L5)

*From Phelps DL, et al: *J Pediatr* 1972; 81:336. Used by permission.

Technique
    Central ray: Perpendicular to plane of film.
    Position: Anteroposterior.
    Target-film distance: Immaterial.

Measurements (Table 6–26)

Source of Material
Data derived from aortograms on 15 newborn infants, of whom 5 had congenital heart disease, 7 had renal anomalies, and 5 had nonvascular related disease. Gestational age ranged from 24 to 44 weeks.

Ref: Phelps DL, et al: *J Pediatr* 1972; 81:336.

ANATOMIC LEVEL OF ORIGIN
OF AORTIC BRANCHES

In Adults* (Table 6–27)

TABLE 6–27.

Relationship Between Vertebral Bodies and Origin of Aortic Branches*†

Artery	Range	Mean	Range for 85% of Patients
Celiac	UT11 to UL2	UL1	MT12 to DL1–2
Superior mesenteric	MT12 to DL2–3	LL1	UL1 to UL2
Right renal	LT12 to ML4	UL2	LL1 to ML2
Left renal	MT12 to ML4	UL2	LL1 to ML2
Inferior mesenteric	ML2 to LL4	LL3	UL3 to UL4
Aortic bifurcation	ML3 to LL5	LL4	UL4 to UL5

*Adapted from Caldwell EW, Anson BJ: *Am J Anat* 1943; 73:27.
† U = upper; m = middle; L = lower portions of the thoracic (T) and lumbar (L) vertebrae. Discs (D) are designated in reference to the vertebral bodies they separate.

Source of Material

The data are based on dissections of 300 consecutive cadavers of American whites and blacks, ranging in age from 18 to 79 years. Twenty-three were females. The data are useful for catheter positioning in selective and nonselective abdominal aortography.

*Ref: Seitchik MW, et al: Surg *Gynecol Obstet* 1960; 160:192.

MEASUREMENT OF THE ABDOMINAL AORTA

In Children[*]

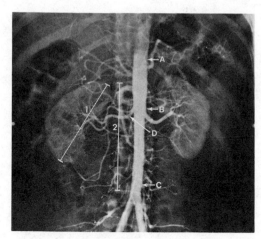

FIG 6–38.

Measurements obtained from abdominal aortograms. A = aortic diameter at the level of the pedicles of the eleventh thoracic vertebra; B = aortic diameter at the level of renal arteries; C = aortic diameter at bifurcation; D = diameter of renal artery; 1 = renal length at greatest longitudinal axis; 2 = distance between the first and fourth lumbar vertebrae. (From Taber P, et al: *Radiology* 1972; 102:129. Used by permission.)

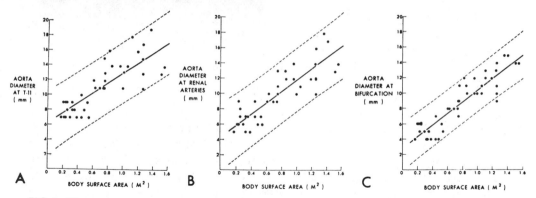

FIG 6–39.

Aortic diameter related to body surface area. **A,** at eleventh thoracic vertebra. **B,** at renal arteries. **C,** at aortic bifurcation. The *dotted lines* represent the 95% confidence limits of the regression curve. (From Taber P, et al: *Radiology* 1972; 102:129. Used by permission.)

Ref: Taber P, et al: *Radiology* 1972; 102:129.

MEASUREMENT OF THE ABDOMINAL AORTA

FIG 6–40.
Diameter of the renal artery related to ipsilateral kidney
length. (From Taber P, et al: *Radiology* 1972; 102:129. Used
by permission.)

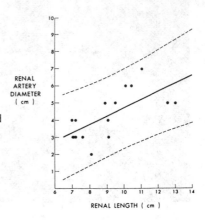

Technique
    Central ray: Perpendicular to plane of film.
    Position: Anteroposterior.
    Target-film distance: 40 inches.

Measurements (Fig 6–38)
    Aortic diameter was measured in three sites. Site A is at the level of the
pedicles of the eleventh thoracic vertebra, Site B just above the renal arteries,
and Site C, at the aortic bifurcation. The renal arteries were measured between 1 and 2 cm from their aortic origin. Renal lengths were measured from
the nephrographic phase of the arteriograms. The measurements were correlated with body surface areas from the known height and weight of the patients (see page 414). Results are shown in Figures 6–39 and 6–40.

Source of Material
    Data derived from aortograms of 45 patients, ranging in age from 1 day to
15 years.

MEASUREMENT OF THE ABDOMINAL AORTA

In Adults*

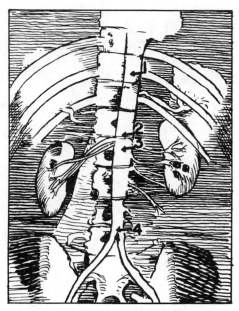

FIG 6–41.
(From Steinberg CR, et al: *AJR* 1965; 95:703. Used by permission.)

*Ref: Steinberg CR, et al: *AJR* 1965; 95:703.

TABLE 6–28.

Average Age and Diameter (in mm) of Abdominal Aorta at Sites Measured*

Sex and Diagnosis	No. of Cases	Age	At 11th Rib	Above Renal Arteries	Below Renal Arteries	At Bifurcation of Aorta	Difference between 11th Rib and Bifurcation of Aorta
Male							
Normal	29	53.9±13.7	26.9±3.96	23.9±3.92	21.4±3.65	18.7±3.34	8.14±2.14
Hypertensive	49	48.6±15.1	27.7±4.62	24.5±4.43	21.3±4.37	19.5±3.08	8.16±3.70
Occlusive	109	56.8±9.9	27.2±3.42	23.6±3.29	20.5±3.30	18.2±3.68	9.08±3.72
Abdominal aneurysm	90	63.6±7.1	33.5±6.05	31.2±8.36	34.3±12.56	31.8±10.53	1.76±10.23
Female							
Normal	44	56.9±14.3	24.4±3.45	21.6±3.16	18.7±3.36	17.5±2.52	6.80±4.54
Hypertensive	45	53.8±13.0	25.6±2.85	21.7±3.02	19.5±3.29	17.5±2.92	8.09±2.22
Occlusive	48	57.0±8.5	24.7±2.96	20.7±2.71	17.6±2.74	15.7±3.02	8.92±3.48
Abdominal aneurysm	18	67.2±7.3	30.5±6.05	28.5±6.94	32.2±14.00	25.4±6.21	5.05±6.40

*From Steinberg CR, et al: AJR 1965; 95:703. Used by permission.

MEASUREMENT OF THE ABDOMINAL AORTA

Technique
   Central ray: Perpendicular to plane of film centered over midabdomen.
   Position: Anteroposterior.
   Target-film distance: 48 inches.

Measurements (Fig 6–41)
Measurements were made at the following sites:

1. The eleventh rib, the level where the aorta pierces the diaphragm.
2. Above the renal arteries, at a site that is almost at one-half the length of the abdominal aorta and is below the celiac axis.
3. Below the renal arteries.
4. At the bifurcation of the abdominal aorta.

The values for male and female normals, hypertensives, and patients with occlusive arterial disease and abdominal aneurysms are given in Table 6–28. Hypertension and thrombotic occlusive disease do not alter the mean diameter. In arteriosclerotic aneurysmal disease, there is enlargement of the aorta at each site, suggesting that aortic dilatation is a significant accompaniment of the aneurysm.

Source of Material
Measurements are based on a study of 500 consecutive patients referred for intravenous abdominal aortography.

MEASUREMENT OF THE ABDOMINAL AORTA BY CT (ALSO APPLICABLE TO ULTRASONOGRAPHY)*

Technique

1. Studies performed on a Siemens Somatom 2 CT system.
2. Images were obtained:
   A. Immediately caudal to the origin of the superior mesenteric artery.
   B. Approximately midway between the superior mesenteric artery and the bifurcation.
   C. Immediately cranial to the bifurcation.

Measurements (Fig 6–42)

An average aortic diameter is calculated by taking the mean of the three measurements.

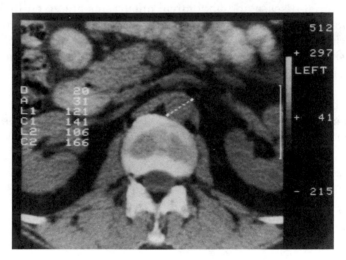

FIG 6–42.
Normal aorta shown by CT: no calcification. Electronic calipers traverse the aorta to give measurement of diameter of 20 mm (L + 41). (From Dixon AK, et al: *Clin Radiol* 1984; 35:33–37. Used by permission.)

Ref: Dixon AK, et al: *Clin Radiol* 1984; 35:33–37.

MEASUREMENT OF THE ABDOMINAL AORTA BY CT (ALSO APPLICABLE TO ULTRASONOGRAPHY)

The mean "aortic diameters" are shown in Figure 6−43.

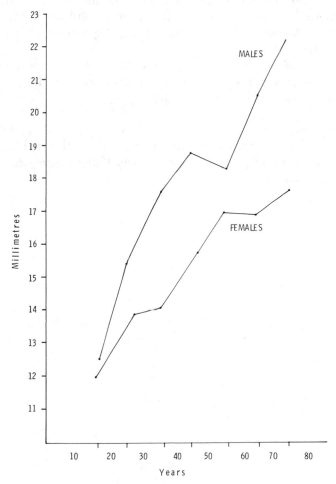

FIG 6−43.
Graph of mean 'aortic diameter' in males and females of each group plotted against age. (From Dixon AK, et al: *Clin Radiol* 1984; 35:33−37. Used by permission.)

MEASUREMENT OF THE ABDOMINAL AORTA BY CT (ALSO APPLICABLE TO ULTRASONOGRAPHY)

The aortic diameter increases with advancing age. In females the diameter varies from 12.3 mm in the second decade to 16.9 mm in the sixth decade. In men the diameter increases from 12.2 mm in the second decade to 22.8 mm in the sixth decade. An aortic diameter greater than 30 mm on ultrasound is considered abnormal.[*]

Note: Studies correlating measurements obtained on cross-table lateral radiographs, made at a 40-inch tube-to-film distance, are larger than sonographic measurements by a factor of 1.3.[†]

Source of Material

Data based on CT examinations of 257 patients with a variety of clinical problems but without suspected aortic disease. Patient ages ranged from the second to eighth decade.

[*]Ref: Sarti DA: *Diagnostic Ultrasound: Text and Cases,* ed. 2. Chicago, Year Book Medical Publishers, 1987, pg 284.

[†]Ref: Handy DC, et al: *Radiology* 1981; 141:821–823.

MEASUREMENT OF SIZE
OF MESENTERIC VESSELS*

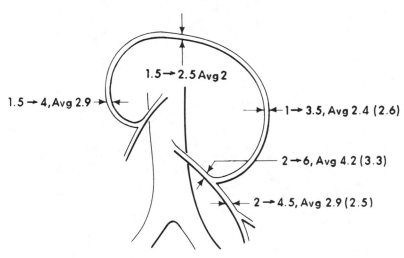

FIG 6–44.

Measurement of mesenteric vessels to the colon beyond the mid-transverse-colon. (From Wittenberg J, et al: *AJR* 1975; 123:287. Used by permission.)

Technique
Central ray: Perpendicular to plane of film.
Position: Anteroposterior.
Target-film distance: 40 inches.

Measurements (Fig 6–44)
The numbers represent the width of the vessels in millimeters as measured at points designated by the *arrows*. Both range and averages are given. The numbers in parentheses represent the average in millimeters for the same vessel as determined by Kahn and Abrams.†

Source of Material
Data based on a study of 19 patients, 11 females and 8 males. The ages ranged from 56 to 89; the average age was 73.

*Ref: Wittenberg J, et al: *AJR* 1975; 123:287.
†Ref: Kahn and Abrams: *Radiology* 1964; 82:429.

CHAPTER 7

The Gastrointestinal System

MEASUREMENT OF THE LOWER
ESOPHAGEAL RING*

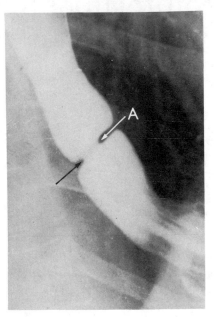

FIG 7–1.
(From Schatzki R: *AJR* 1963; 90:805. Used by permission.)

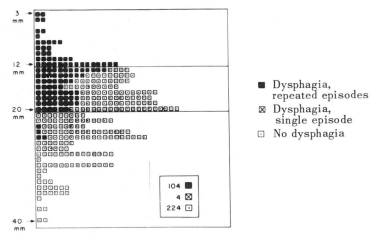

FIG 7–2.
Relationship between dysphagia and diameter of esophageal rings of various patients. The measurement refers to the maximal diameter of the ring at the time of first demonstration as measured on spot roentgenogram. (From Schatzki R: *AJR* 1963; 90:805. Used by permission.)

*Ref: Schatzki R, Gary JW: *AJR* 1953; 70:911.

MEASUREMENT OF THE LOWER
ESOPHAGEAL RING

Technique
   Central ray: Spot roentgenograms are used.
   Position: Erect or recumbent.
   Target-film distance: Variable. Target-table top distance: 18 inches.

Measurements (Figs 7–1 and 7–2)
Maximum diameter of the ring in a barium-filled esophagus. Measured on spot films without consideration of magnification.
Schatzki states that the lower esophageal ring:

1. Is not an abnormal contraction.
2. Lies at the junction of esophageal and gastric mucosa and is the junction of esophagus and stomach.
3. Has always been symptomatic in his experience if it has an original diameter of less than 13 mm.

Source of Material
The data are based on measurements of 104 patients with repeated episodes of dysphagia, 4 patients with one episode of dysphagia, and 224 patients without dysphagia.
Note: This does not include all asymptomatic patients with lower esophageal ring who were seen in this study.

MEASUREMENT OF ESOPHAGEAL DIAMETER*

TABLE 7−1.

Measurement Made at the Level of the
Cricopharyngeus Muscle*

Age	Anatomic Diam. (MM)
9 days to 4 weeks	6
1−9 months	7−8
10 months to 7 years	8−11
7−16 years	9−13

*From Haase FR, Brenner A: *Arch Otolaryngol* 1963; 77:119. Used by permission.

Technique

Central ray: Spot roentgenograms are used.

Position: Lateral neck. Erect or recumbent position. Barium-filled esophagus.

Target-film distance: Variable. Roentgenographic measurements must be corrected before comparison is made with Table 7−1.

Measurements

The cricopharyngeal diameter was found to be the narrowest point. Range of measurements is shown in Table 7−1.

Source of Material

Fresh esophageal specimens were obtained from 28 cadavers. Direct measurement of mucosa was made. In no case was the cause of death due to an abnormality of the esophagus.

Ref: Haase FR, Brenner A: *Arch Otolaryngol* 1963; 77:119.

MEASUREMENTS OF THE PYLORUS IN INFANCY BY ULTRASOUND FOR INVESTIGATION OF HYPERTROPHIC PYLORIC STENOSIS*

Technique

1. High resolution real-time equipment (Picker Microview) was used with a 10 MHz transducer.
2. Examination was performed in the right decubitus position for evaluation of fluid passage through the pyloric canal and antral distension (Fig 7–3) and in the left decubitus position for detection of gas passage through the canal (Fig 7–4).

Measurement

The following measurements were recorded: the maximal anteroposterior diameter of the pylorus, the thickness of one pyloric muscle wall, and the length of the pylorus.

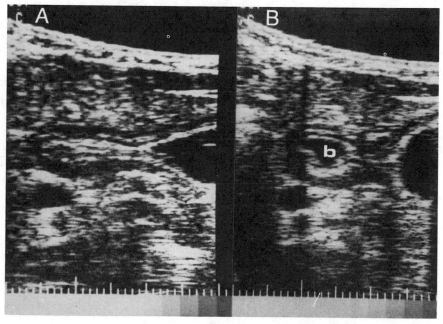

FIG 7–3.
Ultrasonic image of normal pylorus in longitudinal axis, contracted phase (**A**) and during fluid passage (**B**). Note fluid bolus *(b)*. (From Graif M, et al: *Pediatr Radiol* 1984; 14:14–17. Used by permission.)

Ref: Graif M, et al: *Pediatr Radiol* 1984; 14:14–17.

MEASUREMENTS OF THE PYLORUS IN INFANCY
BY ULTRASOUND FOR INVESTIGATION
OF HYPERTROPHIC PYLORIC STENOSIS

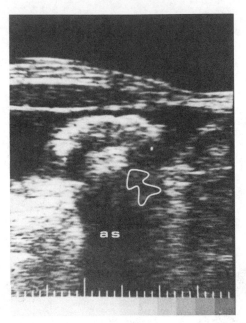

FIG 7–4.
Ultrasonic image of normal pylorus scanned in left decubitus position. The echogenic area *(arrow)* represents pyloric musoca and gas interface, causing acoustic shadow *(as)*. (From Graif M, et al: *Pediatr Radiol* 1984; 14:14–17. Used by permission.)

The mean pyloric length in the hypertrophied condition was 84% longer than the mean length in the normal. The mean and standard deviation (SD) for the transverse diameter and pyloric wall thickness in the normals were 745 ± 2.2 mm and 2.3 ± 0.7 mm respectively, while the corresponding measurements for the mean and SD in hypertrophic pyloric stenosis were 13.4 ± 1.6 mm and 4.5 ± 0.9 mm. In most of the hypertrophic pyloric stenosis cases the known morphological changes of the antropyloric region were observed, such as impingement on the fluid filled antrum, prepyloric antral thickening, extension of fluid into the proximal portion of the pyloric canal, and the angle formed between antral peristaltic wave and pyloric mass. Detection of these changes furnished further criteria for highly accurate diagnosis of hypertrophic pyloric stenosis even of borderline cases.

Source of Material
Data are based on sonographic examinations of a control group of 24 infants ranging in age from 2 days to 32 weeks and a second group of 22 patients ranging in age from 2 to 10 weeks in whom the clinical impression was hypertrophic pyloric stenosis.

MEASUREMENT OF THE ADULT STOMACH AND DUODENUM*

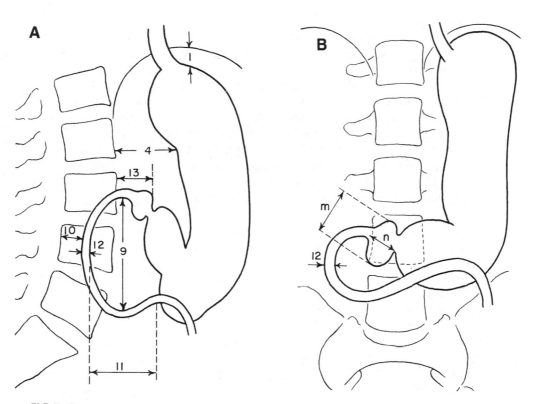

FIG 7–5.

A, stomach and duodenum in right lateral recumbent or left lateral erect positions. **B,** stomach and duodenum in posteroanterior recumbent position. (Adapted from Meschan I, et al: *South Med J* 1953; 46:878.)

Technique

Central ray: Posteroanterior recumbent: to second lumbar vertebra. Right lateral recumbent: 3 inches anterior to midcoronal plane at level of second lumbar vertebra. Left lateral erect: same as right lateral recumbent. Stomach may be lower in position than for recumbent, and fluoroscopic observation is recommended for accurate centering.

Position: Posteroanterior recumbent; right lateral recumbent; left lateral erect.

Target-film distance: 36 inches.

Stomach contained approximately 8 oz of barium sulfate in water. Films obtained in suspended respiration.

*Ref: Meschan I, et al: *South Med J* 1953; 46:878.

MEASUREMENT OF THE ADULT
STOMACH AND DUODENUM

Measurements (Fig 7–5 and Table 7–2)

1 = Distance between top of stomach fundus and diaphragm.

4 = Stomach to anterior spine. See measurements on retrogastric space, page 489.

9 = Maximum vertical internal diameter of the duodenal loop.

10 = Minimum measurement of the outer margin of the second portion of the duodenum to the posterior margin of the vertebral bodies.

11 = Maximum horizontal internal diameter of the duodenal loop.

12 = Maximum outer diameter of the second portion of the duodenum.

13 = Distance between pylorus and the outer margin of the spine.

m = Width of base of duodenal bulb.

n = Height of duodenal bulb from apex to pylorus.

Figure 7–5,A, dimension 1: average = 0.5 cm; maximum = 1.5 cm.

Diameter of second portion of duodenum, Figure 7–5,A and B, dimension 12: average = 2.0 cm; minimum = 1.0 cm; maximum = 2.5 cm.

Width of gastric and duodenal rugae: upper stomach, 0.5 cm; lower stomach, 0.3–0.5 cm; midduodenum, 0.2–0.3 cm.

Size of duodenal bulb (Fig 7–5,B) width at base *(m)*: average = 3.0 cm; maximum = 3.5 cm; height *(n): average = 3.0 cm; maximum = 4.0 cm.*

Types of stomachs

1. J-shaped or eutonic stomach: pylorus and incisura angularis are at the same level.

2. Cascade stomach: fundus has a posterior pouchlike projection that overlaps the body of the stomach.

3. Fishhook or hypotonic-type stomach: Incisura angularis is considerably lower than pylorus.

4. Steer-horn stomach: Incisura angularis lies above the level of the pylorus.

Weight Groups (Table 7–2)

Meschan et al. divided the patients into three groups according to weight. The Equitable Life Assurance Society standards for height and weight were used to establish whether patients were normal weight (plus or minus 10%), overweight or underweight.

TABLE 7-2.

Relationships of Stomach and Duodenum to the Spine in Different Weight and Stomach Type Groups (Both Asymptomatic and Symptomatic Summated)*

Weight Group	Stomach Type	No. of Cases (211 Total)	9 Rt. Lat.		10 Rt. Lat.		11 Rt. Lat.		13 Rt. Lat.	
			Avg. of Medians	Range	Avg. of Medians	Range	Avg. of Medians	Range	Avg. of Medians	Range
Normal	J-shape	58	6.5	4.0–9.5	3.0	1.0–9.0	3.0	0.0–12.5	4.0	0.5–8.0
	Fishhook	10	6.0	4.0–8.0	3.0	2.5–4.0	5.6	3.5–8.0	4.5	2.5–9.0
	Cascade	13	6.0	4.5–6.0	4.3	2.0–9.5	6.6	1.0–11.0	5.0	2.5–9.0
	Steer-horn	9	6.5	5.5–8.0	3.5	0.5–5.0	5.5	1.5–9.0	5.0	2.5–10.0
Underweight	J-shape	56	5.5	2.0–11.0	3.0	0.5–7.0	4.0	0.0–9.0	3.0	0.5–6.5
	Fishhook	21	5.5	3.5–8.0	2.5	0.0–5.0	3.0	1.5–5.0	2.5	1.0–4.0
	Cascade	5	6.0	5.5–6.5	2.5	2.0–3.5	4.5	4.0–5.0	3.0	2.0–5.0
	Steer-horn	3	8.0	8.0	4.5	2.0–6.0	7.0	6.5–8.0	4.0	1.5–5.0
Overweight	J-shape	13	6.5	4.0–9.0	3.3	2.0–7.0	4.5	3.5–9.0	3.5	1.5–9.5
	Fishhook	5	5.0	3.0–7.5	2.5	0.0–4.0	4.5	2.0–9.5	4.6	3.0–6.5
	Cascade	10	7.0	4.0–9.0	4.0	1.0–7.5	5.0	1.5–10.0	5.6	3.0–12.0
	Steer-horn	8	6.0	5.5–8.0	4.0	3.5–5.5	5.0	3.0–7.5	4.5	3.0–7.5

*Data from Meschan I, et al: *South Med J* 1953;46:878.

MEASUREMENT OF THE ADULT STOMACH AND DUODENUM

Source of Material

The data are based on a study of 211 adult individuals of all ages between the third and the seventh decade, chosen at random from patients at two Veterans Administration hospitals, the University of Arkansas Hospital, and University of Arkansas medical students.

Of these adults, 107 were asymptomatic, and 104 were symptomatic with no apparent radiographic abnormality in stomach or duodenum.

Sex and age distribution were random.

More than 10,000 measurements were made for this study.

Note: Gastrocolic space (measurement made from inferior aspect of the greater curvature of the stomach to the adjacent transverse colon) has been measured by Moreno* and by Seymour.[†] Moreno proposed a normal limit of 3 cm for the gastrocolic space, but Seymour, who examined 50 patients, found that the 3 cm limit was exceeded in 36% of the patients, in whom the gastrocolic space averaged 8.7 cm.

*Ref: Moreno G, Rivera HH: *Radiology* 1976; 118:535.
†Ref: Seymour EQ: *Radiology* 1977; 123:527.

MEASUREMENT OF RETROGASTRIC
AND RETRODUODENAL SPACES*

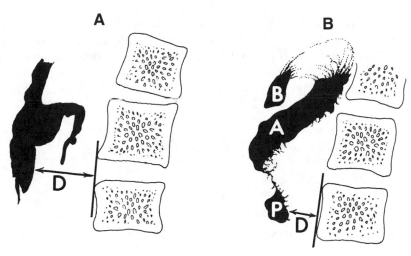

FIG 7–6.
(Adapted from Poole GJ: *Radiology* 1970; 97:71.)

Technique

Central ray: To barium-filled stomach and duodenum during fluoroscopic examination.

Position: Left lateral erect. Patient's left shoulder toward fluoroscopic screen, right shoulder against table top.

Target-film distance: Varies with thickness of patient. A coin marker, i.e., a nickel, is placed on the skin for purposes of magnification correction.

Measurements (Fig 7–6)

A barium mixture of 3 parts Intropaque, 2 parts Barosperse, and 5 parts water (all by volume) was used by Poole. In the upright posteroanterior position the patient swallows ½ oz of barium.

Antrum-to-Spine Measurement (Fig 7–6,A): The fluoroscopic pressure cone is used to flatten the column of barium in the antrum. Adequate compression is denoted by displacement of the barium column to both sides of the midline.

The patient is then turned laterally with arms raised so that his right side is against the table top and the spot-film device is against his left side. A compression device (Poole used a plunger-type device with a padded head 3½ inches in diameter) is placed over the same spot on the anterior abdominal

*Ref: Poole GJ: *Radiology* 1970; 97:71.

wall as was used in splaying the folds in the posteroanterior projection. The patient is fluoroscoped, and the abdominal wall is pressed with the compression device until the midline viscus strikes the retroperitoneal structures. A lateral spot-film is taken. Distance D is measured as shown in Figure 7–6,A from the posterior stomach wall to the anterior vertebral body surface. Distance is corrected for magnification according to the following ratio:

$$\frac{D_t}{D_m} = \frac{C_t}{C_m}; D_t = \frac{D_m C_t}{C_m}$$

where:

D_t = True antrum- or duodenum-to-spine distance.
D_m = Magnified distance from antrum or duodenum to spine measured on the spot-film.
C_t = True marker diameter (nickel coin).
C_m = Magnified marker's greatest diameter measured on the spot-film.

Corrected antrum-to-spine distance is plotted against weight as shown in Figure 7–7.

MEASUREMENT OF RETROGASTRIC
AND RETRODUODENAL SPACES

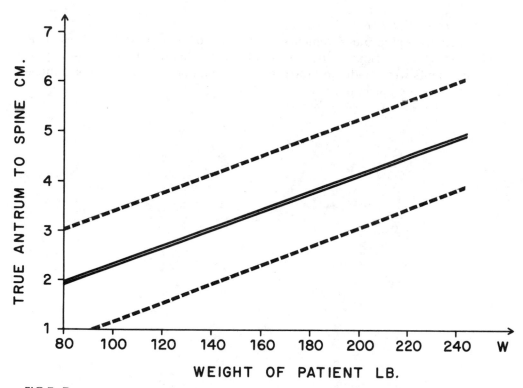

FIG 7–7.
Body weight versus corrected antrum-to-spine distance. Regression line and 95% confidence limits are shown. (From Poole GJ: *Radiology* 1970; 97:71. Used by permission.)

Duodenum-to-Spine Measurement (Fig 7–6,B): Following the antrum-to-spine spot-film, the patient is placed in the right lateral decubitus position to allow barium to enter the horizontal duodenum. The patient is placed erect in the posteroanterior position. When the midline duodenum is identified the patient is turned to a left lateral position. When the horizontal duodenum is seen on end, a spot-film is made without pressure. The duodenum-to-spine distance is measured from the posterior aspect of the midline duodenum to the spine (measurement D, Fig 7–6,B) If hypertrophic spurs are present, the measurement is taken to the anterior aspect of the spurs. Measurement D is corrected for magnification as described for antrum-to-spine measurement.

Mean value is 1.3 cm (SD 5 mm). Upper limit of normal is 2.3 cm (1.3 cm + 2 SD). The duodenum-to-spine measurement showed no relationship to body weight.

MEASUREMENT OF RETROGASTRIC
AND RETRODUODENAL SPACES

Source of Material

Antrum-to-spine measurements were made on 141 patients who had no radiographic or clinical evidence of retrogastric mass. Duodenum-to-spine measurements were made on 96 patients who had no radiographic or clinical evidence of retrogastric mass.

DETERMINATION OF LIVER SIZE
IN INFANCY AND CHILDHOOD*

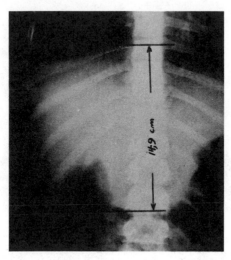

FIG 7–8.
Measurement of vertical axis of the liver. The lower horizontal line is drawn from the lowest right border of the liver. (From Deligeorgis D, Yannakos D, Doxiadis S: *Arch Dis Child* 1973; 48:790. Used by permission.)

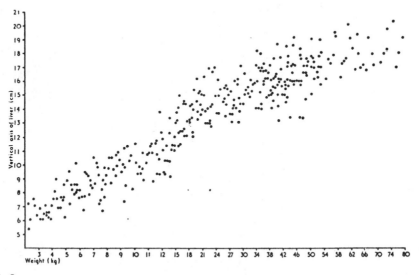

FIG 7–9.
Vertical axis of the liver related to weight. (From Deligeorgis D, Yannakos D, Doxiadis S: *Arch Dis Child* 1973; 48:790. Used by permission.)

*Ref: Deligeorgis D, Yannakos D, Doxiadis S: *Arch Dis Child* 1973; 48:790.

DETERMINATION OF LIVER SIZE
IN INFANCY AND CHILDHOOD

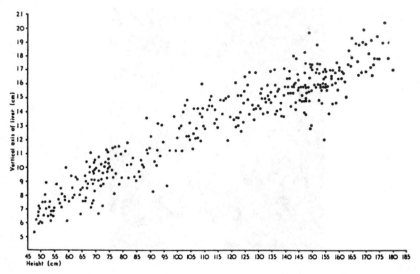

FIG 7–10.
Vertical axis of the liver related to height. (From Deligeorgis D, Yannakos D, Doxiadis S: *Arch Dis Child* 1973; 48:790. Used by permission.)

FIG 7–11.
Vertical axis of the liver related to age. (From Deligeorgis D, Yannakos D, Doxiadis S: *Arch Dis Child* 1973; 48:790. Used by permission.)

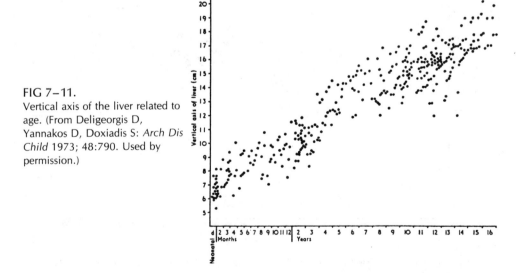

DETERMINATION OF LIVER SIZE IN INFANCY AND CHILDHOOD

Technique
   Central ray: Perpendicular to plane of film.
   Position: Anteroposterior supine, filmed at end of expiration.
   Target-film distance: 140 cm.

Measurements (Fig 7−8)
   A horizontal line is drawn across the uppermost region of the liver, just below the dome of the diaphragm, and another is drawn parallel to the first across the lowest right border of the liver. The vertical distance between the two lines is the vertical axis of the liver. Normal values are given in Figures 7−9 to 7−11.

Source of Material
   Data derived from studies of 350 healthy Greek infants and children between birth and 16 years.

LIVER SIZE DETERMINATION IN PEDIATRICS USING SONOGRAPHIC AND SCINTIGRAPHIC TECHNIQUES*

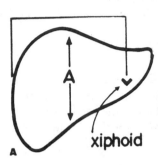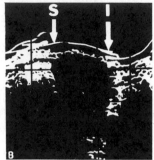

FIG 7–12.

A, both the ultrasound and the radionuclide image measurements are made in the plane halfway between the xiphoid and right lateral liver margin. **B,** an example of a longitudinal B-mode scan along the plane described in **A.** The superior point of the measurement (S) is defined by the echoes of the liver lung interface. The inferior part of the measurement (I) is defined by the intra-abdominal echoes below the liver. (From Holder LE, et al: *Radiology* 1975; 117:349. Used by permission.)

FIG 7–13.

Anterior view liver image. Costal margin (CM), xiphoid (X) and size marker (10 cm) are located on each image. (From Holder LE, et al: *Radiology* 1975; 117:349. Used by permission.)

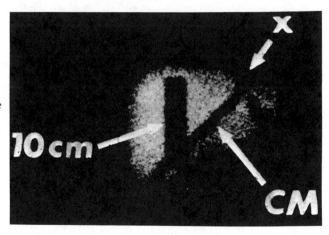

Ref: Holder LE, et al: *Radiology* 1975; 117:349.

LIVER SIZE DETERMINATION IN PEDIATRICS USING SONOGRAPHIC AND SCINTIGRAPHIC TECHNIQUES

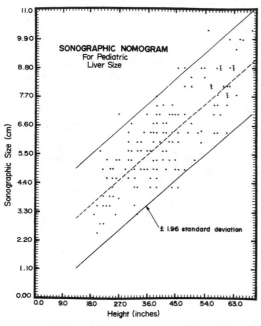

FIG 7–14.
Sonographic liver size in centimeters versus height of patient in inches. (From Holder LE, et al: *Radiology* 1975; 117:349. Used by permission.)

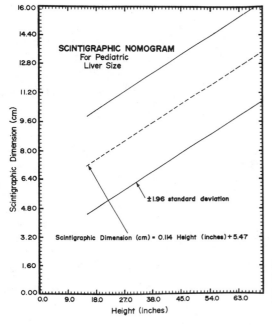

FIG 7–15.
Scintigraphic liver size in centimeters versus height of patient in inches. (From Holder LE, et al: *Radiology* 1975; 117:349. Used by permission.)

LIVER SIZE DETERMINATION IN PEDIATRICS USING SONOGRAPHIC AND SCINTIGRAPHIC TECHNIQUES

Technique

1. Scintigraphic: Liver scintiscan using technetium-99m sulfur colloid; Ohio-Nuclear Series 100 gamma camera. Anterior view with xiphoid and costal margins marked and 10 cm or 5 cm marker (Fig 7–13) placed against the collimator face. A Polaroid picture was taken of the oscilloscope display, and the scintiscan measurement was taken from the Polaroid picture.
2. Sonographic: Longitudinal, supine ultrasound scan of liver using Picker Echoview VI: ultrasonic B-scan imaging using a 2 MHz collimated scanning transducer. The longitudinal ultrasound measurement was made halfway between xiphoid and right lateral liver margin (Fig 7–12).

Measurements (Figs 7–14 and 7–15)

Source of Material
Data based on a normally distributed population of 185 children ranging in age from 6 days to 17 years, in weight from 7 to 166 pounds, in height from 19 to 69 inches, and in surface area from 0.21 to 1.88 square meters.

DETERMINATION OF LIVER VOLUME*†

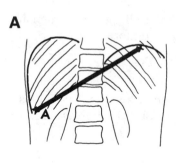

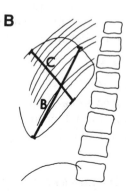

FIG 7–23.
(Adapted from Walk L: *Acta Radiol* 1961: 55:49.)

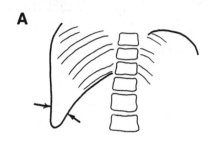

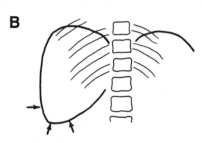

FIG 7–24.
A, thin border of liver. **B,** rounded border of liver. (Adapted from Walk L: *Acta Radiol* 1961; 55:49.)

Technique
Central ray: Centered over upper abdomen.
Position: Exposure 1 is taken anteroposterior with patient supine (Fig 7–23,A). Exposure 2 is taken in right posterior oblique position of 50° to 60° (Fig 7–23,B).
Target-film distance: 120 cm.

Measurements (Fig 7–23)
Dimension A (Fig 7–23,A) is the distance from the right border of the liver to the middle of the left cupola of the diaphragm. Use Exposure 1.

Dimension B (Fig 7–23,B) is the distance from the anteroinferior border of the liver to the most distal part of its posterior surface as outlined by the diaphragm. Use Exposure 2.

Dimension C (Fig 7–23,B) is the distance from the posterior surface of the liver, where it lies close to the upper pole of the kidney, to the upper anterior surface. Use Exposure 2.

*Ref: Walk L: *Acta Radiol* 1961; 55:49.
†Ref: Walk L: *Acta Radiol Diagn* 1967; 6:369.

DETERMINATION OF LIVER VOLUME

For a target-film distance of 120 cm the A, B, and C dimensions taken from the two exposures are used in the following formula:

$$\text{Liver volume} = A \cdot B \cdot C \text{ index}$$

Indices to be used for children and adults are shown in Tables 7−4 and 7−5 for normal border, in Figure 7−24,A for thin border, and in Figure 7−24,B for round border.

TABLE 7−4.

Indices to be Used for Children in Calculation of Liver Volume*

Age of Patient	Liver Configuration		
	Round Border	Normal Border	Thin Border
1 year	0.242	0.217	0.204
2−3 yr	0.227	0.204	0.191
4−6 yr	0.215	0.193	0.181
7−11 yr	0.204	0.183	0.172
12−17 yr	0.197	0.177	0.166

*From Walk L: *Acta Radiol Diagn* 1967; 6:369. Used by permission.

TABLE 7−5.

Indices to be Used for Adults in Calculation of Liver Volume

Rounded border	0.19
Normal configuration	0.17
Thin border	0.16

Liver volume per square meter of body surface is clinically useful. Surface area is calculated according to the formula of DuBois and DuBois* as follows:

$$\text{BSA (m}^2\text{)} = \frac{\text{weight (kg)}}{2.35} \times \frac{\text{height (cm)}}{1.38} \times 6$$

This formula may be simplified according to Von Behrens,[†] as follows:

$$\text{BSA(m}^2\text{)} = 0.176 \sqrt{\text{Wt(kg)Ht(m)}}$$
$$\text{or}$$
$$\text{BSA(m}^2\text{)} = 0.1035 \, [\text{Wt(kg)}]^{2/3}$$

Normal liver volume = 850 cc/m^2.

*Ref: DuBois D, DuBois EF: *Proc Soc Exp Biol Med* 1916; 13:77.
†Ref: Von Behrens WE: *Australas Radiol* 1972; 16:180.

Borderline liver volume $= 800-900$ cc/m^2.
Liver volume more than 900 cc/m^2 is definitely pathologic.

Source of Material

Roentgenologic measurements of liver were compared with the postmortem specimen measurements in 80 autopsies. Error was $\pm$ 16%.

MEASUREMENT OF LIVER AND SPLEEN VOLUME BY CT*

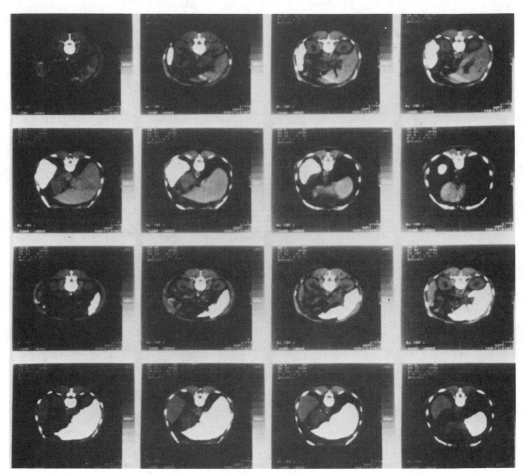

FIG 7–25.
CT scan of the upper abdomen for measurement of liver and spleen size. The first eight panels show the liver blanked out with a light pen, while the next eight illustrate splenic measurement. (From Henderson JM, et al: *Radiology* 1981; 141:525. Used by permission.)

Ref: Henderson JM et al: *Radiology* 1981; 141:525.

MEASUREMENT OF LIVER AND SPLEEN VOLUME BY CT

Technique

1. A GE 8800 CT/T scanner was used to make 10-mm thick slices at 2-cm intervals through the liver and spleen, beginning at the level of the diaphragm.
2. Breath holding was in comfortable inspiration. No intravenous contrast was used.

Measurement (Fig 7–25 and Table 7–6)

Each slice was displayed, the organ of interest outlined by the cursor, and the enclosed area calculated by the CT computer.

Areas of each organ were added and multiplied by 2 to estimate total organ volume.

TABLE 7–6.

Mean Liver and Spleen Volumes on Two Different Days as Read by Two Observers*

	Liver Volume (cm³)				Spleen Volume (cm³)			
	Observer 1		Observer 2		Observer 1		Observer 2	
	Scan 1	Scan 2	Scan 1	Scan 2	Scan 1	Scan 2	Scan 1	Scan 2
Mean	1,445	1,500	1,468	1,557	215	228	216	217
S.D.	±166	±295	±199	±270	±77	±85	±76	±72

*From Henderson JM, et al: *Radiology* 1981; 141:525. Used by permission.

Source of Material

Eleven normal subjects 20 to 30 years of age were studied on two occasions, 1 week apart.

MEASUREMENT OF THE NORMAL LIVER, SPLEEN, AND PANCREAS BY ULTRASOUND*

Technique

1. A high resolution real-time scanner (Siemens Imager) was used with a 3.5-MHz transducer.
2. Subjects were examined supine, with the right side elevated to demonstrate the porta hepatis, and with the left side elevated to show the longitudinal axis of the spleen. Length was measured to the nearest millimeter with dividers.

Measurement

Longitudinal scans of the liver were obtained in the midclavicular line and midline, measuring the longitudinal and anteroposterior diameters (Figs 7–16 to 7–20).

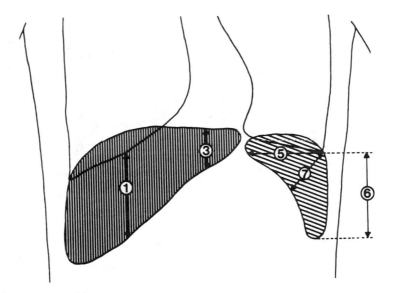

FIG 7–16.
AP view. *1* = midclavicular longitudinal diameter of the liver; *3* = midline longitudinal diameter of the liver; *5* = transverse diameter of the spleen; *6* = longitudinal diameter of the spleen; *7* = diagonal diameter of the spleen. The upper regions of the liver and the spleen are located in the dome of the diaphragm and hidden by the air in the lung, so that their longitudinal diameters can be measured only as far as the margin of the lung. (From Niederau C, et al: *Radiology* 1983; 149:537–540. Used by permission.)

Ref: Niederau C, et al: *Radiology* 1983; 149:537–540.

MEASUREMENT OF THE NORMAL LIVER, SPLEEN, AND PANCREAS BY ULTRASOUND

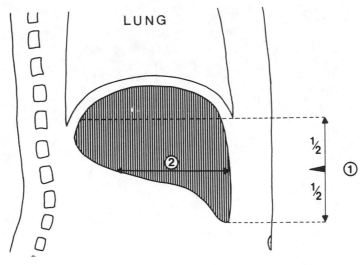

FIG 7–17.
Lateral view of the liver in the midclavicular plane. *1* = midclavicular longitudinal diameter; *2* = midclavicular AP diameter, measured at the midpoint of the longitudinal diameter. The upper region of the liver is masked by the air in the lung. (From Niederau C, et al: *Radiology* 1983; 149:537–540. Used by permission.)

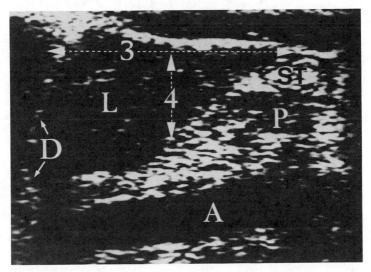

FIG 7–18.
Midline longitudinal scan of the liver. *3* = midline longitudinal diameter; *4* = midline AP diameter, measured at the midpoint of the longitudinal diameter; *D* = diaphragm; *L* = Liver; *ST* = stomach (target); *P* = pancreas; *A* = aorta. The upper margin of the liver, under the dome of the diaphragm, served as the upper limit of the longitudinal diameter. (From Niederau C, et al: *Radiology* 1983; 149:537–540. Used by permission.)

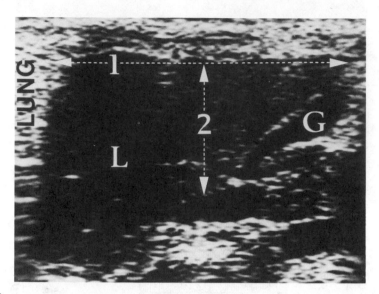

FIG 7–19.
Longitudinal scan of the liver in the right midclavicular plane. *1* = midclavicular longitudinal diameter; *2* = midclavicular AP diameter measured at the midpoint of the longitudinal diameter; *L* = liver; *G* = gallbladder. The margin between the lung and liver was used as the upper limit of the longitudinal diameter, since the upper region of the liver was partly masked by the air in the lung. (From Niederau C, et al: *Radiology* 1983; 149:537−540. Used by permission.)

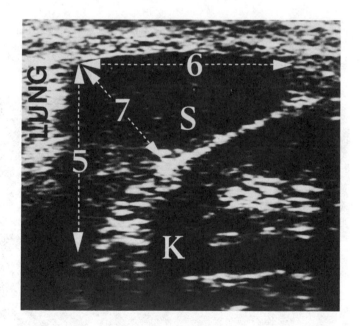

FIG 7–20.
Longitudinal scan of the spleen. *5* = transverse diameter; *6* = longitudinal diameter; *7* = diagonal diameter; *S* = spleen; *K* = kidney. The margin between the lung and spleen served as both the transverse diameter and the upper limit of the longitudinal diameter. (From Niederau C, et al: *Radiology* 1983; 149:537−540. Used by permission.)

MEASUREMENT OF THE NORMAL LIVER, SPLEEN, AND PANCREAS BY ULTRASOUND

In the midclavicular line, the upper portion of the liver was partly masked by the air inside the lung, and the margin between the lung and liver was used as the upper limit of the longitudinal diameter. In the midline, the upper margin of the liver under the dome of the diaphragm served as the upper limit of the longitudinal diameter. The AP diameters were measured at the midpoint of the longitudinal diameters. Both the liver and spleen were measured during deep inspiration. The cross-sectional area of the liver was calculated from the longitudinal and AP diameters using the equation:

$$(\text{Longitudinal diameter} \times \text{AP diameter})/2 = \text{cross-sectional area}$$

The spleen was viewed along its longitudinal axis. Transverse, longitudinal, and diagonal diameters were measured from the image showing the maximum cross-sectional areas (Figs 7–21 and 7–22). The margin between lung and spleen served as both the transverse diameter and the limit of the longitudinal diameter. The cross-sectional diameter was calculated using all three diameters:

$$\frac{\text{Diagonal X}}{\sqrt{(\text{Transverse}^2 + \text{longitudinal}^2)/2}} = \text{area}$$

The maximum AP diameter of the pancreas was measured on a transverse/oblique scan, using the upper abdominal blood vessels as landmarks. The portal and splenic veins, which comprise the regular posterior (dorsal) boundaries of the body of the pancreas, were not included (Figs 7–21 and 7–22), nor was the tail of the pancreas measured since it is not often visible and varies widely in shape. The maximum diameter of the portal vein and the diameter at the porta hepatis were measured, with the inner dimensions being used for sonographic assessment.

Statistics

Statistical calculations were performed on a Telefunken TR 440 computer using a routine program. Linear regression analysis was carried out for age, sex, weight, height, surface area, and all diameters. The 95th percentile was considered the upper limit of normal, i.e., 95% of all measurements were below this point. Results of the X^2 test were evaluated using Yates' correction.

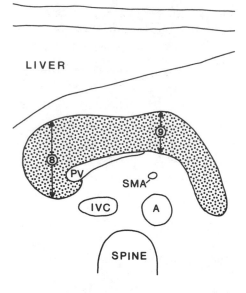

FIG 7–21.
Transverse scan. *8* = maximum AP diameter of the head of the pancreas; *9* = maximum AP diameter of the body of the pancreas; *PV* = portal vein; *SMA* = superior mesenteric artery; *IVC* = inferior vena cava; *A* = aorta. The portal and splenic veins, which represent the posterior (dorsal) boundaries of the pancreas, are not included. (From Niederau C, et al: *Radiology* 1983; 149:537–540. Used by permission.)

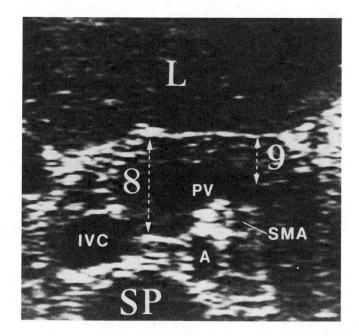

FIG 7–22.
Transverse scan. *8* = maximum AP diameter of the head of the pancreas; *9* = maximum AP diameter of the body of the pancreas; *L* = liver; *PV* = portal vein; *IVC* = inferior vena cava; *SMA* = superior mesenteric vein; *A* = aorta; *SP* = spine. The upper abdominal vessels served as pancreatic landmarks. The portal and splenic veins are not included. (From Niederau C, et al: *Radiology* 1983; 149:537–540. Used by permission.)

MEASUREMENT OF THE NORMAL LIVER, SPLEEN, AND PANCREAS BY ULTRASOUND

Mean organ diameters are given in Table 7–3.

TABLE 7–3.

Mean Organ Diameters*

	Diameter (cm) (mean ± SD)	95th Percentile (cm)
Midclavicular longitudinal diameter of the liver	10.5±1.5	12.6
Midclavicular AP diameter of the liver	8.1±1.9	11.3
Midline longitudinal diameter of the liver	8.3±1.7	10.9
Midline AP diameter of the liver	5.7±1.5	8.2
Transverse diameter of the spleen	5.5±1.4	7.8
Longitudinal diameter of the spleen	5.8±1.8	8.7
Diagonal diameter of the spleen	3.7±1.0	5.4
Maximum diameter of the head of the pancreas	2.2±0.3	2.6
Maximum diameter of the body of the pancreas	1.8±0.3	2.2
Maximum diameter of the portal vein	1.2±0.2	1.4
Diameter of the portal vein at the porta hepatis	1.0±0.2	1.2

*From Niederau C, et al: *Radiology* 1983; 149:537–540. Used by permission.

Source of Material

Data are based on a study of 1,000 healthy subjects, 160 women and 840 men between the ages of 18 and 65 years. Eighty-five subjects were excluded.

MEASUREMENT OF NEONATAL BILIARY SYSTEM BY REAL-TIME ULTRASOUND*

Technique

1. A 6.0- or 7.5 MHz transducer and a mechanical sector real-time scanner were used and images recorded on Polaroid or multiformat transparencies.
2. Scans were in the transverse and sagittal projections and in the supine and left lateral decubitus positions.
3. Subjects were scanned immediately prior to next feeding or fasting state.

Measurements (Fig 7–26; Tables 7–7 and 7–8)

Measurements were made from prints or film and corrected for magnification.

*Ref: Carroll BA, et al: *Radiology* 1982; 145:437.

MEASUREMENT OF NEONATAL BILIARY SYSTEM
BY REAL-TIME ULTRASOUND

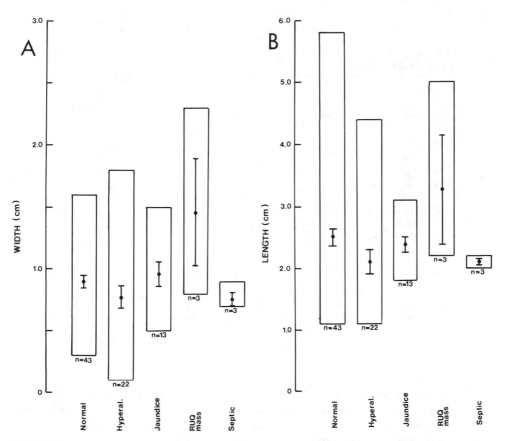

FIG 7–26.
Graphs display the range of neonatal gallbladder measurements and the mean ± SEM. **A,** width. **B,** length. (From Carroll BA, et al: *Radiology* 1982; 145:437. Used by permission.)

TABLE 7–7.

Infant Ages*

Age (Wk Gestation or Postpartum)	Number of Infants
25–29	6
30–34	25
35–39	16
40–42	23
1–2 wk	8
3 wk–3 mo	7
Total	85

*From Carroll BA, et al: *Radiology* 1982; 145:437. Used by permission.

MEASUREMENT OF NEONATAL BILIARY SYSTEM BY REAL-TIME ULTRASOUND

TABLE 7−8.

Sludge in Infant Gallbladders*

Medical Status of Neonate		Number of Neonates Involved
Hyperalimented	(HA)	6
HA only	(2)	
HA + jaundice	(2)	
HA + sepsis	(1)	
HA + sepsis + jaundiced	(1)†	
Jaundiced only		1
Prior history of HA, sepsis, and jaundice. Now clinically normal at discharge		1
Never HA, no sepsis or jaundice		4
Congenital heart disease	(1)	
Meconium aspiration	(2)	
Severe hypotension	(1)	
Total		12(14%)

*From Carroll BA, et al: *Radiology* 1982; 145:437. Used by permission.
†Sludge persisted after hyperalimentation ceased and jaundice and sepsis resolved.

Source of Material

Eighty-five neonates were studied, 29 female and 56 males; 43 were normal and nonjaundiced; 42 had potential biliary tract abnormalities, including 22 on hyperalimentation, 14 with jaundice, 3 with right upper quadrant masses, and 3 with sepsis only.

MEASUREMENT OF THE COMMON BILE DUCT IN CHILDREN*

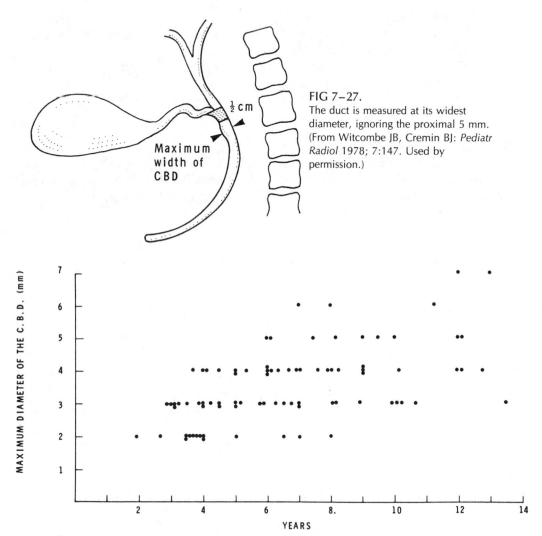

FIG 7–27.
The duct is measured at its widest diameter, ignoring the proximal 5 mm. (From Witcombe JB, Cremin BJ: *Pediatr Radiol* 1978; 7:147. Used by permission.)

FIG 7–28.
Normal range of measurements. (From Witcombe JB, Cremin BJ: *Pediatr Radiol* 1978; 7:147. Used by permission.)

*Ref: Witcombe JB, Cremin BJ: *Pediatr Radiol* 1978; 7:147.

MEASUREMENT OF THE COMMON BILE DUCT
IN CHILDREN

Technique
Intravenous cholangiography by drip infusion of 20 cc of 50% meglumine iodipamide.
Central ray: Perpendicular to plane of film centered over right upper abdomen.
Position: 15° prone oblique.
Target-film distance: 100 cm.

Measurement (Fig 7–27)
The widest diameter of the common bile duct was measured to the nearest millimeter. Measurements were not taken within 5 mm because of overlapping of the cystic duct and common hepatic duct near their junction.
Normal measurements are given in Figure 7–28.

Source of Material
Data based on study of 44 females and 41 males of African, European, and mixed parentage.

MEASUREMENT OF NORMAL PEDIATRIC GALLBLADDER AND BILIARY TRACT BY ULTRASOUND*

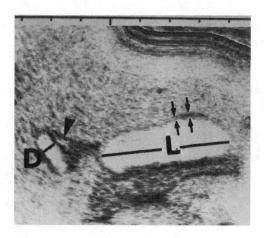

FIG 7–29.
Parasagittal scan of the right upper quadrant, showing the common hepatic duct *(arrowhead)*, right portal vein *(D)*, and gallbladder. The length *(L)*, AP dimension, and wall thickness of the gallbladder *(arrows)* were measured on this scan. (From McGahan JP, et al: *Radiology* 1982; 144:873. Used by permission.)

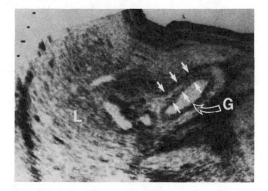

FIG 7–30.
Longitudinal scan of the right upper quadrant in an 8-year-old boy with serum hepatitis. Note increased thickness *(arrows)* giving a "tram-track" appearance to the gallbladder wall. G = gallbladder lumen; L = liver. (From McGahan JP, et al: *Radiology* 1982; 144:873. Used by permission.)

*Ref: McGahan JP et al: *Radiology* 1982; 144:873.

MEASUREMENT OF NORMAL PEDIATRIC GALLBLADDER AND BILIARY TRACT BY ULTRASOUND

Technique

1. Either static sector or linear-array real-time scanners with 3.5- or 5-MHz transducers were used.
2. Younger subjects fasted about 3 hours and older ones 8 hours or more.
3. Sagittal, transverse, and oblique images were used to optimally outline the gallbladder and ducts.

Measurement (Figs 7–29 and 7–30)

Length, AP diameter, and width (coronal size) of the gallbladder were measured on images that gave greatest dimensions. All measurements were made intraluminally, except gallbladder wall thickness (Table 7–9).

Portal vein and common hepatic duct were measured as internal diameters.

Source of Material

Fifty-one patients aged 1 month to 16 years were evaluated. None had signs, symptoms, or laboratory evidence of gallbladder or biliary tract disease.

TABLE 7–9.

Sonographic Measurements of the Normal Pediatric Gallbladder and Biliary Tract

Age Range (yr)	AP Diameter (cm)		Coronal Diameter (cm)		Length (cm)		Wall Thickness (mm)		Common Hepatic Duct Size (mm)		Right Portal Vein Size (mm)	
	Mean	Range	Mean	Range	Mean	Range	Mean	Range	Mean	Range	Mean	Range
0–1 (8 patients)	9.9	0.5–1.2	0.9	0.7–1.4	2.5	1.3–3.4	1.7	1.0–3.0	1.3	1.0–2.0	3.8	3.0–5.0
2–5 (10 patients)	1.7	1.4–2.3	1.8	1.0–3.9	4.2	2.9–5.2	2.0	None	1.7	1.0–3.0	4.8	3.0–7.0
6–8 (11 patients)	1.8	1.0–2.4	2.0	1.2–3.0	5.6	4.4–7.4	2.2	2.0–3.0	2.0	None	5.7	6.0–9.0
9–11 (12 patients)	1.9	1.2–3.2	2.0	1.0–3.6	5.5	3.4–6.5	2.0	1.0–3.0	1.8	1.0–3.0	6.8	4.0–9.0
12–16 (10 patients)	2.0	1.3–2.8	2.1	1.6–3.0	6.1	3.8–8.0	2.0	1.0–3.0	2.2	1.0–4.0	7.8	6.0–10.0

*From McGahan JP et al: *Radiology* 1982; 144:873. Used by permission.

MEASUREMENT OF NORMAL PEDIATRIC GALLBLADDER AND BILIARY TRACT BY ULTRASOUND*

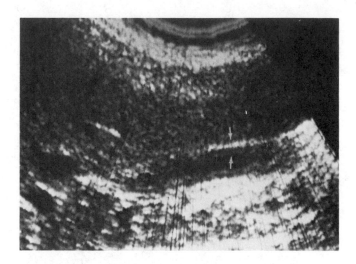

FIG 7–31.
Measurement of the gallbladder wall *(arrows)* made along the axis of the ultrasound beam using the portion of the gallbladder contiguous with the liver and including all identifiable layers. Note the distinguishable, less echodense zone adjacent to the lumen. (From Finberg HJ, et al: *Radiology* 1979; 133:693. Used by permission.)

Technique

1. All subjects were studied with an electronic sector scanner (Varian 3000) using a 2.25-mHz fixed focus transducer. Additional views optionally taken with a manual sector scanner (Searle Phosonic).
2. Standard viewing is via an intercostal transhepatic portal, but additional decubitus or upright views were used.

Measurement (Fig 7–31 and Table 7–10)

TABLE 7–10.
Pathologic Findings in 40 Patients: Type of Cholecystitis*

Ultrasound Wall (mm)	Chronic	Chronic Active	Chronic and Acute	Subacute	Acute
1–2†	15	1	3	0	0
3	3	0	0	0	1
4	6	1	1	1	0
≥5	3	0	4	0	1

*From Finberg HJ, et al: *Radiology* 1979; 133:693. Used by permission.
†1–2 different from ≥5 at $P < 0.05$.

Ref: Finberg HJ, et al: *Radiology* 1979; 133:693.

MEASUREMENT OF NORMAL AND ABNORMAL GALLBLADDER WALL THICKNESS BY ULTRASOUND

The gallbladder wall is measured between the fluid-filled lumen and the nearer subhepatic wall with the ultrasound beam perpendicular to the wall. Measurements are rounded to the nearest millimeter as measured on the prints or transparencies.

Wall thickness greater than 2 mm was seen in only 3.5% of 368 patients with otherwise normal scans.

Wall thickness was greater than 2 mm in 21 of 40 pathologically confirmed cholecystitis cases and 47 of 103 sonographically diagnosed cases of cholelithiasis.

Raghavendra et al.† showed 70% of patients with acute cholecystitis had gallbladder wall measurements of 5 mm or greater, gallbladder wall anechoicity, a gallbladder AP diameter of 4 cm or greater (external width), and cholelithiasis.

Other causes of increased thickness of the gallbladder wall measurements include ascites, hypoalbuminemia, hepatitis, heart failure, renal disease, and multiple myeloma.

Source of Material
Finberg et al.* data based on 47 surgical patients.

Raghavendra et al.† data based on 30 patients without biliary tract symptoms and 24 patients with proved acute cholecystitis.

Lewandowski et al.‡ data based on 8 patients with ascites.

Ralls et al.§ data based on 40 patients with hypoalbuminemia.

Shlaer et al.# data based on a study of 20 patients with thickened gallbladder walls. Only eight had cholecystitis.

*Ref: Finberg HJ et al: Radiology 1979; 133:693.
†Ref: Raghavendra BN, et al: AJR 1981; 137:327.
‡Ref: Lewandowski BJ, et al: AJR 1981; 137:519.
§Ref: Ralls PW, et al: AJR 1981; 137:165.
#Ref: Shlaer WJ, et al: AJR 1981; 136:337.

MEASUREMENT OF COMMON BILE DUCT DIAMETER BY INTRAVENOUS CHOLANGIOGRAPHY

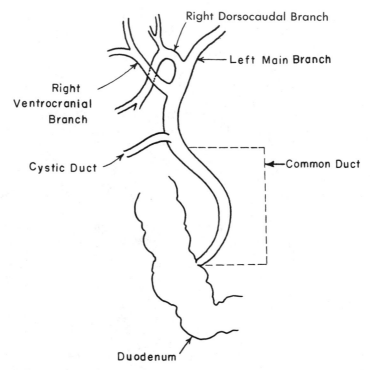

FIG 7–32.

Technique

Central ray: To twelfth thoracic vertebra on median plane.

Position: Posteroanterior, rolled up 15° toward the right; additional projections obtained as necessary after inspection of scout film. Posteroanterior tomograms may be necessary. First tomogram is taken by setting the fulcrum point on a centimeter scale at one third of the AP centimeter measurement of the patient. Tomographic exposures are taken posteriorly from the level at 0.5 cm levels to a depth of 2 cm.

Target-film distance: 36 inches.

Measurements (Fig 7–32 and Table 7–11)

Maximum width of the common duct is measured in the supra-ampullary portion.

MEASUREMENT OF COMMON BILE DUCT DIAMETER BY INTRAVENOUS CHOLANGIOGRAPHY

TABLE 7–11.

Common Duct Size

Normal	
Average diameter (mm)	5.5
Range (mm)	3–9
Diameter greater than 10 mm is abnormal.	
Postcholecystectomy	
Average diameter (mm)	9
Range (mm)	3–30

Source of Material

Numerous articles have been published on the subject of common duct size. The measurements shown above have been selected as most representative. For further information, see Anderson,* Beargie,† Edmunds,‡ and Wise.§

*Ref: Anderson FG: *AJR* 1957; 78:623.

†Ref: Beargie RJ, et al: *Surg Gynecol Obstet* 1962; 115:143.

‡Ref: Edmunds R, Rucker C, Finby N: *Arch Surg* 1965; 90:73.

§Ref: Wise RE, Johnston DO, Salzman FA: *Radiology* 1957; 68:507.

MEASUREMENT OF DISTAL COMMON BILE DUCT AND PANCREATIC HEAD BY CT CHOLANGIOGRAPHY*

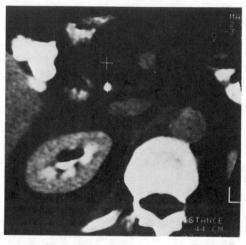

FIG 7–33.
Magnified view (×2) of the distal common bile duct illustrating its measurement (0.44 cm) using electronic cursors. (From Greenberg M: *Radiology* 1982;144:363. Used by permission.)

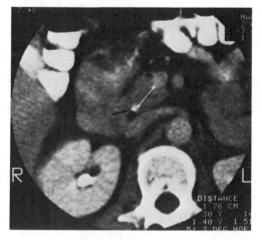

FIG 7–34.
Typical case illustrating measurements for the uncinate process. Line drawn between the common bile duct *(arrow)* and superior mesenteric vein *(arrowhead)* represents true transverse diameter of the uncinate process (1.76 cm). (From Greenberg M: *Radiology* 1982; 144:363.)

*Ref: Greenberg M: *Radiology* 1982; 144:363.

MEASUREMENT OF DISTAL COMMON BILE DUCT AND PANCREATIC HEAD BY CT CHOLANGIOGRAPHY*

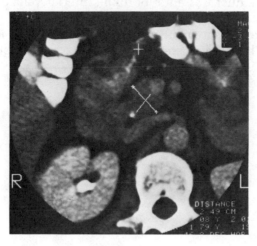

FIG 7–35.
Line drawn perpendicular to figure on left represents true ventral-dorsal measurement of the uncinate process (2.49 cm). (From Greenberg M: *Radiology* 1982; 144:363. Used by permission.)

Technique

1. GE CT/T 8800 scanner was used to scan 5- or 10-mm sections at a scan speed of 9.6 seconds. Sections were usually at 1-cm intervals, with 5-mm sections through the pancreas.
2. The night before the scan, the patient was given 3 gm of copanoic acid (Telepaque) and kept on a clear liquid diet. The next morning the patient was given calcium ipodate granules (Oragrafin, 2 packages) and scanned about 1.5 hours later, after oral administration of dilute Gastrografin or barium.
3. Opacification of the biliary tree is better seen if intravenous contrast is not given. Repeat studies with intravenous contrast may be used to better show vascular structures.

Measurement (Figs 7–33 to 7–35)

In 84 of 97 patients, the gallbladder and/or biliary tree were visualized well.

The distal common bile duct measured 4.7 ± 1.2 mm in 56 normal patients and 6.8 ± 1.1 mm in 10 patients postcholecystectomy ($P < 0.001$). The

*Ref: Greenberg M: *Radiology* 1982; 144:363.

MEASUREMENT OF DISTAL COMMON BILE DUCT AND PANCREATIC HEAD BY CT CHOLANGIOGRAPHY

distal common bile duct was anterior to the inferior vena cava in 55 patients, lateral in 8, and medial in 5.

The transverse measurement of the uncinate process in 44 patients was 2.06 ± 0.53 cm. The AP diameter was 2.34 ± 0.51 cm in 28 patients.

Source of Material
Data based on a study of 97 patients.

MEASUREMENT OF THE BILIARY DUCTS BY ENDOSCOPIC RETROGRADE CHOLANGIOGRAPHY*

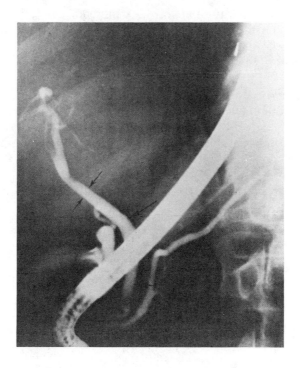

FIG 7–36.

The normal cholangiogram and pancreatogram. The *short arrow* points to the intrapancreatic portion of the common bile duct. The *long arrow* points to the prepancreatic portion of the common bile duct, and the *double arrows* point to the common hepatic duct. These are the areas measured. (From Lasser RB, et al: *Am J Dig Dis* 1978; 23:586–590. Used by permission.)

Technique

Endoscopic retrograde cholangiopancreatography with Olympus JF-B endoscope.

Central ray: Perpendicular to plane of film.

Position: Anteroposterior supine.

Target-film distance: Immaterial. Measurements were corrected for magnification relative to the size of the endoscope.

Measurements (Fig 7–36)

The widest diameter of the intrapancreatic portion of the common duct was measured. This is defined as the portion of the common bile duct that

*Ref: Lasser RB, et al: *Am J Dig Dis* 1978; 23:586–590.

MEASUREMENT OF THE BILIARY DUCTS BY ENDOSCOPIC RETROGRADE CHOLANGIOGRAPHY

runs parallel to the ascending part of the pancreatic duct. The widest part of the prepancreatic portion of the common bile duct was also measured. This region started at the upper border of the intrapancreatic common bile duct and ended at the origin of the cystic duct. The common hepatic duct that extends from the end of the cystic duct to the bifurcation of the common hepatic duct was also measured.

Normal measurements were as follows:

1. The common hepatic duct: 4.6 mm (range, 2.1 to 9.2 mm).
2. The prepancreatic portion of the common bile duct: 4.9 mm (range, 2.3 to 8.5 mm).
3. The intrahepatic portion of the common bile duct: 4.3 mm (range, 2.3 to 6.9 mm).

Source of Material

Data based on study of 49 normal patients, 36 males and 13 females, aged 18 to 72 years. The mean age was 50.5 years.

MEASUREMENT OF EXTRAHEPATIC BILE DUCTS IN HEALTHY SUBJECTS, PATIENTS WITH GALLSTONES, AND POSTCHOLECYSTECTOMY PATIENTS BY ULTRASOUND*

Technique

1. Patients imaged with a 3.5-MHz real-time or static scanner.
2. Supine or right-side elevated position. All subjects imaged after an overnight fast. The lumen of the duct was measured in the porta hepatis where it parallels the main portal vein, and at the widest point, generally more distal than the first measurement. Electronic cursors were used.

Measurement (Table 7–12)

TABLE 7–12.

Diameter of Common Duct Size (mm) in 830 Normal Subjects, 73 Patients With Gallstones, and 55 Patients After Cholecystectomy Without Signs of Biliary Obstruction*

	Mean ± SD	Range	95th Percentile
Normal subjects			
Porta hepatis	2.5±1.1	1–7	4
Widest point	2.8±1.2	1–7	4
Patients with gallstones			
Porta hepatis	3.8±2.0	1–10	8
Widest point	4.8±2.2	2–12	9
Patients after cholecystectomy			
Porta hepatis	5.2±2.3	1–11	10
Widest point	6.2±2.5	3–13	11

*From Niederau D, et al: *J Clin Ultrasound* 1983; 11:23. Used by permission.

Healthy subjects had diameters 4 mm or less, while patients with gallstones or postcholecystectomy had significantly larger diameters.

Source of Material

Eight hundred thirty normal volunteers were recruited from blood donors. In addition, 73 patients with gallstones and 55 who had undergone cholecystectomy were studied. Patients with jaundice or stones in the extrahepatic ducts were excluded.

An ultrasonographic study by Mueller et al.† of pre- and postcholecystectomy patients has indicated that postcholecystectomy dilatation of the common bile duct does not occur in most normal patients.

*Ref: Niederau D, et al: *J Clin Ultrasound* 1983; 11:23.
†Ref: Mueller PR, et al: *AJR* 1981; 136:355–358.

MEASUREMENT OF THE WIDTHS OF THE PORTAL AND SPLENIC VEIN*

Technique
 Central ray: Centered over spleen.
 Position: Anteroposterior abdomen.
 Target-film distance: 100 cm.
Films taken in deep inspiration.

Thirty cc of Triurol 50% (sodium acetrizoate: specific gravity, 1.3; viscosity at 37° C, 2.1 centipoise) was injected into the spleen at the rate of 6 to 7.5 cc/sec. Films were taken with an automatic film changer at a rate of 1 film per second for 13 seconds after the beginning of the injection; then 1 film every 3 seconds for 20 seconds.

Measurements
Diameter of the splenic vein (measured hepatoproximally, where the vein usually is of uniform width) = less than 16 mm.

Diameter of the portal vein (measured hepatodistally, where the vein is widest) = less than 23 mm.

Note: No correction was made for variation in vessel-film distance with body build.

Source of Material
The data are based on a study of 14 adults with no evidence of portal hypertension. The widths of the splenic vein and the portal vein are often increased in the presence of portal hypertension.

Ref: Bergstrand I, Eckman C-A: *Acta Radiol* 1957; 47:1.

MEASUREMENT OF THE PORTAL VEIN
BY REAL-TIME ULSTRASOUND*

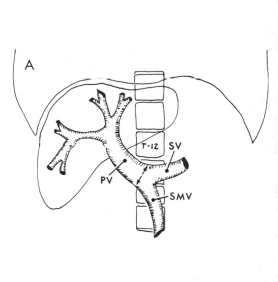

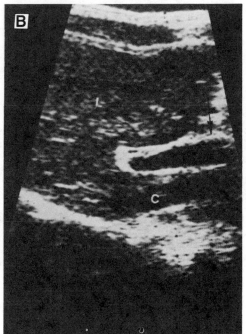

FIG 7–37.
A, main portal vein *(PV)* formed by confluence of splenic vein *(SV)* and superior mesenteric vein *(SMV).*
Arrows indicate site of portal vein measurement. **B,** real-time sagittal sonogram in right anterior oblique
plane. *Arrows* indicate site of portal vein measurement. *L* = liver; *C* = inferior vena cava. (From Weinreb J, et al: *AJR* 1982; 139:497. Used by permission.)

Technique

1. All studies were with a real-time mechanical sector scanner, using a
   3.5-MHz transducer.
2. Patients were examined in the supine, right anterior oblique, and left
   lateral decubitus positions during suspended inspiration.

Measurement (Figs 7–37 and 7–38)

The measurements were obtained at the broadest point of the portal vein,
just distal to the union of the splenic and superior mesenteric veins. There
was no difference between measurements of male and female patients.

The overall mean diameter in patients aged 21 to 40 years was 11 ± 2
mm. Note that the Valsalva maneuver is reported to make the portal vein di-
late.

Ref: Weinreb J, et al: *AJR* 1982; 139:497.

MEASUREMENT OF THE PORTAL VEIN
BY REAL-TIME ULTRASOUND

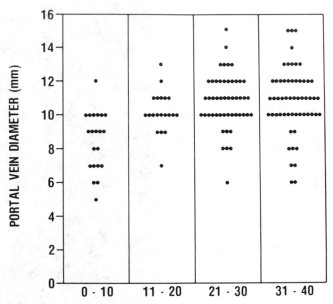

FIG 7–38.
Portal vein measurements in 40 patients. (From Weinreb J, et al: *AJR* 1982; 139:497. Used by permission.)

Source of Material

One hundred forty-eight patients (83 females and 65 males) were studied, aged 0 to 40 years. The sonogram was performed for indications other than to evaluate portal vein size. The only other criterion was that the extrahepatic portal vein be adequately visualized.

MEASUREMENT OF THE VELOCITY OF PORTAL VEIN BLOOD FLOW*

Technique
   Cental ray: Centered over spleen.
   Position: Anteroposterior abdomen.
   Target-film distance: 100 cm.
Films taken in deep inspiration.

Thirty cc of Triurol 50% (sodium acetrizoate: specific gravity 1.3; viscosity at 37° C, 2.1 centipoise) was injected into the spleen at the rate of 6 to 7.5 cc/sec. Films were taken with an automatic film changer at a rate of 1 film per second for 13 seconds after the beginning of the injection; then 1 film every 3 seconds for 20 seconds.

Measurements
The velocity of flow was estimated in four ways:

1. Measurement of the distance that the head of the contrast medium had advanced between two consecutive exposures was assessed in centimeters per second.
2. Spleen-hilum time is equivalent to the interval between the beginning of the injection of contrast medium and the demonstration of the bifurcation of the portal trunk in the liver hilum.
3. Spleen-liver time is equivalent to the interval between the beginning of injection of contrast medium and the moment the contrast filled the smallest observable intrahepatic portal branches in the right liver lobe.
4. Emptying time of the portal branches is equivalent to the interval between the end of the injection and the moment that the intrahepatic portal branches are no longer discernible.

The portal vein blood flow data are summarized in Table 7–13.

TABLE 7–13.

Method	Range	Mean	In Normal Controls	In Patients With Portal Hypertension
Velocity (cm/sec)	8–42	21.6	15 or more	15 or less*
Spleen-hilum time (sec)	.5–3	1.7	2 or less	2 or more
Spleen-liver time (sec)	3–6	4.3	5 or less	5+
Emptying time of portal branches (sec)	3–7	4.3	5 or less	5+

*In one half of the patients.

*Ref: Bergstrand I, Eckman C-A: *Acta Radiol* 1957; 47:1.

MEASUREMENT OF THE VELOCITY OF PORTAL VEIN BLOOD FLOW

Source of Material
Sixteen adults with normal circulation in the portal system were compared with 54 patients with portal hypertension.

Note: Average linear velocity of portal vein flow ranged from 15.5 to 24.1 cm/sec in six patients studied by Sovak et al.†

---

†*Ref:* Sovak M, Soulen RL, Reichle FA: Radiology 1971; 99:531.

MEASUREMENT OF THE DUODENAL MAJOR PAPILLA OF VATER*

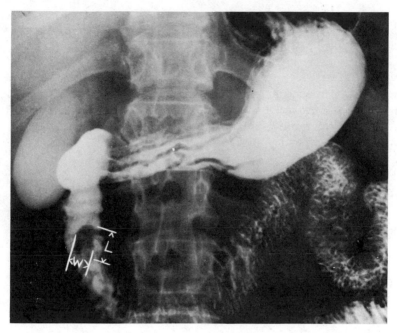

FIG 7–39.

Technique

Central ray: To second lumbar vertebra.
Position: Posteroanterior abdomen for stomach and duodenum.
Target-film distance: 36 inches.

Measurements (Fig 7–39 and Table 7–14)

TABLE 7–14.

	Length (cm)	Width (cm)	Height (cm)
Measurements of major papilla from anatomic specimens			
Average size	1.5	0.5	0.5
Minimum size	0.1	0.1	0.1
Maximum size	3.0	1.2	1.2
Measurements from series of gastrointestinal films			
Average size (cm)	1.5	0.7	

*Ref: Poppel MH, Jacobsen HG, Smith RW: *The Roentgen Aspects of the Papilla and Ampulla of Vater.* Springfield, Ill, Charles C Thomas, Publisher, 1953.

MEASUREMENT OF THE DUODENAL
MAJOR PAPILLA OF VATER

The papilla position is most frequently on the medial duodenal wall toward the posterior portion of the middescending duodenum.

Source of Material

The anatomic measurements were made on 100 specimens described as normal, fresh, and unassociated with any history, symptoms, or gross evidence of disease referable to the biliary tract, pancreas, or duodenum.

The measurements of papilla size from the films correspond well to the anatomic measurements.

SMALL BOWEL CALIBER IN CHILDREN AND ADULTS*

Technique
Central ray: Perpendicular to plane of film centered over midabdomen.
Position: Anteroposterior with patient supine.
Target-film distance: Children, 36 inches; adults, 30 inches.

Measurements (Table 7–15)
Nonflocculating media that are complex barium sulphate suspensions are used. A 50% dilution in volume of 2 to 8 oz is used according to age in children and according to size of stomach in adults. Three segments of the small bowel that have clearly defined margins and approximately the same caliber as the rest of the small bowel are selected for measurement. The measurements are made at right angles to the parallel margins of the bowel. The average of the three measurements is used.

TABLE 7–15.
Mean Diameter of Small Bowel*†

Age	Diameter (mm)‡
6 mo	12.0
1 yr	13.0
2 yr	15.0
3 yr	16.7
4 yr	18.9
5 yr	19.0
6 yr	19.9
7 yr	20.5
8 yr	21.0
9 yr	21.4
10 yr	21.8
11 yr	22.1
12 yr	22.3
13 yr	22.5
14 yr	22.7
15 yr	23.0

*From Haworth EM, et al: *Clin Radiol* 1967; 18:417. Used by permission.
†Adult value is 23.1 mm ± 1.9 (1 SD). Upper limit for adult is 25 mm.
‡1 SD = 1.9 mm.

Source of Material
Small bowel measurements were taken from 61 infants and children aged 9 months to 15½ years and from 77 adults (37 males and 40 females) aged 19 to 77 years.

Ref: Haworth EM, et al: *Clin Radiol* 1967; 18:417.

SIZE OF GAS-FILLED BOWEL LOOPS
IN INFANTS*

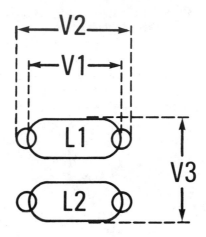

FIG 7–40.

Measurements of the upper lumbar spine elements used in this study. (From Edwards DK: *AJR* 1980; 135:331. Used by permission.)

Technique
    Central ray: Perpendicular to plane of film.
    Position: Anteroposterior supine.
    Target-film distance: Immaterial.

Measurements (Fig 7–40 and Table 7–16)

The width of the largest bowel loop was measured. No attempt was made to distinguish large from small bowel. Three dimensions of the upper lumbar spine were made.

V_1 = Width of the first lumbar vertebral body (L_1).
V_2 = Distance between the outer edges of the pedicles of L_1.
V_3 = Total height of L_1 and L_2, including the disc space. This measurement is the easiest to measure and statistically the most reproducible.

The maximum bowel width is divided by the three vertebral measures to form the three bowel-vertebral ratios.

Ref: Edwards DK: *AJR* 1980; 135:331.

SIZE OF GAS-FILLED BOWEL LOOPS IN INFANTS

TABLE 7–16.

Ratios of Maximum Bowel Width and Vertebral Body Measures*

Population, Age†/Bowel-Vertebral Ratio	Mean Value	SD (σ)	Mean ± 2 σ
Normal (N = 375), 0.9			
B:V1	0.81	0.12	0.56–1.05
B:V2	0.57	0.11	0.36–0.79
B:V3	0.61	0.11	0.40–0.83
Suspected NEC‡ (all) (N = 188), 11.3			
B:V1	1.27	0.27	
B:V2	0.90	0.21	
B:V3	0.96	0.20	
Proved NEC (N = 48), 17.1			
B:V1	1.40	0.31	
B:V2	0.97	0.23	
B:V3	1.05	0.23	
NEC suspected, not proved (N = 140), 9.3			
B:V1	1.23	0.24	
B:V2	0.87	0.19	
B:V3	0.93	0.18	
Congenital obstruction (N = 24), 3.4			
B:V1	2.16	0.51	
B:V2	1.59	0.38	
B:V3	1.63	0.40	

*From Edwards DK: *AJR* 1980; 135:331. Used by permission.
†Mean age at radiograph (days).
‡NEC = necrotizing enterocolitis.

Source of Material
Normal data based on a study of 375 normal patients (Table 7–16).

MEASUREMENT OF THE ILEOCECAL VALVE*

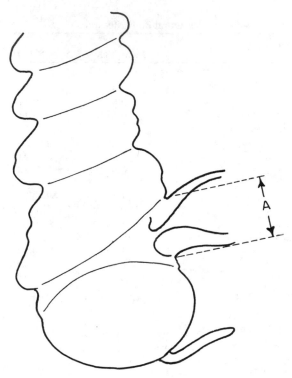

FIG 7–41.

Technique
 Central ray: Spot roentgenograms made during fluoroscopy.
 Position: Posterior and oblique views (found to best demonstrate the valve during fluoroscopy), using graduated pressure over ileocecal valve region.
 Target-film distance: Depends on patient thickness.

Measurements (Fig 7–41)
Average vertical diameter (A) = 2.5 cm.
 Vertical diameter (A) of 4.0 cm or more is considered abnormal by Hinkel.*

Source of Measurement
Five hundred consecutive routine barium enema examinations.

*Ref: Hinkel CL: AJR 1952; 68:171.

MEASUREMENT OF CECAL DIAMETER*

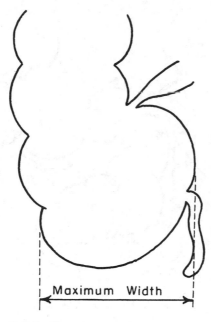

FIG 7–42.

Technique
　Central ray: On median plane at level of iliac crests.
　Position: Posteroanterior.
　Target-film distance: 36 inches.

Measurements (Fig 7–42)
The greatest transverse diameter is measured on the prone film of the abdomen.

Average diameter = 5–7 cm.

A width of 9 cm or greater is a critical diameter beyond which danger of perforation exists.

Source of Material
Artificial distention of the cecum with barium and air was performed on 100 selected patients without intrinsic cecal disease or distal large bowel obstruction. Nineteen cases of cecal distention with distal large-bowel obstruction were studied for comparison.

Ref: Davis L, Lowman RM: *Radiology* 1957; 68:542.

MEASUREMENT OF THE PRESACRAL SPACE IN CHILDREN AND ADULTS

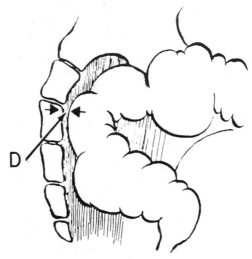

FIG 7–43.
Measurement of the presacral space in children and adults. (From Kattan KR, King AY: *AJR* 1979; 132:437. Used by permission.)

Technique
Central ray: Spot roentgenograms made during fluoroscopy.
Position: Lateral view obtained during barium enema examination.
Target-film distance: Variable; depends on width of patient.

Measurements (Fig 7–43)
The shortest distance between the posterior rectum and the sacrum is indicated by *D*.

In children aged 1 to 15 years the average distance is 3 mm (range, 1 to 5 mm). Measurements over 5 mm should be considered abnormal.

In adults the average distance is 7 mm (range, 2 to 16 mm). Measurements over 20 mm should be considered abnormal. However, in some normal patients older than 45 years, the presacral space is wider than 15 mm and may even exceed 20 mm.

MEASUREMENT OF THE PRESACRAL SPACE IN CHILDREN AND ADULTS

Source of Material

Eklof and Gierup† studied 85 boys and 75 girls in the 1- to 15-year age group who had no evidence of inflammatory bowel disease.

Chrispin and Fry‡ studied 100 patients, selected at random, in whom no bowel abnormality could be demonstrated.

Kattan and King* studied 100 men and 87 women, aged 17 to 89.

*Ref: Kattan KR, King AY: *AJR* 1979; 132:437.
†Ref: Eklof O, Gierup J: *AJR* 1970; 108:624.
‡Ref: Chrispin AR, Fry IK: *Br J Radiol* 1963; 36:319.

THE RECTOSIGMOID INDEX FOR THE EARLY DIAGNOSIS OF HIRSCHSPRUNG'S DISEASE*

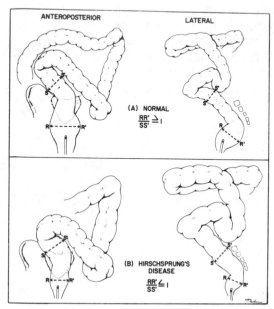

FIG 7–44.

The rectosigmoid index. (From Pochaczevsky R, Leonidas JC: *AJR* 1975; 123:770. Used by permission.)

Technique

Central ray: Perpendicular to plane of film.

Position: Anteroposterior lateral and left posterior oblique.

Target-film distance: Immaterial.

Measurements (Fig 7–44)

The widest diameter of the rectum (RR^1) was obtained at any level below the third sacral vertebra. The largest measurement of the sigmoid (SS^1) was also measured. All measurements were obtained along a transverse axis, vertical to the longitudinal axis of the colon at that point. The rectosigmoid index was obtained by dividing the widest diameter of the rectum by the widest margin of the sigmoid loop when the colon was fully distended.

The data indicate that a rectosigmoid index less than 1 indicates Hirschsprung's disease. An index higher than 1 may indicate a normal colon or a condition mimicking Hirschsprung's disease, such as meconium plug syndrome.

*Ref: Pochaczevsky R, Leonidas JC: *AJR* 1975; 123:770.

THE RECTOSIGMOID INDEX FOR THE EARLY DIAGNOSIS OF HIRSCHSPRUNG'S DISEASE

Source of Material

Based on a study of 21 infants with biopsy-proved cases of Hirschsprung's disease, 10 infants with meconium plug syndrome, 12 term newborns considered normal, and 25 infants with other bowel disorders.

FAT THICKNESS IN THE NEONATAL SMALL LEFT COLON SYNDROME*

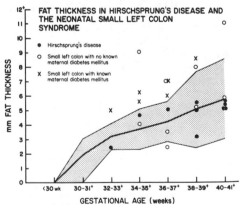

FIG 7–45.
Measurement of flank fat thickness. (From Kuhns LR, et al: *AJR* 1976; 126:538. Used by permission.)

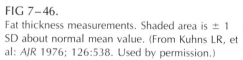

FIG 7–46.
Fat thickness measurements. Shaded area is ± 1 SD about normal mean value. (From Kuhns LR, et al: *AJR* 1976; 126:538. Used by permission.)

Technique
  Central ray: Perpendicular to plane of film centered over midabdomen.
  Position: Anteroposterior supine.
  Target-film distance: 40 inches.

*Ref: Kuhns LR, et al: *AJR* 1976; 126:538.

FAT THICKNESS IN THE NEONATAL SMALL LEFT COLON SYNDROME

Measurements (Fig 7–45)

Fat thickness was measured in the flank from chest or abdominal films. Gestational age was assessed by tooth mineralization, thoracic spine length, humeral head ossification, and knee ossification (see Chapter 4B, Skeletal Maturation, p 94-98).

Figure 7–46 shows results. Note that fat thickness is increased in two thirds of patients with small left colon syndrome, whereas neonates with Hirschsprung's disease have normal fat thickness for gestational maturity.

Source of Material

Based on a study of 15 neonates with neonatal small colon syndrome and 10 with Hirschsprung's disease.

CHAPTER 8

The Spleen, the Pancreas, the Adrenal Glands, and the Retroperitoneum

MEASUREMENT OF SPLEEN POSITION AND SIZE*

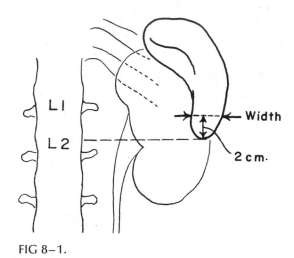

FIG 8–1.

Technique
   Central ray: At level of iliac crests on median plane.
   Position: Anteroposterior.
   Target-film distance: 36 inches.

Measurements (Fig 8–1 and Table 8–1)
   The transverse diameter of the lower pole of the spleen was determined at a point 2 cm above the tip of the lower pole.

TABLE 8–1.

No. of Cases (288 Total)	Age (Yr)	Level of Lower Pole Tip	Width (CM) at 2 CM Above Tip of Spleen
16	Under 5	L1-L3 (usually L2)	2.0–3.6 (avg. 3.0)
37	5–10	L1-L3 (usually L1-L2)	2.5–3.8 (avg. 3.3)
36	11–20	L1-L3 (usually L1-L2)	2.5–3.8 (avg. 3.2)
82	21–30	T12-L2 (usually L1)	2.0–4.2 (avg. 3.5)
117	Over 30	T12-L2 (usually L1)	2.0–4.6 (avg. 3.5)

Ref: Wyman AC: *AJR* 1954; 72:51.

MEASUREMENT OF SPLEEN POSITION
AND SIZE

Enlargement of the splenic shadow occurs in a significantly large number of cases of ruptured spleen. Because the spleen outline is not demonstrated in 58% of abdominal roentgenograms, absence of this sign does not exclude the diagnosis of ruptured spleen.

Source of Material
Five hundred consecutive cases with films of the abdomen were evaluated regardless of the diagnostic problem.

MEASUREMENT OF SPLEEN LENGTH*

Technique
   Central ray: Centered over spleen.
   Position: Anteroposterior abdomen.
   Target-film distance: 100 cm.
Film taken in deep inspiration.

Measurements
The spleen length is the distance between the level of the most cranial part of the diaphragmatic arch and the lower pole of the spleen.
Mean length = 12.4 ± 2.2 cm (range, 8–19 cm). If the spleen length exceeds 16 cm, there is 97% probability that the spleen is enlarged.

Source of Material
Studies were made of 50 adults (23 men, 27 women) without known symptoms or signs of liver or spleen disease.

Ref: Bergstrand I, Eckman C-A: *Acta Radiol* 1957; 47:1.

MEASUREMENT OF SPLEEN VOLUME BY CT

See entry on liver and spleen volume in gastrointestinal chapter, pp 502–503.

SPLEEN LENGTH RELATED TO
VERTEBRAL HEIGHT*

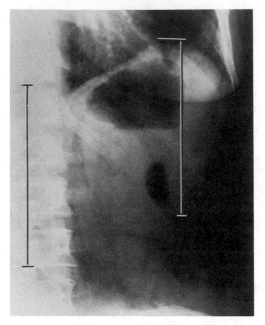

FIG 8–2.
Measurement of the spleen. (From Schlindler G, et al: *Radiologe* 1976; 16:166. Used by permission.)

*Ref: Schindler G, et al: *Radiologe* 1976; 16:166.

SPLEEN LENGTH RELATED TO VERTEBRAL HEIGHT

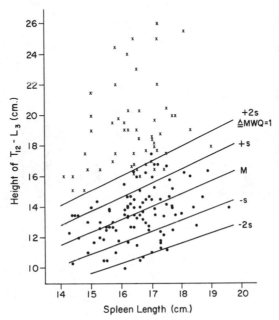

FIG 8–3.

Normal range of the measurements of the spleen related to height of T12-L3. The *dots* are normals. The *x's* are patients with splenomegaly. (From Schindler G, et al: *Radiologe* 1976; 16:166. Used by permission.)

Technique
   Central ray: Perpendicular to plane of film.
   Position: Anteroposterior upright.
   Target-film distance: Immaterial.

Measurements (Fig 8–2)

The spleen is measured from its most superior extent under the diaphragm to its caudal tip. This is compared with the distance from the upper margin of T12 to the lower margin of L3. Normal values are given in Figure 8–3. The normal ratio of spleen length to the vertebral height T12-L3 is 0.82 ± 0.09. Two standard deviations are represented by ratios from 0.64 to 1.0. Spleen length greater than vertebral height T12-L3 indicates pathologic enlargement of the spleen.

Source of Material

Based on a study of 97 healthy adult patients.

THE NORMAL ENDOSCOPIC PANCREATOGRAMS*

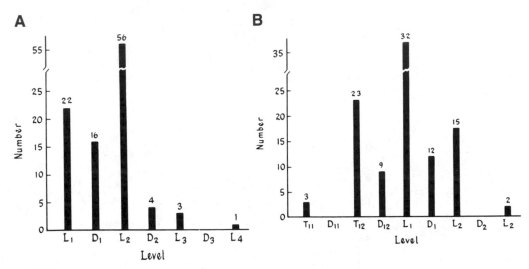

FIG 8−4.

A, level of the ampulla with respect to the lumbar spine. L = lumbar vertebra; D = intervening disc space. **B,** level at which the main pancreatic duct crosses the spine. (From Varley PF et al: *Radiology* 1976; 118:295. Used by permission.)

TABLE 8−2.

Main Pancreatic Ductal Dimensions (mm)*†

	No.	Mean	Range	SD
Diameter				
Head	93	3.1	1.5−6.9	±0.9
Body	88	2.0	1.3−3.6	±0.7
Tail	83	0.9	0.6−2.3	±0.4
Length	80	169	107−223	±27

*From Varley PF, et al: *Radiology* 1976; 118:295. Used by permission.
†Corrected for magnification.

Technique

Central ray: Perpendicular to plane of film.

Position: Anteroposterior supine.

Target-film distance: Immaterial. Magnification corrected using the dimension of the endoscope as a standard.

Ref: Varley PF, et al: *Radiology* 1976; 118:295.

THE NORMAL ENDOSCOPIC PANCREATOGRAM

Measurements

See Figure 8−4 and Table 8−2 for normal position and caliber of ducts.

The ampulla was found at the level of L2 in 75% of cases; the pancreatic duct crossed the spine at L1 in most cases. Mean ductal diameters were 3.1, 2.0, and 0.9 mm in the head, body, and tail respectively.

Source of Material

Based on a study of 102 normal endoscopic pancreatograms in 68 men and 34 women from 11 to 81 years of age; 47% of the patients were between 40 and 60 years of age.

MEASUREMENT OF THE PANCREAS WITH ULTRASONOGRAPHY*

Technique

1. Conventional, commercially available compound B-scan diagnostic ultrasound equipment with grey scale capability was employed. The transducer was nonfocused, operating at 2.25 megahertz with a lead zirconate/titanate piezo-electric element.
2. *Position:* Supine and prone with particular attention to the region of the pancreas.
3. *Scan procedure:* Longitudinal scan at midline to demonstrate caudad and cephalad boundaries of the pancreas. Lateral movements in 1 cm increments to right and left to demonstrate these boundaries over entire length of pancreas. Scanning repeated in transverse direction over the same area of pancreas.

Measurements

TABLE 8–3.
Sonographic Size of the Normal Pancreas in cm in 382 Patients (p<0.05)*

	Head	Body	Tail
Anteroposterior measurement	2.7 ± 0.7 cm	2.2 ± 0.7 cm	2.4 ± 0.4 cm
Craniocaudad measurement	3.6 ± 1.2 cm	3.0 ± 0.6 cm	2.9 ± 0.4 cm

*From Haber K, et al: Am J Roentgenol 1976; 126:624. Used by permission.

MEASUREMENT OF THE PANCREAS WITH COMPUTED TOMOGRAPHY†

Haga et al. have related the width of the pancreas to the transverse diameter of the adjacent vertebral body. The ranges of these ratios are shown below.

Measurements	Range
AP measurement of head of pancreas Transverse diameter of vertebral body	0.5 to 1.0
AP measurement of body or tail of pancreas Transverse diameter of vertebral body	0.33 to 0.66

MEASUREMENT OF THE PANCREATIC HEAD BY CT CHOLANGIOGRAPHY

See entry by Greenberg M, in gastrointestinal chapter, p 522.

*Ref: Haber K, et al: *Am J Roentgenol* 1976; 126:624.
†Ref: Haga JR, et al: *Radiology* 1976; 120:589.

MEASUREMENT OF THE NORMAL PANCREAS BY CT*

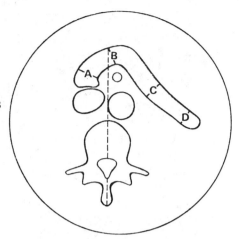

FIG 8–5.
Schematic representation of a section showing normal values (mean ± SD) as seen on CT. ($A = 23 ± 3.0$ mm, $B = 19 ± 2.5$ mm, $C = 20 ± 3.0$ mm, $D = 15 ± 2.5$ mm.) (From Kreel L, et al: *J Comput Assist Tomogr* 1977; 1:290. Used by permission.)

Technique

1. The measurements are based on 15 postmortem pancreas studies and 50 patients studied on a prototype EMI scanner using 15-mm slices generated in 20 seconds. The postmortem measurements were made on radiographs of formalin-fixed glands injected with a barium suspension in the pancreatic duct.
2. An anticholinergic drug was used to reduce artifact from bowel movement. Dilute oral contrast helped to identify bowel.

Measurement
See Figure 8–5.

Radiographs and hard copy images of CT were measured to determine ventrodorsal diameter of the head, neck, body, and tail. The autopsy specimens were also measured in the craniocaudal diameter. Comparison of the in vivo and postmortem studies demonstrated close correlation of measurements.

TABLE 8–4.

Normal Pancreas (postmortem) in 15 Patients (5 Males and 10 Females) Aged 25 to 65 Yr (Mean, 45.4 Yr)*

Localization in Pancreas	Mean Ventrodorsal Diameter (mm)	Mean craniocaudal Diameter (mm)
Head	24	44
Neck	17	34
Body	20	35
Tail	15	30

*From Kreel L, et al: *J Comput Assist Tomogr* 1977; 1:290. Used by permission.

Source of Material
Fifty patients without evidence of pancreatic disease, aged 25 to 65 (mean 45.8), and 15 patients with normal pancreases, aged 25 to 65 (mean 45.4), studied at autopsy.

*Ref: Kreel L, et al: *J Comput Assist Tomogr* 1977; 1:290.

MEASUREMENT OF NORMAL PANCREATIC DUCT USING REAL-TIME ULTRASOUND*

Technique

1. Patients were imaged with a linear array real-time scanner using a 3.5-MH2 focused transducer.
2. Images were stored on an analogue freeze-frame device.
3. Most patients fasted overnight and received a laxative the previous day. If the pancreas was nonvisualized because of overlying bowel gas, the patient was given water to drink and rescanned in the erect position.

Measurement (Tables 8–5 and 8–6)

In 65 patients, the pancreatic duct was identified as a tabular structure. Only a single line could be identified in 21 patients.

There was a tendency for younger patients to have smaller ducts, but this was not statistically significant.

TABLE 8–5.

Appearance of the Pancreatic Duct*

Single line	21
1 mm	47
2 mm	17
3 mm	1
Not seen	14
Total	100

*From Bryan PJ: *J Clin Ultrasound* 1982; 10:63. Used by permission.

TABLE 8–6.

Segment of the Pancreatic Duct Seen*

Body alone	64
Head and body	20
Head alone	2
Not seen	14

*From Bryan PJ: *J Clin Ultrasound* 1982; 10:63. Used by permission.

Source of Material

One hundred patients having abdominal sonograms for reasons other than biliary or pancreatic disease, in whom at least a portion of the pancreas was seen.

*Ref: Bryan PJ: *J Clin Ultrasound* 1982; 10:63.

MEASUREMENT OF ADRENAL GLAND SIZE

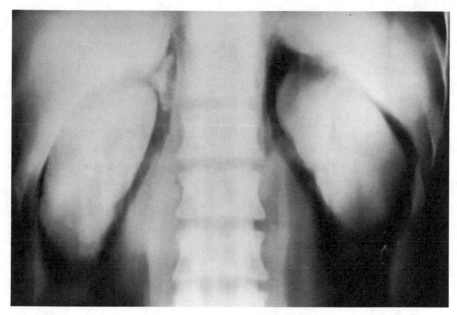

FIG 8–6.
Normal extraperitoneal pneumogram. The right adrenal is triangular, and the left is semilunar. (From Steinbach HL, Smith DR: *Arch Surg* 1955; 70:161. Used by permission.)

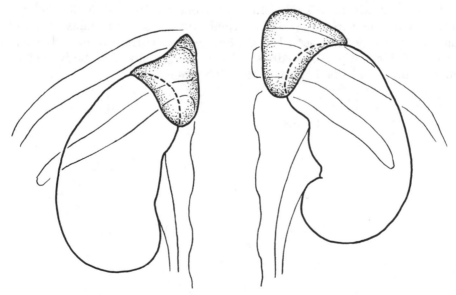

FIG 8–7.
Diagram to illustrate shape of adrenal glands.

MEASUREMENT OF ADRENAL GLAND SIZE

Technique
  Central ray: At level of iliac crests on median plane.
  Position: Anteroposterior abdomen.
  Target-film distance: 40 inches.

Measurements (Figs 8–6 and 8–7; Table 8–7)
The cross-sectional area of the gland was obtained by tracing the gland contour with a compensating planimeter. The same results may be obtained by tracing the contour of the gland on 1 mm graph paper and counting the enclosed squares.

TABLE 8–7.

Average Adrenal Cross-Sectional Area

Right	4.2 cm^2
Left	4.3 cm^2
Range, right	2.0 — 7.8 cm^2
Range, left	2.0 — 8.7 cm^2

Holmes et al.* have shown that the weight of the adrenal is related to body weight and surface area. The weight of adrenals in males was greater than in females by 11%, but when the figures were corrected for body size, the females had slightly more adrenal tissue per kilogram of body weight or square centimeter of body surface than the males.

Source of Material
Study of 25 normal adults.

Ref: Holmes RO, Moon HD, Rinehart JF: *Am J Pathol* 1951; 27:724.

MEASUREMENT OF NORMAL SIZE AND SHAPE
OF ADRENAL GLANDS BY CT*

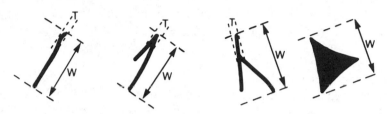

FIG 8–8.
Method of measuring width *(W)* and thickness *(T)* of adrenal glands. (From Montagne JP, et al: *AJR* 1978; 130:963. Used by permission.)

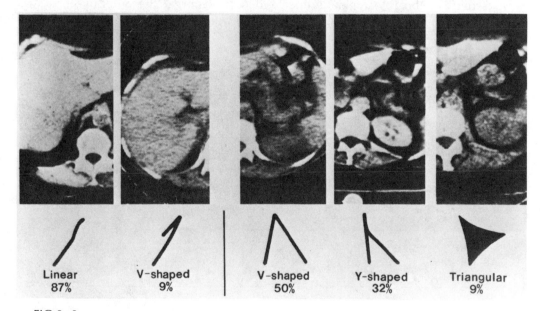

FIG 8–9.
Most frequent shapes of normal adrenal glands. (From Montagne JP, et al: *AJR* 1978; 130:963. Used by permission.)

Technique

1. EMI 5000 scanner with 160 × 160 matrix or GE 8800 CT/T scanner with 320 × 320 matrix.
2. Slice thickness 1 cm. Use of intravenous contrast not noted.

Ref: Montagne JP, et al: *AJR* 1978; 130:963.

MEASUREMENT OF NORMAL SIZE AND SHAPE
OF ADRENAL GLANDS BY CT

Measurement (Figs 8–8 and 8–9; Tables 8–8 to 8–9)

The right adrenal is located just posterior to the inferior vena cava as it enters the liver. The left adrenal is somewhat more anterior than the right, lateral to the left crus of the diaphragm, posterior to the tail of the pancreas.

Shape of the right adrenal is usually linear, and the left is usually "V" or "Y" (Fig 8–10).

The length of each adrenal gland was estimated by counting the number of transverse cross sections on which each was visualized (Table 8–8). The width of each gland was determined on the section in which the adrenal appeared largest during the examination (Fig 8–8). The thickness of the adrenal gland was defined as its dimension perpendicular to the long axis of the gland or one of its limbs. The greatest thickness at any site was the measurement recorded. In the linear glands this tended to occur at the anterior portion, while in the V- and Y-shaped glands the site was usually at the junction of the limbs.

TABLE 8–8.

Length of Adrenal Glands*

	Right		Left	
No. Sections†	No.	%	No.	%
1	3	6	. . .	. . .
2	20	43	16	34
3	23	49	29	62
4	1	2	2	4

*From Montagne JP, et al: *AJR* 1978; 130:963. Used by permission.
†Nonoverlapping adjacent slices either 10 or 13 mm thick.

TABLE 8–9.

Width of Adrenal Glands*

	Right		Left	
Cm	No.	%	No.	%
1.0	2	4	1	2
1.5	3	6	4	9
2.0	21	45	25	53
2.5	15	32	16	34
3.0	6	13	1	2

*From Montagne JP, et al: *AJR* 1978;130:963. Used by permission.

MEASUREMENT OF NORMAL SIZE AND SHAPE
OF ADRENAL GLANDS BY CT

TABLE 8–10.

Thickness of Adrenal Glands*†

Cm	Right		Left	
	No.	%	No.	%
<1.0	35	72	10	23
1.0	12	26	33	77
1.5	1	2	. . .	. . .

*From Montagne JP, et al: *AJR* 1978; 130:963. Used by permission.
†Measurements not made in 4 left and 1 right triangular-shaped glands.

Source of Material

Sixty random patients were reviewed who had complete studies of the adrenal region and who had no clinical evidence of adrenal disease. Thirty-three men and 27 women ranged in age from 27 to 80 years (mean 56 years).

MEASUREMENT OF NORMAL RETROPERITONEAL LYMPH NODES BY LYMPHOGRAPHY FOR CORRELATION WITH CT*

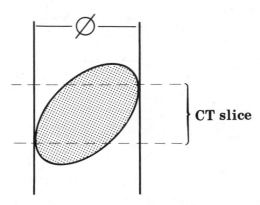

FIG 8–10.
(From Magnusson A: *Acta Radiol Diagn* 1983; 24:315. Used by permission.)

Technique

1. Lymphography with Lipodol. Measurements on anteroposterior and posterior oblique films taken 24 hours after injection.
2. Measure the largest transverse diameters of the largest lymph node at each vertebral body level. Where the node lies oblique to the longitudinal axis of the body, the measurement is between the two lymph node tangents that are parallel to the longitudinal planes of the body (Fig 8–10).
3. Correct for magnification in the imaging system.

Measurement (Table 8–11)

The measurement is performed to determine the apparent node size when imaged in the transaxial plane by CT.

No correction was possible for potential node swelling from the contrast material.

*Ref: Magnusson A: *Acta Radiol Diagn* 1983; 24:315.

MEASUREMENT OF NORMAL RETROPERITONEAL LYMPH NODES BY LYMPHOGRAPHY FOR CORRELATION WITH CT

TABLE 8–11.

Distribution of the 95 Patients With Normal Lymphographic Findings According to the Maximum Lymph Node Diameter at Different Vertebral Body Levels*

	No Contrast-Filled Nodes	<4 mm	4–5 mm	6–7 mm	8–9 mm	10–11 mm	12–13 mm	14–15 mm	16–17 mm
Th12	51	15	11	14	4				
L1	30	25	11	22	7				
L2	1	5	11	33	28	16		1	
L3				20	37	28	10		
L4			2	13	34	30	14	2	
L5				10	19	28	27	8	3

*From Magnusson A: *Acta Radiol Diagn* 1983; 24:315. Used by permission.

Source of Material

Ninety-five patients undergoing lymphography for various diseases, whose studies were judged to be normal. Twenty-seven of these had normal histopathology or had Hodgkin's disease other than in the abdomen and were in remission for 3 to 7 years. No difference was found in measurements from these 27 patients and the other 68 in the series.

CHAPTER 9

The Urinary Tract

SIZE OF NORMAL KIDNEYS*

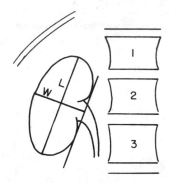

FIG 9–1.
(From Friedenberg MJ, et al: *Radiology* 1965; 84:1022. Used by permission.)

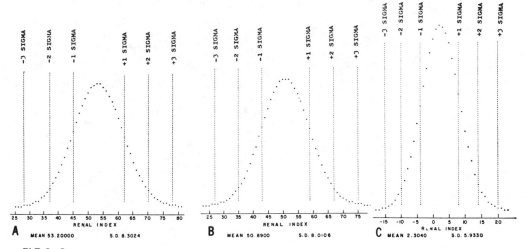

FIG 9–2.
Frequency plot of theoretical normal distribution. **A,** left renal index—children. **B,** right renal index—children. **C,** left minus right renal index—children. (From Friedenberg MJ, et al: *Radiology* 1965; 84:1022. Used by permission.)

Ref: Friedenberg MJ, et al: *Radiology* 1965; 84:1022.

SIZE OF NORMAL KIDNEYS

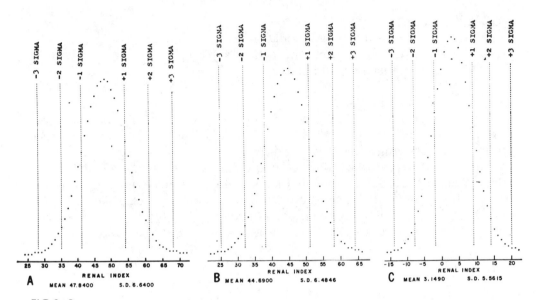

FIG 9–3.
Frequency plot of theoretical normal distribution. **A,** left renal index—adult males. **B,** right renal index—adult males. **C,** left minus right renal index—adult males. (From Friedenberg MJ, et al: *Radiology* 1965; 84:1022. Used by permission.)

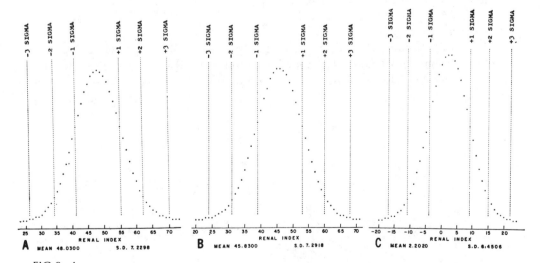

FIG 9–4.
Frequency plot of theoretical normal distribution. **A,** left renal index—adult females. **B,** right renal index—adult females. **C,** left minus right renal index—adult females. (From Friedenberg MJ, et al: *Radiology* 1965; 84:1022. Used by permission.)

Technique
  Central ray: Centered over midabdomen.
  Position: Anteroposterior with patient supine.
  Target-film distance: 40 inches.

Measurements (Fig 9–1)
The length of each kidney was determined by measuring the maximum distance from the cephalad to the caudad margin. The medial margin was determined by drawing a line between the most medial aspects of the upper and lower poles. The width was then ascertained by measuring the maximum distance from the lateral to the medial margin along a line perpendicular to the length line. The body surface area of each patient was obtained from his height and weight by use of the DuBois nomogram (p 414). A renal index was calculated for each kidney, defined according to the following formula:

$$RI = \frac{L \times W}{BSA}$$

where RI is the renal index, L is the length of the kidney in centimeters, W is the width of the kidney in centimeters, and BSA is the body surface area of the patient in square meters. The values obtained and the left minus the right renal indices are given in Figures 9–2 to 9–4).

Source of Material
The data are based on a study of 1,286 persons, white and black (322 children, 363 male adults, and 601 female adults), from the general population of a large hospital. These individuals had no evidence of renal disease, as determined by history, physical examination, and routine laboratory findings.

SIZE OF NORMAL KIDNEYS RELATED
TO VERTEBRAL HEIGHT

In Children*

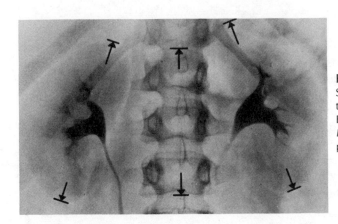

FIG 9–5.
Supine films demonstrating technique of measurement. (From Eklöf O, Ringertz II: *Acta Radiol Diagn* 1976; 17:617. Used by permission.)

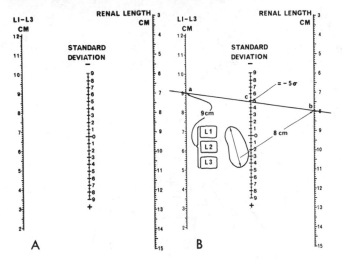

FIG 9–6.
A, nomogram for length of any given kidney in standard deviations. **B,** the method in practice. The length of the selected kidney is at the level of −5SD. (From Eklöf O, Ringertz H: *Acta Radiol Diagn* 1976; 17:617. Used by permission.)

Technique
    Central ray: Perpendicular to plane of film centered over midabdomen.
    Position: Anteroposterior with patient supine.
    Target-film distance: Immaterial.

Ref: Eklof O, Ringertz H: *Acta Radiol Diagn* 1976; 17:617.

SIZE OF NORMAL KIDNEYS RELATED
TO VERTEBRAL HEIGHT*

Measurements

A linear correlation exists between the length of the kidney and that of the lumbar vertebra L1-L3, including the intervertebral spaces comprised by these vertebrae. The left kidney appears, as a rule, approximately 2% longer than the right one. The procedure of measurement appears in Figure 9–5. A nomogram (Fig 9–6,A) is used to determine the mean of the kidney at any length of the lumbar spine. Figure 9–6,B illustrates the method applied in practice. The kidney in the example given has a length of about −5SD.

The right-to-left kidney length ratio may be determined to make comparison of consecutive examinations easier. This ratio has a 96% probability interval between 1.12 and 0.84. It is independent of the length of the lumbar segment L1-L3.

Source of Material

Based on a series of 135 patients in the pediatric age group. The material comprised 15 patients for every centimeter of lumbar length. The sexes were equally represented.

In Adults

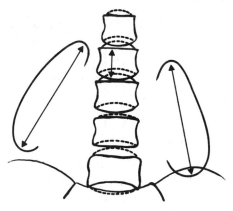

FIG 9–7.
(Adapted from Simon AL: *AJR* 1964; 92:270. Used by permission.)

*Ref: Simon AL: *AJR* 1964; 92:270.

SIZE OF NORMAL KIDNEYS RELATED
TO VERTEBRAL HEIGHT

TABLE 9−1.*

Age (Decade)	Mean Weight (gm)	Mean Length (cm)	Mean Ratio (Kidney Length/ Height of L2)	Mean Ratio (Kidney Length/ Height of L2 Plus Disc)
2nd	210	12.4	4.1	3.6
3rd	170	12.2	3.5	3.0
4th	155	11.2	3.5	3.0
5th	135	12.2	3.8	3.1
6th	145	11.8	3.7	3.1
7th	125	11.5	3.6	3.1
8th	120	11.3	3.7	3.1
9th	100	11.4	3.7	3.1

*From Simon AL: *AJR* 1964; 92:270. Used by permission.

In Adults

Technique
Central ray: Perpendicular to plane of film centered over midabdomen.
Position: Anteroposterior supine.
Target-film distance: Immaterial.

Measurements (Fig 9−7)
The length of each kidney was determined in its longest axis. The height of the second lumbar vertebral body was determined with and without the L2-L3 disc. The measurements were made at the posterior margins of the body. These are then used to create two sets of ratios: kidney length/height of L2 and kidney length/height of L2 plus disc. The normal values are given in Table 9−1.

Source of Material
The data were derived from a study of roentgenograms of 100 consecutive patients with autopsy-proved kidneys of normal weight and normal gross and microscopic appearance. There were 55 females and 45 males, ranging in age from 23 to 86 years. About half of the patients were in the sixth and seventh decades.

MEASUREMENT OF NORMAL RENAL DIMENSIONS BY ULTRASOUND*

Technique

1. All studies were performed with static-image scanners using 3.5-MHz or 5-MHz focused transducers. In many examinations, a 3-MHz mechanical real-time sector scanner was also used.
2. Kidneys were measured in longitudinal plane parallel to the longest renal axis. When possible, the height (ventral dorsal dimension) and transverse width were also measured.
3. Measurements were obtained in prone and oblique positions.

Measurement (Tables 9–2 and 9–3)

TABLE 9–2.

Right Renal Dimensions in Sample Groups
of Patients Examined Retrospectively*

	Mean (cm)	SD
Length		
Oblique (n = 52)	10.646	1.345
Prone (n = 51)	10.743	1.349
Width†		
Oblique (n = 35)	4.920	0.638
Prone (n = 32)	5.047	0.764
Depth†		
Oblique (n = 19)	3.947	0.812
Prone (n = 9)	4.167	0.507

*From Brandt TD, et al: *J Ultrasound Med* 1982; 1:49.
  Used by permission.
†Approximate values.

Ref: Brandt TD, et al: *J Ultrasound Med* 1982; 1:49.

MEASUREMENT OF NORMAL RENAL DIMENSIONS BY ULTRASOUND

TABLE 9−3.

Left Renal Dimensions in Sample Groups
of Patients Examined Retrospectively*

	Mean	SD
Length		
Oblique (*n* = 50)	10.130	1.165
Prone (*n* = 50)	11.096	1.152
Width†		
Oblique (*n* = 36)	5.303	0.744
Prone (*n* = 31)	5.300	0.802
Depth†		
Oblique (*n* = 18)	3.578	0.912
Prone (*n* = 10)	4.140	0.844

*From Brandt TD, et al: *J Ultrasound Med* 1982; 1:49.
  Used by permission.
†Approximate values.

Source of Material

Fifty-two patients with normal renal function referred for nonrenal illnesses and 10 normal volunteers were studied. Sonographic renal dimensions
are smaller than those obtained by radiography, because there is no geometric
magnification or osmotic diuresis.

MEASUREMENT OF RENAL VOLUME
BY ULTRASOUND*

Technique

1. Images were obtained with ATL real-time and Picker 80L static scanner, using 3.5-MHz transducers.
2. Kidneys were sonographically measured within 24 hours of nephrectomy. Renal length was the maximal midsagittal measurement. Transverse scans at right angles to the axis of the midsagittal plane 1 cm above the hilum, at the hilum, and 1 cm below the hilum were measured to give average width. Anteroposterior diameter was measured on the midsagittal scan.
3. Mass and water displacement of the kidneys were determined after nephrectomy.

Measurement (Figs 9−8 to 9−10)
Volume by ultrasound was calculated by the equation for an ellipsoid:

$$V = 0.53 \times L \times W \times AP$$

Based on the water displacement measurements, the equation was modified:

$$V = 0.49 \times L \times W \times AP$$

The correlation was better between displacement and sonographic volume than between renal mass and sonographic volume. Hricak and Lieto* suggest that the diseased kidney does not have a specific gravity of 1.0.

Ref: Hricak H, Lieto RP: *Radiology* 1983; 148:311.

MEASUREMENT OF RENAL VOLUME
BY ULTRASOUND

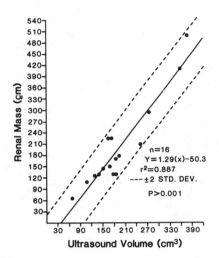

FIG 9–8.
Linear correlation of ultrasound volume vs. renal mass. (From Hricak H, Lieto RP: *Radiology* 1983; 148:311. Used by permission.)

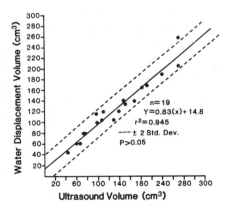

FIG 9–9.
Linear correlation of ultrasound volume vs. renal volume, as measured by water displacement. (From Hricak H, Lieto RP: *Radiology* 1983; 148:311. Used by permission.)

MEASUREMENT OF RENAL VOLUME
BY ULTRASOUND

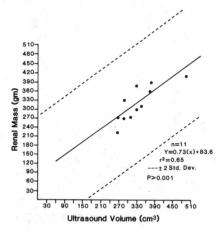

FIG 9–10.
Linear correlation of ultrasound volume vs. renal mass, as measured by different personnel than those who determined the correlation shown in Figure 9–8. (From Hricak H, Lieto RP: *Radiology* 1983; 148:311. Used by permission.)

Source of Material
Thirty-four human kidneys to be removed for transplantation were studied.

KIDNEY LENGTH CORRELATED
WITH AGE IN CHILDREN*

Technique
   Central ray: Centered over midabdomen.
   Position: Anteroposterior supine.
   Target-film distance: 40 inches.

Measurement
The length of the kidney was determined by measuring the maximum distance from the cephalad to the caudad margin. The measurements of length vs. age with 3 SD is shown in Figure 9–11.

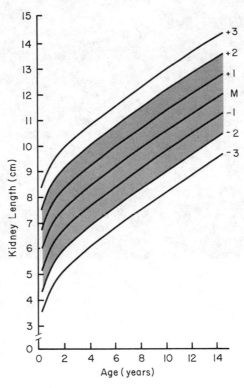

FIG 9–11.
Graph of kidney length vs. age, including 3 SD above and below the mean: 1 SD = 0.785 cm. (From Currarino G, et al: *Radiology* 1984; 150:703. Used by permission.)

Source of Material
Data obtained from excretory urograms of 262 children ranging in age from birth to 14.5 years. Four hundred twenty-two kidneys were measured.

*Ref: Currarino G, et al: *Radiology* 1984; 150:703.

MEASUREMENT OF RENAL LENGTH IN CHILDREN BY ULTRASOUND*

Technique

Images obtained with a real-time mechanical sector scanner, either a Diasonics Wide-vue using a 3.5, 5, or 7.5 MHz transducer, or a Diasonics Neonatal unit using a 6 MHz transducer.

Measurement (Fig 9–12)

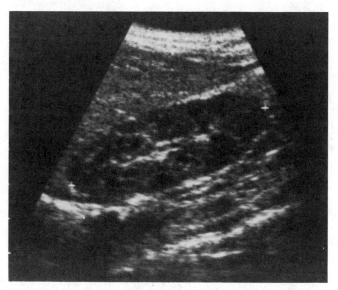

FIG 9–12.
Length of kidney can be measured with electronic calipers, as on this image of right kidney in 5-month-old baby. For purpose of this study, measurements were done with mechanical calipers. (From Rosenbaum DM, et al: *AJR* 1984; 142:467–469. Used by permission.)

Ref: Rosenbaum DM, et al: *AJR* 1984; 142:467–469.

MEASUREMENT OF RENAL LENGTH
IN CHILDREN BY ULTRASOUND

The transducer was positioned to image the kidney in its longest dimension and the renal length was measured with mechanical calipers from the hard-copy transparencies. Sonographic renal length plotted against age is shown in Figure 9–13.

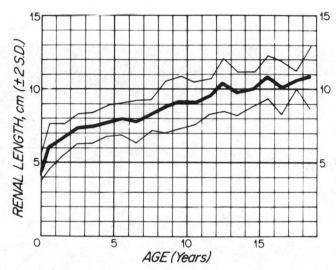

FIG 9–13.

Sonographic renal length plotted against age. (From Rosenbaum DM, et al: *AJR* 1984; 142:467–469. Used by permission.)

Source of Material

Data derived from sonographic examination of 203 children ranging in age from several hours to 19 years.

MEASUREMENT OF KIDNEY LENGTH AND VOLUME IN CHILDREN BY ULTRASOUND*

Technique
Sonographic examinations were performed with a 3.5 MHz mechanical Combison 100 scanner equipped with a freeze frame, calibration setting and a water display. Examinations performed in the prone position.

Measurements (Figs 9–14 and 9–15)

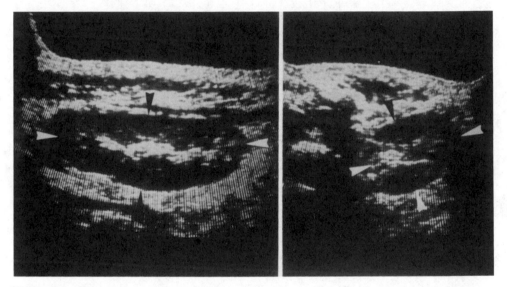

FIG 9–14.
The maximum longitudinal and transverse section of the left kidney is indicated by arrows. (From Dinkel E, et al: *Pediatr Radiol* 1985; 15:38–43. Used by permission.)

*Ref: Dinkel E, et al: *Pediatr Radiol* 1985; 15:38–43.

MEASUREMENT OF KIDNEY LENGTH AND VOLUME IN CHILDREN BY ULTRASOUND

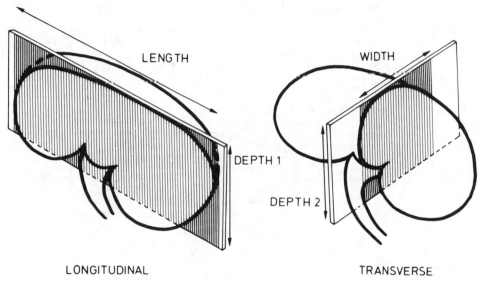

LONGITUDINAL   TRANSVERSE

FIG 9–15.
Standardized planes in renal biometry. Sonographic measurements performed in the maximum longitudinal and transverse kidney section. The latter were obtained in the kidney hilar region. Volume formula for an ellipsoid:

$$\text{Kidney volume (ml)} = L \times W \times \frac{D1 + D2}{2} \times 0.523$$

L = maximum bipolar length; W = maximum width in the hilar region; D = maximum depth in the longitudinal *(depth 1)* and transverse section *(depth 2)*. (From Dinkel E, et al: *Pediatr Radiol* 1985; 15:38–43. Used by permission.)

The normal lengths of the kidneys related to body height are shown in Figure 9–16.

MEASUREMENT OF KIDNEY LENGTH AND VOLUME IN CHILDREN BY ULTRASOUND

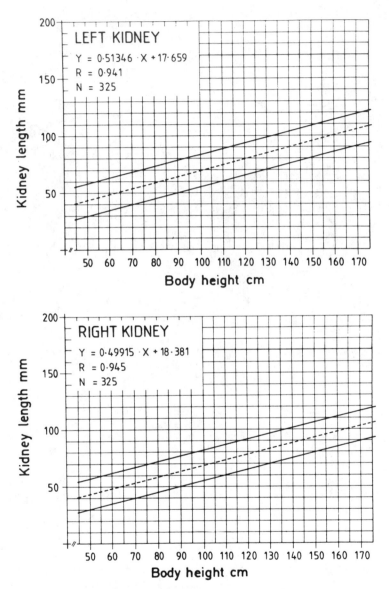

FIG 9–16.

Length of both kidneys related to body height. Mean values and the 95% regions of tolerance are determined by routine statistical analysis of 325 children. (From Dinkel E, et al: *Pediatr Radiol* 1985; 15:38–43. Used by permission.)

The kidney volumes related to body weight are shown in Figure 9–17.

MEASUREMENT OF KIDNEY LENGTH AND VOLUME IN CHILDREN BY ULTRASOUND

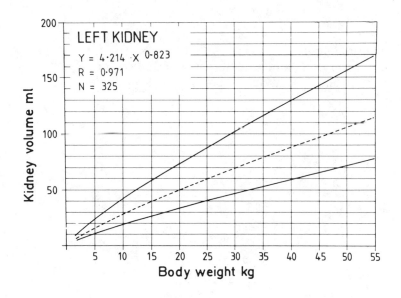

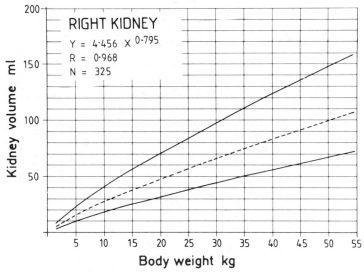

FIG 9–17.
Volume of left and right kidney correlated to body weight. Median values and the 95% regions of toler-ance are determined by statistical analysis of 325 children. Regression line and tolerance limits were computed after logarithmic transformation of volume and weight and then retransformed. There is only a slight difference between the left and right kidneys. (From Dinkel E, et al: *Pediatr Radiol* 1985; 15:38–43. Used by permission.)

MEASUREMENT OF KIDNEY LENGTH AND VOLUME IN CHILDREN BY ULTRASOUND

Source of Material

Data derived from sonographic study of 325 children without kidney disease, 188 boys and 137 girls aged between 3 days and 15 years 11 months.

THE RADIOGRAPHIC SIZE
OF RENAL TRANSPLANTS*

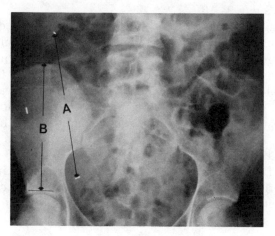

FIG 9–18.
Technique of measurements. (From Burgener FA, Schabel SJ: *Radiology* 1975; 117:547. Used by permission.)

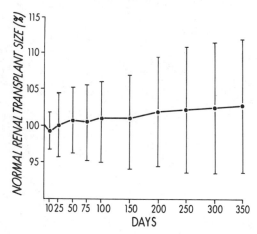

FIG 9–19.
(From Burgener FA, Schabel SJ: *Radiology* 1975; 117:547. Used by permission.)

Technique
  Central ray: Perpendicular to plane of film.
  Position: Anteroposterior.
  Target-film distance: Immaterial.

Ref: Burgener FA, Schabel SJ: *Radiology* 1975; 117:547.

THE RADIOGRAPHIC SIZE
OF RENAL TRANSPLANTS

Measurements (Fig 9–18)

The renal length was estimated by measurement of the distance between the upper- and lower-pole clips *(A)*; this size was compared to the height of the ilium *(B)*. Parallel lines were drawn through the superior portion of the acetabular roof and the iliac crest, and the distance between the two lines was measured. The ratio between the two measurements *(A/B)* was calculated and defined as 100% on the first available radiograph. On follow-up, the transplants were measured in the same way and compared to the baseline value (100%), with any change expressed as a percentage increase or decrease. The changes in size in normal transplants is shown in Figure 9–19. The normal maximum rate of increase was 0.5% per day, found only in the immediate postoperative period. Sixty percent of transplants, with severe rejection, had an abnormal length and/or growth rate. In chronic rejection, size and growth rates were rarely abnormal.

Source of Material

Data based on a study of 50 patients, 29 males and 21 females, 13 to 57 years of age. All patients were followed for up to 3 years.

MEASUREMENT OF RENAL SIZE IN CHILDREN WITH MYELODYSPLASIA BY ULTRASOUND*

Technique

Sonograms were performed with real-time equipment and a 3.5, 5, or 7.5 MHz transducer.

Measurements

Maximum renal lengths were measured. In general, mean renal length for each age group was below mean values for normal children. A normal renal growth curve for children with spina bifida is presented in Figure 9–20.

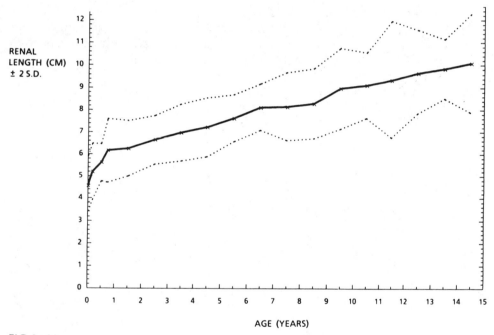

FIG 9–20.
Sonographic renal length versus age for spina bifida children. (From Gross GW, Boal DK: *J Urol* 1988; 140:784–786. Used by permission.)

Source of Material

Data are based on sonographic examination of 145 patients with spina bifida, 69 males and 76 females ranging in ages from 3 days to 33 years.

Ref: Gross GW, Boal DK: *J Urol* 1988; 140:784–786.

EVALUATION OF RENAL TRANSPLANT REJECTION BY DUPLEX DOPPLER EXAMINATION USING THE RESISTIVE INDEX*

Technique

1. Duplex Doppler sonographic examinations were performed with 3.5 and/or 5-MHz transducers.
2. The pulsed examinations were performed in the areas of the arcuate arteries. The tracings were recorded on film and/or a strip chart recorder.

Measurement (Figs 9–21 to 9–24)

Measurements of peak systolic and lowest diastolic frequency shifts were calculated by using a caliper and measured against the baseline. A resistive index (RI) was determined by using the following formula:

$$RI = \frac{\text{Peak systolic frequency shift} - \text{lowest diastolic frequency shift}}{\text{Peak systolic frequency shift}}$$

*Ref: Rifkin MD, et al: *AJR* 1987; 148:759–762.

EVALUATION OF RENAL TRANSPLANT REJECTION BY DUPLEX DOPPLER EXAMINATION USING THE RESISTIVE INDEX

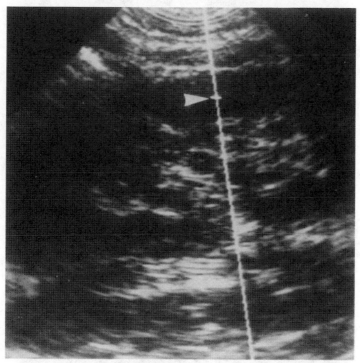

FIG 9–21.
Doppler examination of a renal transplant. Longitudinal sonogram of transplanted kidney shows Doppler line of information and specific area of sampling *(arrowhead)* at level of arcuate artery adjacent to medullary pyramid. (From Rifkin MD, et al: *AJR* 1987; 148:759–762. Used by permission.)

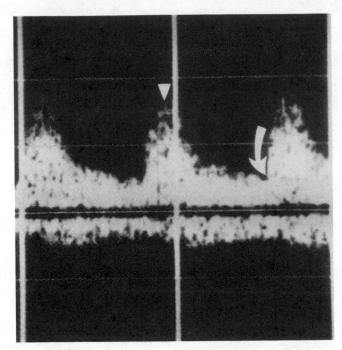

FIG 9–22.
Normal renal transplant. Doppler waveform shows peak systole *(arrowhead)* and end diastole *(curved arrow)*. Resistive index is 0.64. (From Rifkin MD, et al: *AJR* 1987; 148:759–762. Used by permission.)

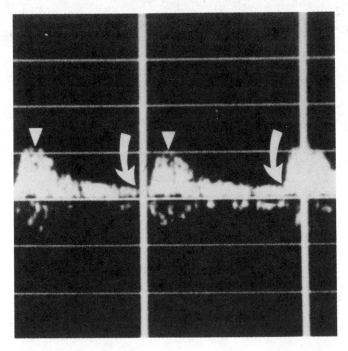

FIG 9–23.
Renal transplant rejection. Doppler waveform shows peak systolic frequency shift *(arrowheads)* and end-diastolic frequency shift *(curved arrows)*. Resistive index is 0.83. (From Rifkin MD, et al: *AJR* 1987; 148:759–762. Used by permission.)

EVALUATION OF RENAL TRANSPLANT REJECTION BY DUPLEX DOPPLER EXAMINATION USING THE RESISTIVE INDEX

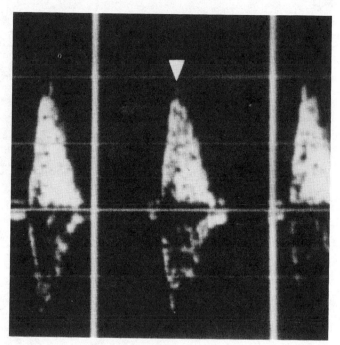

FIG 9–24.
Renal transplant rejection. Doppler waveform shows peak systole *(arrowhead)* and no end-diastolic flow. Resistive index is 1.0. (From Rifkin MD, et al: *AJR* 1987; 148: 759–762. Used by permission.)

EVALUATION OF RENAL TRANSPLANT REJECTION BY DUPLEX DOPPLER EXAMINATION USING THE RESISTIVE INDEX

The results are given in Table 9–4.

TABLE 9–4.

Resistive Index in Renal Transplant Patients With Normal Kidney Function and in Those With Renal Failure*†

Resistive Index	Normal	Causes of Renal Failure			
		Rejection	Acute Tubular Necrosis	Toxic Reactions to Cyclosporine	Glomerulo- nephritis
0.50–0.54	1	0	2	1	0
0.55–0.59	7	0	3	1	0
0.60–0.64	9	0	2	0	2
0.65–0.69	8	3	6	3	0
0.70–0.74	9	7	4	3	1
0.75–0.79	9	7	5	1	1
0.80–0.84	1	23	7	0	0
0.85–0.89	1	7	4	0	0
0.90–0.94	0	3	0	0	0
0.95–0.99	0	0	0	0	0
1.00	0	4	0	0	0
Total	45	54	33	9	4

*From Rifkin MD, et al: *AJR* 1987; 148:759–762. Used by permission.
†Data are for 145 studies in 81 patients. Resistive indexes were determined from results of duplex Doppler examinations. Causes of renal failure were determined by biopsy and/or clinical evaluation.

Criteria for diagnosis of transplant rejection are shown in Table 9–5.

TABLE 9–5.

Criteria for Diagnosis of Transplant Rejection*

Resistive Index	Interpretation
≥0.9	Rejection highly likely
0.80–0.89	Rejection likely
0.70–0.79	Indeterminate†
<0.7	Rejection unlikely

*From Rifkin MD, et al: *AJR* 1987; 148:759–762. Used by permission.
†Rejection is possible but less likely than other diagnoses.

Source of Material

Data based on a study of 81 patients with renal transplants, including 41 with acute rejection.

DETERMINATION OF RENAL CORTICAL INDEX*

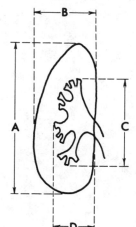

FIG 9–25.
(Adapted from Vuorinen P, et al: *Acta Radiol* 1962; suppl 211.)

Technique
Central ray: Perpendicular to plane of film centered over midabdomen.
Position: Anteroposterior supine.
Target-film distance: Immaterial.

Measurements (Fig 9–25)
The upper and lower poles are marked. The lateral and medial borders are marked. The renal calyceal system is outlined and the superior, inferior, and lateral calyces are marked. The distances between the marked lines are measured in millimeters.

$$\text{Renal cortical index (RCI)} = \frac{C(\text{mm}) \times D(\text{mm})}{A(\text{mm}) \times B(\text{mm})}$$

RCI (mean value of both kidneys of a patient) = 0.35; SD = 0.04.
RCI/D (difference in RCI between the two kidneys of the same patient) = 0.02; SD = 0.02.

Source of Material
One hundred six normal patients.

*Ref: Vuorinen P, et al: *Acta Radiol* 1962; suppl 211.

DETECTION OF NONFUNCTIONAL UPPER SEGMENT OF DUPLICATED KIDNEY IN INFANTS AND CHILDREN*

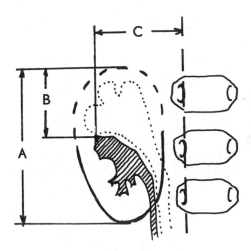

FIG 9–26.
Method of measurement of a kidney with a dilated and nonfilled upper pelvis. (From Lundin E, Riggs W: *Acta Radiol* 1968; 7:13. Used by permission.)

Technique
Central ray: Perpendicular to plane of film.
Position: Anteroposterior supine.
Target-film distance: Immaterial.

Measurements (Fig 9–26)
The letter A indicates renal length; B the distance from the upper pole to the most cephalad of the contrast-filled calyces. The dimension C is not used in this entry.

In normal cases, without duplication, the ratio is more than 3.3:1. In 29 of the cases of Lundin and Riggs,* with duplication and nonfunctioning upper pole, the ratio was less than 2.6:1. A ratio of less than 2.6 to 1 is highly indicative of duplication and nonfunctioning upper pole.

Source of Material
Data based on 31 cases of duplication with nonfunctioning or only slightly functioning upper pole, with upper renal systems associated with ectopic ureterocele, in patients aged 2 months to 11 years, and 31 cases of complete duplication, without ureterocele, with both systems functioning.

*Ref: Lundin E, Riggs W: *Acta Radiol* 1968; 7:13.

NORMAL POSITION OF RENAL PELVES AND URETERS ON THE LATERAL UROGRAM*

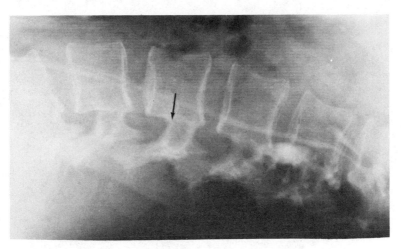

FIG 9–27.
(From Cook IK, Keats TE, Seale DL: *Radiology* 1971; 99:499. Used by permission.)

Technique

Central ray: Perpendicular to plane of film centered to lateral midabdomen in cross-table lateral projection.

Position: Patient supine. Cross-table lateral.

Target-film distance: 40 inches.

Measurements (Fig 9–27)

Measure the distance from the posterior margin of the renal pelvis to the midpoint of the posterior surface of the adjacent vertebral body (Tables 9–6 to 9–8).

TABLE 9–6.

Distance of the Posterior Margin of the Renal Pelvis From the Posterior Surface of the Adjacent Vertebral Body*

Vertebral Level	No. of Renal Pelves	Mean Distance (mm)	Standard Deviation
D12	7	1.6	8.2
L1	79	8.6	9.7
L2	91	9.0	8.8
L3	6	−1.00	5.9

*From Cook IK, Keats TE, Seale DL: *Radiology* 1971; 99:499. Used by permission.

*Ref: Cook IK, Keats TE, Seale DL: *Radiology* 1971; 99:499.

NORMAL POSITION OF RENAL PELVES AND URETERS ON THE LATERAL PROGRAM

TABLE 9–7.

Distance of the Posterior Margin of the Ureter From the Posterior Surface of the Adjacent Vertebral Body*

Vertebral Level	No. of Ureters	Mean Distance (mm)	Standard Deviation	Distances That Would Occur <1% of the Time (mm)
L1	4	16.8	7.4	33.0
L2	54	24.2	9.3	45.9
L3	116	29.7	10.1	53.2
L4	116	38.8	9.7	61.4
L5	116	49.2	9.5	71.3

*From Cook IK, Keats TE, Seale DL: *Radiology* 1971; 99:499. Used by permission.

TABLE 9–8.

Distance of the Posterior Margin of the Ureter From the Posterior Surface of the Adjacent Vertebral Body Expressed in Vertebral Widths

Vertebral Level	No. of Ureters	Mean Vertebral Width	Standard Deviation
L3	116	0.75	0.23
L4	116	0.99	0.20
L5	116	1.25	0.31

*From Cook IK, Keats TE, Seale DL: *Radiology* 1971; 99:499. Used by permission.

Source of Material

One hundred five patients with normal excretory urograms. Thirty-five were men and 70 were women. Ages ranged from 14 to 76 years.

MEASUREMENT OF THE NORMAL POSITION OF THE KIDNEYS IN RELATION TO THE CORONAL PLANES OF THE BODY FOR DETERMINATION OF TOMOGRAPHIC PLANE*

Technique

Central ray: Perpendicular to plane of film.

Position: Center posterior supine, expiratory phase of respiration without compression.

Target-film distance: 40 inches.

Measurements

This study shows that the distance from the table top to the kidneys in the supine position varies greatly. A 2-cm thick tomographic cut at 8 cm will include only 41% of the kidneys. A 3-cm cut at 8.5 cm will include 56% of the kidneys. The study also shows that the depth of the kidneys can be predicted with greater accuracy in relation to one third of the body thickness. One third of the body thickness in this study is the plane that is one third of the distance from the table top to the anterior abdominal wall at the inferior margin of the rib cage. The kidneys usually lie anterior to this plane, and a 2-cm thick tomographic cut 1.5 cm anterior to the one-third plane will include 61% of the kidneys, while a 3-cm thick cut 1 cm anterior to the one-third plane will include 79% of the kidneys. Of the few kidneys not included in these cuts, approximately half will be found farther anterior and half farther posterior.

The left kidney usually lies in the plane anterior to the right. As a general rule, therefore, if one kidney is in a tomographic cut and the other is not, the left will be found in a more anterior plane, and the right will be found in a more posterior plane. The difference in level is not great, and a 2-cm thick tomographic cut will include both kidneys in 81% of persons.

Source of Material

Data obtained from measurement of 61 kidneys.

Ref: McConnell F: *J Can Assoc Radiol* 1972; 23:241.

MEASUREMENT OF RENAL ARTERY SIZE*

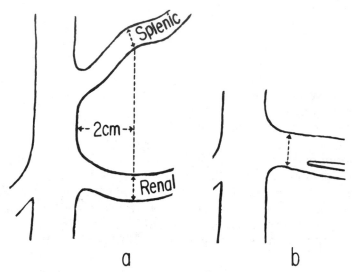

FIG 9–28.
(Adapted from Maluf NSR: *Surg Gynecol Obstet* 1958; 107:415.)

TABLE 9–9.

Internal Diameter of Renal Artery

	Diameter (mm)	SD
Two normal kidneys	6.5–6.7	0.75–0.88
One healthy hyper-trophied kidney	8.4–8.6	0.71–0.83

*Ref: Maluf NSR: Surg Gynecol Obstet 1958; 107:415.

MEASUREMENT OF RENAL ARTERY SIZE

Technique
 Central ray: Perpendicular to plane of film centered over the interspace
 between the first and second lumbar vertebral bodies.
 Position: Anteroposterior.
 Target-film distance: 32 inches. Measurements are reduced by 10% for
 distortion.

Measurements (Fig 9–28 and Table 9–9)

1. The renal and splenic arteries are measured where they intersect a
 line 2 cm from and parallel to the lateral border of the aorta. The
 measurements are made at right angles to the longitudinal axis of the
 vessel at the 2-cm intersection.
2. When the renal artery bifurcates at a point closer than 2 cm from the
 aorta, it is measured proximal to this bifurcation. When a kidney re-
 ceives more than one artery from the aorta, the equivalent diameter
 (D) is obtained from the equation:

$$D = 4 \sqrt{D_1^4 + D_2^4 + \ldots D_n^4}$$

in which D_1 and D_2 are the diameters of two such arteries and D_n the
diameter of the nth such artery.

 Of greater value is the ratio (see below) of internal diameter of the renal
artery to the splenic artery. This is typically greater than unity when the kidney is normal. The ratio rises in renal hypertrophy and falls in renal hypoplasia or reduced renal function. A narrow renal artery is always indicative of
reduced renal function, but an artery of normal caliber does not necessarily
imply normal renal function. Normal ratio:

$$\frac{\text{Diameter of renal artery}}{\text{Splenic artery}} = {>}1$$

Source of Material
 The data are based on measurements of 18 young patients with normal
kidneys, 9 young patients with only one healthy hypertrophied kidney, and
32 patients with unilateral or bilateral renal abnormality.

RELATIONSHIP OF RENAL SURFACE AND PARENCHYMAL AREAS TO RENAL ARTERY SIZE*

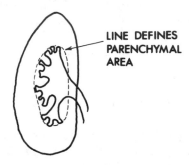

LINE DEFINES
PARENCHYMAL
AREA

FIG 9–29.
(From Wojtowicz J: *Invest Radiol* 1967; 2:231. Used by permission.)

Technique

Central ray: Perpendicular to plane of film centered over the interspace between the first and second lumbar vertebral bodies.
Position: Anteroposterior.
Target-film distance: 95 cm.

Measurements (Figs 9–29 to 9–31)

Study performed using selective renal or abdominal aortography. Serial angiographic films and urographic films were obtained in moderate inspiration. Measurements made as follows:

1. Renal area is determined with a planimeter from the nephrographic phase.
2. Renal parenchymal area is defined by a line drawn through the calyceal fornices and the intrarenal part of the renal pelvis. The parenchymal area is calculated as the difference between the renal area and the area of the pyelocalyceal system.
3. Renal artery diameter is measured at a distance 1 cm from the origin of the artery. Cross-sectional area of the artery is expressed as the square of the artery radius (the constant π is omitted).

Ref: Wojtowicz J: *Invest Radiol* 1967; 2:231.

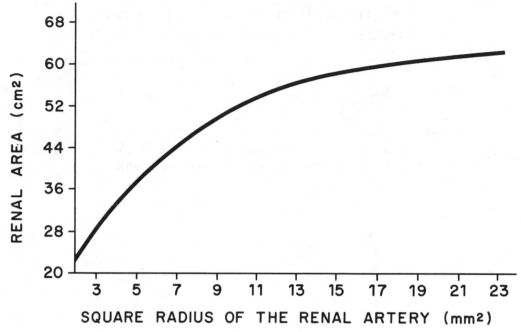

FIG 9–30.
Renal area vs. artery cross-section area. (From Wojtowicz J: *Invest Radiol* 1967; 2:231. Used by permission.)

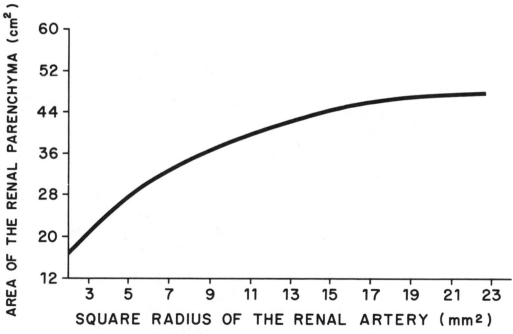

FIG 9–31.
Renal parenchyma area vs. artery cross-section area. (From Wojtowicz J: *Invest Radiol* 1967; 2:231. Used by permission.)

RELATIONSHIP OF RENAL SURFACE AND PARENCHYMAL AREAS TO RENAL ARTERY SIZE

Source of Material

One hundred twenty-four renal angiograms in patients with a single arterial blood supply to each kidney. Some selected cases with pathology were included.

MEASUREMENT OF BLADDER VOLUMES BY ULTRASONOGRAPHY FOR DETERMINING RESIDUAL URINE*

Technique

1. Picker 80-L unit with a 2.25 MHz focused transducer was used.
2. Determinations of bladder volumes were made following measured instillation of saline.
3. Bladders were scanned longitudinally and transversely.

Measurement (Figs 9–32 and 9–33)

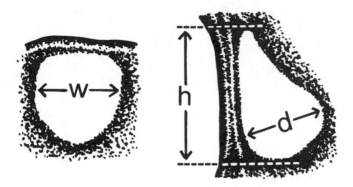

FIG 9–32.
Width *(w)* is obtained from the transverse scan exhibiting the greatest transverse diameter. A midline longitudinal scan yields both height *(h)* and depth *(d)*; the latter is taken as the longest chord in the anteroposterior plane. The calculated volume (V$_c$) is the product of the three dimensions: V$_c$ = w × h × d. (From McLean GK, Edell SL: *Radiology* 1978; 128:181–182. Used by permission.)

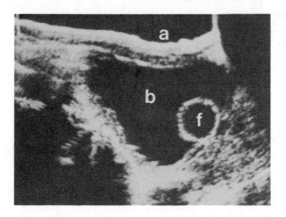

FIG 9–33.
Longitudinal midline scan of patients filled to total bladder volumes of 300 ml. An acceptable scan clearly shows all bladder boundaries. *a* = anterior abdominal wall; *b* = saline-filled bladder; *c* = foley balloon. (From McLean GK, Edell SL: *Radiology* 1978; 128:181–182. Used by permission.)

*Ref: McLean GK, Edell SL: *Radiology* 1978; 128:181–182.

MEASUREMENT OF BLADDER VOLUMES BY ULTRASONOGRAPHY FOR DETERMINING RESIDUAL URINE

Computed volumes are plotted against the volumes of instilled saline (Fig 9–34).

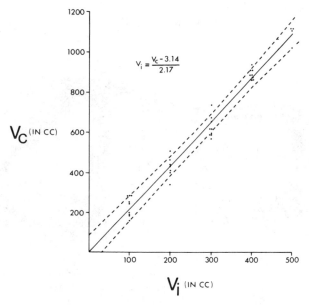

FIG 9–34.
Computed volumes (V_c) are plotted against the volumes of instilled saline (V_i). The calculated linear regression yields the relationship $V_i = (V_c - 3.14)\ 12.17$ with a correlation coefficient of 0.987. *Dashed lines* show the 95% confidence limits. (From McLean GK, Edell SL: *Radiology* 1978; 128:181–182. Used by permission.)

It has been shown that the bladder of a healthy child retains no more than a few millimeters of urine after voiding. Residual urine after normal voiding is abnormal.*

Source of Material
Data are based on a total of 48 scans obtained from 14 patients.

*Ref: Harrison CW, et al: *Br J Urol* 1976; 47:805–814.

MEASUREMENT OF THE NORMAL BLADDER WALL IN CHILDREN BY ULTRASOUND*

Technique

Examinations performed with a real-time ATL unit with 7.5- or 5-MHz probes for children under 5 years of age. A Diasonics unit with a 5-MHz probe was used for older children and adults.

Measurements

The bladder wall thickness was measured on transverse and sagittal cuts, usually in an area of the bladder floor posterolateral to the trigone. The bladder wall thickness varies with the state of filling (Fig 9–35).

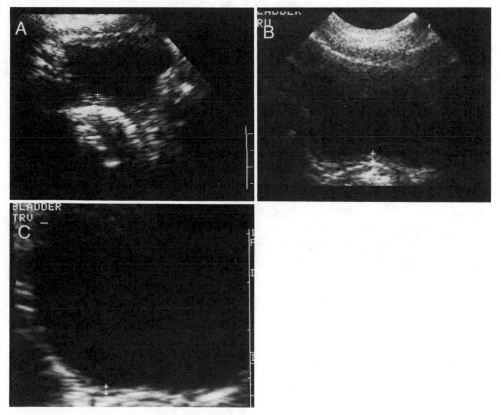

FIG 9–35.

Transverse bladder sonograms: *arrows* outline bladder wall. **A,** "empty" bladder in a 1-month-old boy with hydroceles. Wall is 3 mm thick. **B,** bladder ± full in a 7-year-old boy with remote renal contusion. Wall is 2.9 mm thick. **C,** bladder full. Close-up view in a 9-year-old boy with lactose intolerance. Wall is 1.4 mm thick. (From Jequier S, Rousseau D: *AJR* 1987; 149:563–566. Used by permission.)

*Ref: Jequier S, Rousseau O: *AJR* 1987; 149:563–566.

MEASUREMENT OF THE NORMAL BLADDER WALL IN CHILDREN BY ULTRASOUND

The normal bladder wall thickness is given in Table 9–10.

TABLE 9–10.

Mean Bladder Wall Thickness in Millimeters (±SD) According to Age and State of Bladder Filling*†

Age	Empty	±Full	Full	Full++
<1 mo	2.62±0.51 (8)	2.10±0.31 (10)	1.92±0.51 (12)	1.67±0.57 (3)
1 mo–1 yr	2.61±0.62 (14)	1.93±0.27 (14)	1.65±0.47 (27)	2 (2)
1–6 yr	2.76±0.73 (29)	2.06±0.35 (39)	1.87±0.37 (57)	1.44±0.52 (9)
6–12 yr	2.82±0.46 (36)	2.17±0.32 (43)	1.97±0.42 (49)	1.43±0.53 (7)
>12 yr	2.83±0.51 (18)	2.18±0.32 (14)	1.89±0.39 (22)	1.64±0.74 (7)

*From Jequier S, Rousseau O: *AJR* 1987; 149:563–566. Used by permission.
†Numbers in parentheses indicate numbers of patients in each group. Empty = bladder contained <10% of its normal capacity; ±full = bladder contained 10%–25% of capacity; full = bladder contained 26%–90% of capacity; full ++ = bladder contained >90% of capacity.

The normal bladder wall has a mean thickness of 2.76 mm when the bladder is almost empty and 1.55 mm when it is distended. The upper limits are 3 and 5 mm for a full or empty bladder, respectively.

Source of Material

Data are based on a study of 410 children ranging in age from 1 day to 19 years and 10 adults without urinary tract complaints.

MEASUREMENT OF THE URETHROVESICAL ANGLES IN STRESS INCONTINENCE*

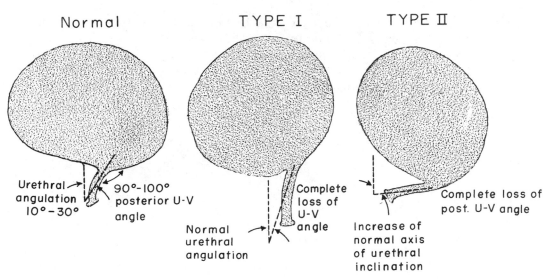

FIG 9–36.
(Adapted from Green TH, Jr: Am J Obstet Gynecol 1962; 83:632.)

Technique
Central ray: At level of greater trochanter perpendicular to plane of film.
Position: Lateral erect straining.
Target-film distance: Immaterial.

Measurements
Angles are determined by chain cystourethrography in the erect position during straining. The angle between the posterior aspect of the urethra and the base of the bladder (posterior urethrovesical angle) normally measures 90°–100°. Loss of this angle alone indicates Type I stress incontinence. The angle of inclination of the urethra is found by extending a line through the direction of the upper urethra to join a line in the vertical axis of the patient. The normal angle is 10° to 30°, and an angle above 45° is definitely abnormal. Loss of this angle plus loss of the posterior urethral angle constitutes Type II stress incontinence.

Source of Material
The data on the posterior urethrovesical angle is based on a study of more than 500 roentgen examinations of the bladder and urethra of 132 nonpreg-

*Ref: Green TH, Jr: Am J Obstet Gynecol 1962; 83:632.

MEASUREMENT OF THE URETHROVESICAL ANGLES IN STRESS INCONTINENCE

nant women.† The data on the angle of inclination of the urethra are based on a study of 350 patients examined by cystourethrography.‡

Green* notes that angle measurements do not apply if a cystocele is present. The chain cystourethrogram is usually abnormal in stress incontinence. However, an abnormal cystourethrogram does not necessarily indicate stress incontinence.

†*Ref*: Jeffcoate TNA, Roberts H: *J Obstet Gynaecol Br Emp* 1952; 59:685.
‡*Ref*: Bailey KV: *J Obstet Gynaecol Br Emp* 1956; 63:663.
*Ref: Green TH, Jr: *Am J Obstet Gynecol* 1962; 83:632.

THE SACROCOCCYGEAL–INFERIOR PUBIC POINT (SCIPP) LINE AND THE LATERAL CYSTOURETHROGRAM*

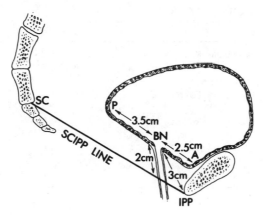

FIG 9–37.
Composite drawing of lateral recumbent film showing average normal adult female measurements. (From Noll LE, Hutch JA: *Obstet Gynecol* 1969; 33:680. Used by permission.

Technique
Central ray: At level of greater trochanter perpendicular to plane of film.
Positions: Lateral recumbent, lateral erect straining, lateral erect voiding.
Target-film distance: 36 inches.

Measurements (Fig 9–37)
The bladder is filled with opaque medium until the patient experiences discomfort. A small chain of metal beads is used to demonstrate the urethrovesical angle. A line *(SCIPP)* is drawn from the sacrococcygeal joint *(SC)* to the inferior point of the pubic bone *(IPP)*. *BN* is the bladder neck, and the flat base of the bladder is the base plate.

Average measurements (cm) in lateral recumbent position are shown in Table 9–11.

Ref: Noll LE, Hutch JA: *Obstet Gynecol* 1969; 33:680.

THE SACROCOCCYGEAL–INFERIOR PUBIC POINT (SCIPP) LINE AND THE LATERAL CYSTOURETHROGRAM

TABLE 9–11.*

	Average (cm)
Base plate: Range 5–7 cm	6.0
Base plate: Anterior to bladder neck	2.5
Base plate: Posterior to bladder neck	3.5
Bladder neck above SCIPP line	2.0
Bladder neck to IPP	3.0

*From Noll LE, Hutch JA: *Obstet Gynecol* 1969; 33:680. Used by permission.

In standing position the bladder neck drops 1 cm from recumbent position.

In standing position with straining the bladder neck drops an additional 1 cm or 2 cm compared with recumbent.

In standing position with voiding the bladder neck drops an additional 0.5 cm to 2.5 cm compared with recumbent.

In patients with stress incontinence the recumbent film showed a rounded base plate for about one half of the patients. The bladder neck averaged 1 cm above the SCIPP line. The drop in the bladder neck upon standing, straining, and voiding was greater in distance than for the normal group.

Source of Material
Ninety-five adult women, of whom 20 were urologically normal.

Note: A data sheet has been designed by Noll and Hutch that enables the radiologist to record readily all pertinent cystourethrogram information.

MEASUREMENT OF THE URETHRA
IN CHILDREN*

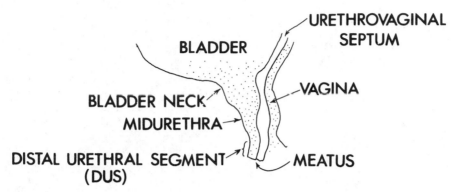

FIG 9–38.
(Adapted from Shopfner CE: *Radiology* 1967; 88:222.)

Technique
    Central ray: Television fluoroscopy and spot roentgenograms made during the voiding cycle.
    Position: Oblique and lateral views obtained during voiding cystourethrography.
    Target-film distance: Variable; Shopfner used a 15% correction for magnification.

Measurements (Fig 9–38 and Table 9–12)
For females the meatus was indicated by barium coating of the mucosa or by identification of the urethrovaginal septum. Diameters of meatus, distal urethral segment, and midurethra were measured on films taken during full voiding.

For males the urethra was measured at the midpart of the membranous and the posterior urethra.

Ref: Shopfner CE: *Radiology* 1967; 88:222.

MEASUREMENT OF THE URETHRA
IN CHILDREN

TABLE 9–12.

Urethrogram Measurements (Percentage of Patients)*†

Diameters (mm)	Females			Males	
	Meatus (%)	DUS (%)	Midurethra (%)	Membranous Urethra (%)	Posterior Urethra (%)
2	4	4		4	
3	16	16		8	
4	20	20	1	16	1
5	31	28	3	26	5
6	25	21	9	24	8
7	4	9	11	16	18
8		2	25	4	24
9			12	2	11
10			4		13
11			5		3
12			17		4
13			4		4
14			1.5		1
15			2		2
16			2		1
17			0.05		1
18			1		1
19			1		1
20			0.05		1
21			0.05		1

*From Shopfner CE: *Radiology* 1967; 88:222. Used by permission.
†Measurements made during full voiding stream.

Source of Material

Fifty-three females and 67 males with no urinary tract abnormality. Ages ranged from less than 1 year to 16 years.

MEASUREMENT OF THE ADULT MALE URETHRA*

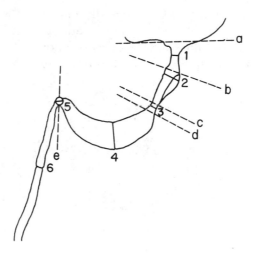

FIG 9–39.
The anatomical landmarks on the micturiton cystourethrogram: a = bladder base; b = upper limit of verumontanum; c = the cone of the prostatic urethra; d = the junction between the membranous and bulbous parts; e = the penoscrotal junction. The sites where the calibers were measured are indicated by *double lines: 1* = SCU; *2* = PRU; *3* = MU; *4* = BU; *5* = PSJ; *6* = PEU. (From Manoliu RA: *Eur J Radiol* 1982; 2:209. Used by permission.)

Technique
Central ray: Voiding cystourethrography using television fluoroscopy and spot roentgenograms made during the voiding cycle.
Position: Anteroposterior and both obliques. Views obtained during voiding.
Target-film distance: All measurements given are corrected for geometric enlargement.

Measurements (Figs 9–39 to 9–41)

1. The narrowest point between the bladder base and the upper limit of the verumontanum (supracollicular urethra [SCU]).
2. The widest diameter of the prostatic urethra (PRU).
3. The narrowest point between the verumontanum and the cone of the bulbous urethra (membranous urethra [MU]).
4. The widest diameter of the bulbous urethra (BU).
5. The diameter of the penoscrotal junction (PSJ).
6. The narrowest caliber of the penile urethra (PEU).

*Ref: Manoliu RA: *Eur J Radiol* 1982; 2:209.

MEASUREMENT OF THE ADULT MALE URETHRA

The measurements were performed with a ruler marked in millimeters. The results were noted as integer numbers. There were three measurements for each segment in Group I and two measurements in Group II. The calibers were corrected for the estimated geometric enlargement (× 1.3 for the obliques and × 1.2 for the anteroposterior projections). For each segment an arithmetic mean was computed. This mean was rounded up to the nearest millimeter.

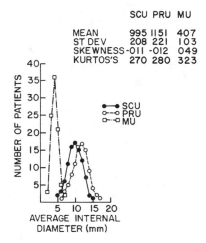

	SCU	PRU	MU
MEAN	995	1151	407
ST DEV	208	221	103
SKEWNESS	-011	-012	049
KURTOS'S	270	280	323

FIG 9–40.
The average internal diameters of the supracollicular, prostatic, and membranous urethra. (From Manoliu RA: *Eur J Radiol* 1982; 2:209. Used by permission.)

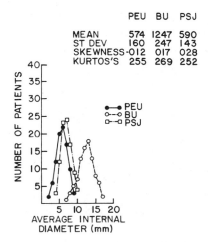

	PEU	BU	PSJ
MEAN	574	1247	590
ST DEV	160	247	143
SKEWNESS	-012	017	028
KURTOS'S	255	269	252

FIG 9–41.
The average internal diameters of the penoscrotal junction, bulbous, and penile urethra. (From Manoliu RA: *Eur J Radiol* 1982; 2:209. Used by permission.)

MEASUREMENT OF THE ADULT MALE URETHRA

Source of Material

Data are based on a study of 92 adult males ranging in age from 18 to 71 years with a mean age of 43.3 years.

MEASUREMENT OF THE NORMAL SEMINAL VESICLES*

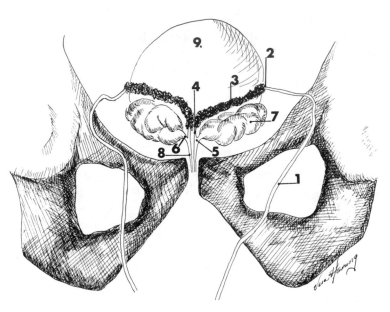

FIG 9–42.
Anatomical drawing of the structures opacified by seminal vesiculography on AP or PA view. Structures are numbered in order of sequential filling by the vasoseminal route. *1* = vas deferens; *2* = deferential-ampullary junction; *3* = ampulla of the vas deferens; *4* = neck of the ampulla; *5* = confluence; *6* = the excretory duct; *7* = the seminal vesicle; *8* = the ejaculatory duct; *9* = the urinary bladder. (From Banner MP, Hessler R: *Radiology* 1978; 128:339. Used by permission.)

Technique
Contrast vesiculography.
Central ray: Perpendicular to plane of film centered 2 cm above the symphysis pubis.
Position: Anteroposterior supine.
Target-film distance: 40 inches.

Measurement (Fig 9–42)
The length of each vesicle was measured from the confluence of the excretory and deferent ducts to the fundus of the vesicle along its main axis. A perpendicular to this line was constructed and the width of the vesicle measured at its widest point. Two vesicles may be asymmetric in size normally within 2 SD.

The ejaculatory ducts were measured from the confluence to their opening in the urethra. The width was measured midway from origin to orifice. Normal measurements are shown in Tables 9–13 and 9–14.

Ref: Banner MP, Hessler R: *Radiology* 1978; 128:339.

MEASUREMENT OF THE NORMAL SEMINAL VESICLES

TABLE 9–13.

Dimensions of the Normal Seminal Vesicle (in cm)*

	Left			Right		
	Length	Width	Luminal Diameter	Length	Width	Luminal Diameter
Greatest	6.6	3.2	1.0	6.1	3.0	1.3
Least	3.2	1.1	0.4	2.7	1.2	0.4
Average	4.6	2.0	0.6	5.0	2.0	0.6
SD	0.8	0.4	0.13	0.6	0.5	0.16

*From Banner MP, Hessler R: *Radiology* 1978; 128:339. Used by permission.

TABLE 9–14.

Dimensions of the Normal Ejaculatory Duct (in mm)*

	Left		Right	
	Length	Width	Length	Width
Greatest	25.0	3.2	25.0	3.8
Least	9.0	0.5	9.0	0.5
Average	16.0	1.5	16.0	1.5
SD	4.0	0.6	3.0	0.7

*From Banner MP, Hessler R: *Radiology* 1978; 128:339. Used by permission.

Source of Material

Data derived from vasoseminal vesiculography performed on 69 asymptomatic men.

MEASUREMENT OF PELVIC ORGANS IN PREMENARCHEAL GIRLS BY ULTRASOUND*

Technique

1. Studies performed with a 3-MHz mechanical sector scanner (SRT L/S GE), with electronic calipers calibrated to a velocity of 1,540 m/sec.
2. The examinations were performed with the bladder distended.
3. Serial longitudinal and transverse scans were obtained in the supine position.

Measurement

When the largest available uterine section was displayed in the longitudinal axis, the image was frozen and the total uterine length (TUL) and AP diameters of the corpus (COAP) and the cervix (CEAP) were measured on the screen. The transducer was then rotated through 90° and scanning was performed in the transverse axis of the uterus to measure the widest transverse diameter of the corpus.

Serial longitudinal scans of the pelvis with the uterus as a landmark were made by tilting the transducer and scanning through the bladder from the contralateral side. The ovaries appeared as oval structures, more transonic than surrounding tissues, about half-way from the uterus to the iliopsoas muscle. The ovarian vessels were useful as additional landmarks.

Ovarian length and longitudinal inclination were evaluated on the scan displaying the largest section of the ovary. Transverse and AP diameters were measured from a transverse scan perpendicular to the longitudinal inclination.

Uterine and ovarian volumes (UV, OV) were determined by the formula for a prolate ellipsoid (Volume = $0.5233 \times D1 \times D2 \times D3$; where D1, D2, D3 are the three maximal longitudinal, AP, and transverse diameters).

Uterine diameters and volumes are given in Table 9–15.

Ref: Orsini LF, et al: *Radiology* 1984; 153:113–116.

TABLE 9–15.

Uterine Diameters and Volume*†

| Age (Yr) | No. of Patients | Uterine Diameters (mm) | | | | Uterine Volume (cm³) | |
| | | TUL | COAP | CEAP | COAP/CEAP | By Chronologic Age | By Bone Age |
		Mean ± SD	Mean ± SD	Mean ± SD	Mean ± SD	Mean ± SD	Mean ± SD
2	7	33.1±4.4	7.0±3.4	8.3±2.0	0.84±0.29	1.98±1.58	1.76±0.72
3	8	32.4±4.3	6.4±1.3	7.6±2.2	0.89±0.29	1.63±0.81	1.80±0.74
4	15	32.9±3.3	7.6±1.8	8.6±1.8	0.90±0.22	2.10±0.57	1.97±0.74
5	7	33.1±5.5	8.0±2.8	8.4±1.6	0.95±0.28	2.36±1.39	2.19±1.16
6	9	33.2±4.1	6.7±2.9	7.5±1.8	0.86±0.18	1.80±1.57	1.65±0.93
7	9	32.3±3.9	8.0±2.2	7.7±2.5	1.08±0.26	2.32±1.07	2.81±1.44
8	11	35.8±7.3	9.0±2.8	8.4±1.7	1.05±0.20	3.12±1.52	2.70±1.43
9	11	37.1±4.4	9.7±3.0	8.8±2.0	1.10±0.24	3.70±1.62	2.69±1.83
10	13	40.3±6.4	12.8±5.3	10.7±2.6	1.17±0.31	6.54±3.78	4.66+3.03
11	13	42.2±5.1	12.8±3.1	10.7±?.6	1.22±0.26	6.66±2.87	6.24±3.07
12	6	54.3±8.4	17.3±5.3	14.3±5.2	1.23±0.16	16.18±9.15	8.88±3.65
13	5	53.8±11.4	15.8±4.5	15.0±2.4	1.03±0.15	13.18±5.64	15.55±5.98

*From Orsini LF, et al: *Radiology* 1984; 153:113–116. Used by permission.
†As determined by ultrasonography in 114 girls from age 2 to 13. TUL = total uterine length; COAP = AP diameter of the corpus; CEAP = AP diameter of the cervix.

Ovarian volumes are given in Table 9–16.

TABLE 9–16.

Ovarian Volume*†

| Age (Yr) | No. of Patients | Ovarian Volume (cm³) | |
| | | By Chronologic Age | By Bone Age |
		Mean ± SD	Mean ± SD
2	5	0.75±0.41	0.78±0.38
3	6	0.66±0.17	0.64±0.18
4	14	0.82±0.36	1.00±0.45
5	4	0.86±0.02	0.95±0.52
6	9	1.19±0.36	1.05±0.65
7	8	1.26±0.59	1.23±0.47
8	10	1.05±0.50	1.29±0.33
9	11	1.98±0.76	1.35±0.71
10	12	2.22±0.69	1.47±0.56
11	12	2.52±1.30	2.45±0.86
12	6	3.80±1.40	3.10±1.29
13	4	4.18±2.30	4.38±2.74

*From Orsini LF, et al: *Radiology* 1984; 153:113–116. Used by permission.
†As determined by ultrasonography in 101 girls from age 2 to 13.

Source of Material

Data are based on study of 114 normal premenarcheal girls ranging in age from 2 to 13 years.

DETERMINATION OF OVARIAN VOLUME
BY ULTRASOUND*

Technique
Ultrasound examination performed with a real-time Diasonics DRF 400 Scanner, using a 3.5-MHz oscillating transducer.

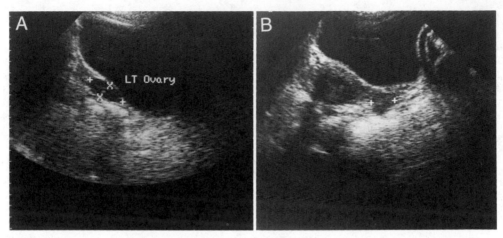

FIG 9–43.
A, longitudinal scan shows typical length and AP thickness measurements. **B,** transverse scan demonstrates measurements of ovarian width. (From Munn CS, et al: *Radiology* 1986; 159:731–732. Used by permission.)

Measurements (Fig 9–43)
The greatest length, transverse dimension (width), and AP thickness were determined. Volumes were calculated using the formula for the volume of an ellipsoid:

$$\text{Volume} = 0.523 \times \text{length} \times \text{width} \times \text{thickness}$$

The derived data show the normal volume ranged as high as 13.84 cm^3 with an average of 6.48 cm^3.

Source of Material
Data are based on ultrasonographic study of 15 women aged 18 to 47 years.

Ref: Munn CS, et al: *Radiology* 1986; 159:731–732.

CHAPTER 10

Pelvimetry and Fetometry

MEASUREMENT OF THE PELVIS
AND THE FETAL CRANIUM

From the many methods of roentgenographic measurement of the pelvis, two were chosen for presentation. One, the Ball method, employs geometric corrections based on target-film and object-film distances; the other, the Colcher-Sussman method, makes corrections by comparing measured diameters with a centimeter scale placed at the same distance from the film as the internal diameters to be measured and projected on the same film.

As Maloy and Swenson* state, "One method is probably as accurate as another if done with the precision advocated by its author. Each radiologist should select a method and learn to use it well, bearing constantly in mind the importance of the shape of the pelvis, which is not necessarily reflected in the measurements of the cardinal diameters alone."

The Ball Method†

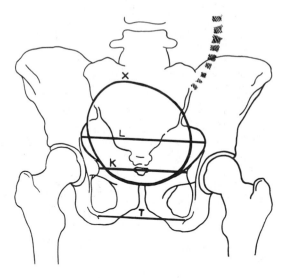

FIG 10–1.
Anteroposterior view of pelvis made near term. (From Maloy HC, Swenson PC, in Golden R (ed): *Diagnostic Roentgenology*. Baltimore, Williams & Wilkins Co, 1952, vol 2. Used by permission.)

*Ref: Maloy HC, Swenson PC, in Golden R (ed): *Diagnostic Roentgenology*. Baltimore, Williams & Wilkins Co, 1952, vol 2.
†Ref: Ball RP, Golden R: *AJR* 1943; 49:731.

MEASUREMENT OF THE PELVIS AND THE FETAL CRANIUM

The Ball Method

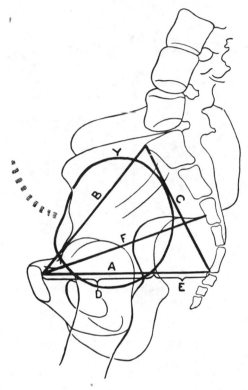

FIG 10–2.
Lateral view of pelvis made near term with patient in erect position. (From Maloy HC, Swenson PC, in Golden R (ed): *Diagnostic Roentgenology*. Baltimore, Williams & Wilkins Co, 1952, vol 2. Used by permission.)

MEASUREMENT OF THE PELVIS
AND THE FETAL CRANIUM

The Ball Method

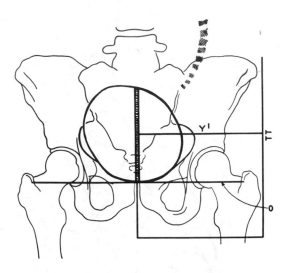

FIG 10–3.
The object-film distance is one-half the true bitrochanteric measurement of the patient plus the distance from table top to film (about 4 cm). The true bitrochanteric measurement is equal to the distance between the mesial margins of the greater trochanters, O, plus 4 cm for a 36-inch target-film distance, or plus 2 cm for a 30-inch target-film distance. Y' extends from the equatorial zone of the fetal cranium (as seen in Figure 10–2) to the table top. (Adapted from Ball RP, Golden R: *AJR* 1943; 49:731 and Maloy HC, Swenson PC, in Golden R (ed): *Diagnostic Roentgenology*. Baltimore, Williams & Wilkins Co, 1952, vol 2. Used by permission.)

MEASUREMENT OF THE PELVIS AND THE FETAL CRANIUM

The Ball Method

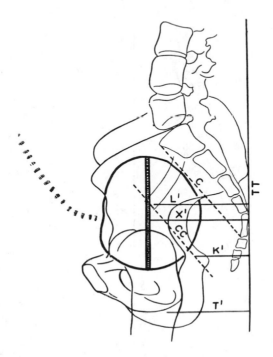

FIG 10–4.
Object-table-top distances are represented by prime letters. Add approximately 4 cm to obtain object-film distance. Line *TT* passes through the most posterior border of the sacrum and parallel to the film edge. The anterior point of *L'* is where a line *CC*, projected through the ischial spines and parallel to *C*, intersects the iliopectineal lines of the pelvic brim. The line *K'* extends from the ischial spine to table top, *TT*. The anterior point of *T'* lies in a vertical plane which intersects the inferior angles of the obturator foramina. The anterior point *X'* is the equatorial zone of the fetal cranium as seen on anteroposterior view (Fig 10–3). (Adapted from Ball RP, Golden R: *AJR* 1943; 49:731 and Maloy HC, Swenson PC, in Golden R (ed): *Diagnostic Roentgenology*. Baltimore, Williams & Wilkins Co, 1952, vol 2. Used by permission.)

Technique

Central ray: Lateral, erect: to 1 inch above the superior margin of the greater trochanter. The central ray should pass through the posterosuperior margin of the greater trochanter. If the centering is correct, the sacroiliac notch shadows will be superimposed.

Anteroposterior, erect: to the median plane of the pelvis. Tube is moved upward 3 inches from the level used for the lateral view.

MEASUREMENT OF THE PELVIS AND THE FETAL CRANIUM

The Ball Method

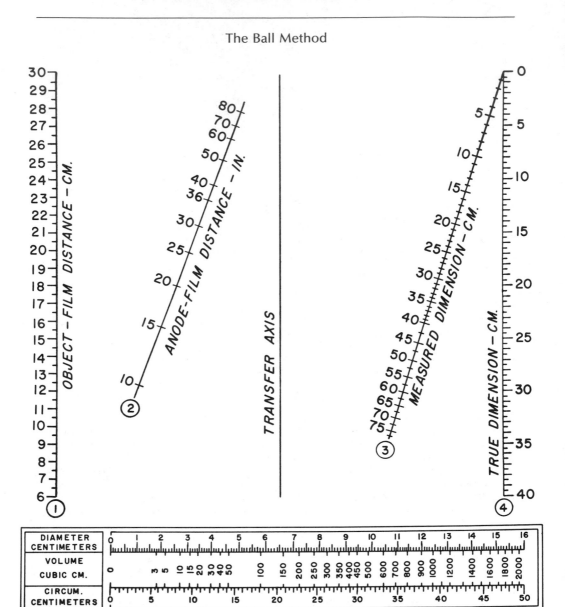

FIG 10–5.
Nomogram (designed by Holmquist) for use with Ball method. Draw a straight line from the object-film distance (1) through the anode-film distance (2) to the transfer axis. Draw a second line from this point on the transfer axis through measured dimension (3) to true dimension (4). Fetal skull volume can be found by using the circumference diameter scale at the bottom. (Adapted from Ball RP, Golden R: *AJR* 1943; 49:731.)

MEASUREMENT OF THE PELVIS AND THE FETAL CRANIUM

The Ball Method

Position: Lateral erect: the patient is placed in the lateral position with the right greater trochanter in contact with the surface of the erect Potter-Bucky diaphragm. Posterior curve of the sacrum falls about 1 inch anterior to posterior margin of the film. The inferior margin of the film should be at the level of the gluteal femoral crease.

Anteroposterior, erect: the patient is positioned with her back to the Potter-Bucky diaphragm, and a compression band is applied.

Target-film distance: 36 inches.

Measurements (Figs 10–1 to 10–5)

1. Pelvis

   Inlet:

Anteroposterior diameter (promontory to pubis, Fig 10–2,B)	11.5 cm
Widest transverse diameter (Fig 10–1,L)	12.5 cm

   Midpelvis:

Anteroposterior diameter (pubic symphysis to lower end of fifth sacral segment, Fig 10–2,A)	12.6 cm

   This diameter is composed of two segments:

The distance from pubic symphysis to interspinous plane (Fig 10–2,D)	8.3 cm
The distance from interspinous plane to fifth sacral segment (Fig 10–2,E)	4.3 cm
Interspinous diameter (Fig 10–1,K)	10.5 cm

   Outlet:

Transverse diameter (bituberal) (Fig 10–1,T)	10.4 cm

2. Fetal Skull

   The perimeter of the fetal skull outline on both the AP and lateral views is traced with a map measure, and each measurement is corrected for magnification. The two corrected measurements are averaged. This is the "mean circumference" of the skull. Two cm is added to the mean circumference for the scalp thickness. This total circumference of the fetal head is translated into cubic centimeters (bottom scale, Fig 10–5).

   The average mean circumference of fetal head (including the scalp), near term, equals 32.5 to 33.5 cm.

   The comparison between fetal head size and the smallest internal pelvic diameter is made by measuring certain pelvic dimensions. Most likely to cause trouble are the inlet diameter and the midplane interspinous diameter.

   The smallest of these two diameters and the total circumference of the fetal head are converted to cubic centimeters.

MEASUREMENT OF THE PELVIS
AND THE FETAL CRANIUM

The Ball Method

When the volume of the fetal head is smaller than the volume of the largest sphere that could pass through the smallest dimension, no disproportion is present.

Source of Material

Studies were made of 349 obstetrical patients examined in the Department of Radiology, Presbyterian Hospital, New York City.

The Ball Method: Friedman-Taylor Nomograhic Aid*

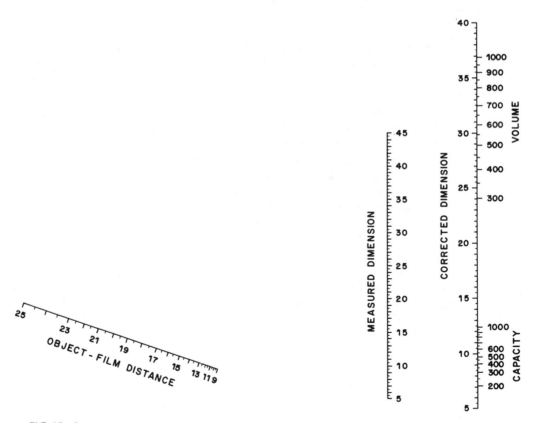

FIG 10–6.
(From Friedman EA, Taylor MB: *Am J Obstet Gynecol* 1969; 105:1110. Used by permission.)

Ref: Friedman EA, Taylor MB: *Am J Obstet Gynecol* 1969; 105:1110.

MEASUREMENT OF THE PELVIS
AND THE FETAL CRANIUM

The Ball Method: Friedman-Taylor Nomographic Aid

Technique

Central ray: Use the Ball Method.

Position: Use the Ball Method.

Target-film distance: 40 inches. To use this nomogram (Fig 10–6), use a target-film distance of 40 inches.

Measurements

Corrections of pelvic and fetal head measurements are made using appropriate object-film distances as follows:

1. Widest transverse diameter of the inlet (measured on AP film): Corrected using the distance from a point representing the widest diameter of the inlet (obtained by drawing a line parallel to the inclination of the sacrum through the ischial spines on the lateral x-ray view) to the posterior sacrum. To the latter measurement one should add an arbitrary figure of 4 cm to take into account distance from the posterior bony aspect of the sacrum through the gluteal soft tissues to the film-holding cassette.
2. Interspinous diameter (measured on AP film): Corrected using distance from spine to posterior sacrum plus factor of 4 cm (obtained from the lateral view).
3. Anteroposterior diameter of the inlet (measured on lateral view): Corrected by using distance from midpoint to greater trochanter plus 4 cm (obtained from AP view).
4. Circumference of fetal head (measured on AP film): Corrected using distance from midpoint of head to posterior sacrum plus 4 cm (obtained from lateral view).
5. Circumference of fetal head (measured on lateral view): Corrected using distance from midpoint to greater trochanter plus 4 cm (obtained from AP view). If AP view head is not in midline, one uses the distance from midpoint of the fetal head to the appropriate greater trochanter. If the correct side is unknown, one measures to both trochanters independently and then uses only the measurement that approaches most closely that obtained after correcting the circumference of the anteroposterior view head.

The final step is the conversion of the corrected pelvic diameters to capacities and skull circumferences to volume. Comparison of capacities and volumes is made to evaluate the cephalopelvic relationship.

The following classification is useful:

1. *Inlet.* If inlet capacities are equal to or greater than fetal head volume, no disproportion exists. Cases in which the inlet capacities are

MEASUREMENT OF THE PELVIS
AND THE FETAL CRANIUM

The Ball Method: Friedman-Taylor Nomographic Aid

smaller than the head volume by 50 cc or less are deemed to have relative or borderline disproportion. Where the negative difference exceeds 50 cc (head volume is more than 50 cc larger than the smallest inlet capacity), "absolute" or high degree of disproportion is considered present.

2. *Midpelvis.* If the interspinous capacity is up to 150 cc smaller than the volume of the head, no disproportion exists; between 150 and 200 cc negative difference, there is relative midpelvic disproportion; if the negative difference exceeds 200 cc at the midplane (head volume more than 200 cc larger than interspinous capacity), interpretation of "absolute" disproportion is warranted.

Source of Measurements

Forty consecutive measurements of 5 pelvic and fetal skull dimensions.

MEASUREMENT OF THE PELVIS
AND THE FETAL CRANIUM

The Colcher-Sussman Method*

POSITIONING

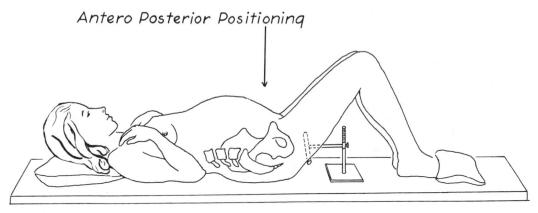

A

Lateral Positioning

B

Antero Posterior Positioning

FIG 10–7.
(From Colcher AE, Sussman W: *AJR* 1944; 51:207. Used by permission.)

Description of Intersecting Diameters (Fig 10–8, **C** and **D**.)
Inlet:
   Anteroposterior diameter *(I-G)*: Extends from upper inner margin of the
   symphysis to the interior surface of the sacrum following the level of
   the iliopectineal line, passing through a midpoint between the brim of
   the pelvis and the apices of the sacrosciatic notches. The apices of the
   notches must approximate each other.

Ref: Colcher AE, Sussman W: *AJR* 1944; 51:207.

MEASUREMENT OF THE PELVIS
AND THE FETAL CRANIUM

The Colcher-Sussman Method

Transverse diameter *(A-A')*: Widest transverse diameter of the inlet *(E)*.
Midpelvis:

Anteroposterior diameter *(P-M)*: Extends from inner lower border of the pubic symphysis through the point halfway between the contours of the two ischial spines to the anterior margin of the sacrum.

Transverse diameter *(B-B')*: Transverse interspinous diameter *(F)*.
Outlet:

Anteroposterior diameter (postsagittal, *S-T*): Extends from the midbituberal point *(T)* to the lower anterior margin of the last sacral segment *(S)*.

MEASUREMENT OF THE PELVIS
AND THE FETAL CRANIUM

The Colcher-Sussman Method

POSITIONING WITH RULER

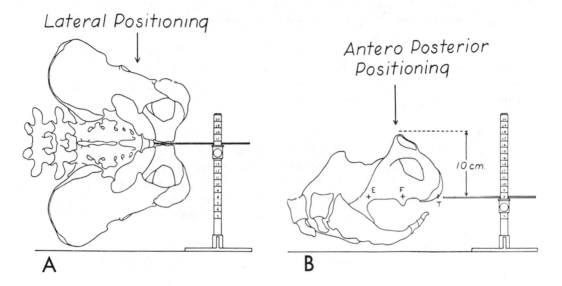

Lateral Positioning

A

Antero Posterior Positioning

10 cm.

B

INTERSECTING DIAMETERS

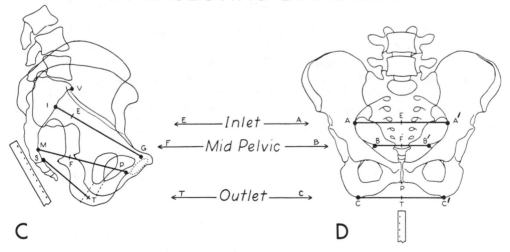

← E ——*Inlet*—— A →

← F —*Mid Pelvic*— B →

← T ——*Outlet*—— C →

C

D

FIG 10–8.
(From Colcher AE, Sussman W: *AJR* 1944; 51:207. Used by permission.)

MEASUREMENT OF THE PELVIS
AND THE FETAL CRANIUM

The Colcher-Sussman Method

Point T is found as follows: On the lateral view, straight lines are projected from the lower border of each obturator foramen to the lowest point on the shadow of the ischial tuberosity. These lowest points (the bituberal points) are connected by a straight line. The midbituberal point T is halfway between these two points.

Transverse diameter (bituberal) $(C\text{-}C')$: On the film, the points C and C' are obtained by projecting a straight line from the lateral margin of the inlet along the lateral wall of the forepelvis, which appears as a dense white line on the film to the lower margin of ischial tuberosity.

Technique
Central ray: Lateral: to greater trochanter of femur;
      Anteroposterior: to superior margin of pubic symphysis.
 Positions: Lateral (Fig 10–7,A): true lateral with patient lying on either right or left side; knees and thighs semiflexed;
      Anteroposterior (Fig 10–7,B): patient supine with knees and thighs semiflexed and separated.
Target-film distance: 36 or 40 inches.
A specially devised ruler* is used to make measurement corrections. When positioned as described below, the ruler will have the same distortion as the diameters on the same level. Therefore, the ruler markings on the film become the centimeter scale. Placement of ruler:

1. *Lateral view* (Fig 10–7,A): The ruler is placed at the midsacral spine parallel with the spine and film. The centimeter rule markings are projected on the film for direct mensuration.
2. *Anteroposterior view* (Fig 10–7,B): The ruler is placed at the level of the tuberosities of the ischium by direct manual palpation or by lowering the ruler 10 cm below the superior border of the symphysis pubis.

Measurements
Diameters of inlet, midpelvis, and outlet (Fig 10–8,C and D and Table 10–1).

---

*This ruler, devised by Colcher and Sussman, may be obtained from the Picker X-ray Corporation.

MEASUREMENT OF THE PELVIS
AND THE FETAL CRANIUM

The Colcher-Sussman Method

TABLE 10–1.

Diameters		Average Normal	Average Total	Low Normal
Actual inlet				
Anteroposterior	I to G	12.5	25.5	22.0
Transverse	A to A'	13.0		
Midpelvis				
Anteroposterior	M to P	11.5	22.0	20.0
Transverse				
(bispinous)	B to B'	10.5		
Outlet				
Anteroposterior				
(post. sagittal)	S to T	7.5	18.0	16.0
Transverse				
(bituberal)	C to C'	10.5		

Source of Material

The number of patients studied is not stated by Colcher and Sussman. However, the measurements are in good agreement with those obtained in other extensive studies.

PELVIMETRY BY MAGNETIC RESONANCE IMAGING*

Technique

1. MRI is performed with a superconducting magnet at 0.35 T. An elliptical body coil with a 50 × 58 cm aperture is used.
2. Position: supine. Spin echo technique using 1.0 sec TR for both sagittal and transverse planes.

Measurement
Sagittal images are centered 5 cm below the maternal umbilicus (Fig 10–9).

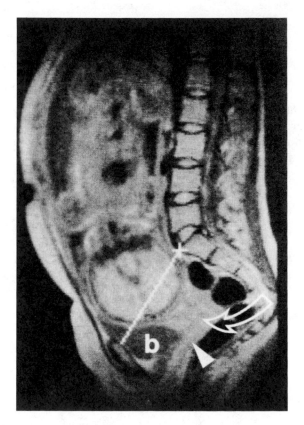

FIG 10–9.
Sagittal, midline MRI. Fetus in vertex presentation with fetal head imaged coronally, maternal pelvis imaged sagittally. Electronic cursor measures distance between inner cortex of symphysis pubis and sacral promontory (+): AP pelvic inlet diameter. Maternal cervix (arrow), vagina (arrowhead), and urinary bladder (b) are well seen. Bony fetal calvaria is of low intensity and is covered by scalp fat of high intensity. (From Stark DD, et al: AJR 1985; 144:947–950. Used by permission.)

*Ref: Stark DD, et al: AJR 1985; 144:947–950.

PELVIMETRY BY MAGNETIC RESONANCE IMAGING

A transverse series of 10 multislice images centered 5 cm above the symphysis pubis includes one section through the widest transverse inlet diameter (Fig 10–10).

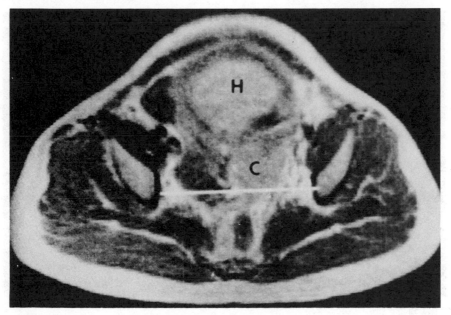

FIG 10–10.
Transverse MRI at pelvic inlet. Vertex of fetal head *(H)* and part of cervix *(C)* are identified. Transverse inlet diameter is measured at its widest point (From Stark DD, et al: *AJR* 1985; 144:947–950. Used by permission.)

PELVIMETRY BY MAGNETIC RESONANCE IMAGING

Another more caudal section obtained through the ischial spines allows measurement of the transverse midpelvis diameter (Fig 10–11). See page 637 for normal pelvic dimensions.

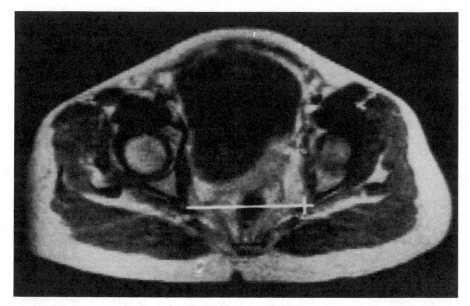

FIG 10–11.
Transverse MRI at midpelvis. Measurement of transverse (bispinous) midpelvis diameter is shown. (From Stark DD, et al: *AJR* 1985; 144:947–950. Used by permission.)

Source of Material
Data are based on MR examination of 10 third trimester women.

MEASUREMENT OF THE GESTATIONAL SAC
BY ULTRASOUND FOR DETERMINATION
OF FETAL MATURITY*

Technique
Contact scanner operating at 2.0 MHz.

Measurement (Figs 10–12 and 10–13)
An average linear measurement is as accurate as a volume measurement and is therefore preferable. The measurement should be performed from inner to inner edge. If the sac is round, only one measurement is needed. If ovoid or teardrop shaped, three measurements are obtained and averaged. Two of these measurements are taken from the long axis of the uterus, the length and AP dimension perpendicular to the length. By turning into a transaxial projection at the point of the AP dimension, the width measurement is obtained.

Ref: Kurtz AB, Goldberg BB: *Obstetrical Measurements in Ultrasound.* Chicago, Year Book Medical Publishers, 1988, pp 3–11. Based on original work of Hellman LF, et al: *Am J Obstet Gynecol* 1969; 103:789–800.

MEASUREMENT OF THE GESTATIONAL SAC
BY ULTRASOUND FOR DETERMINATION
OF FETAL MATURITY

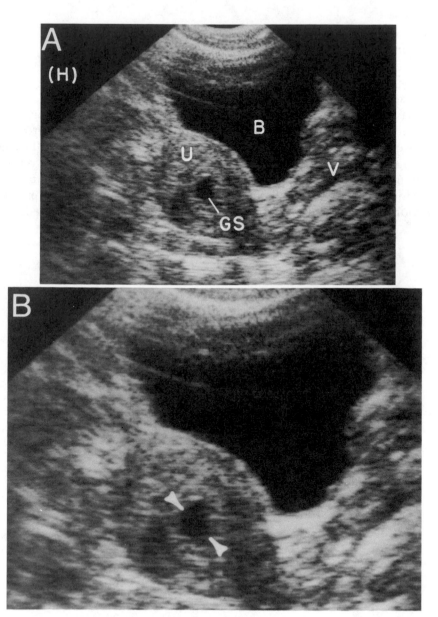

FIG 10–12.
A, long-axis ultrasound image of a round gestational sac *(GS)* within the uterus *(U)* at 5 weeks. Since the sac is round, only one measurement is needed. **B,** same image as **A.** *Arrowheads* denote inner edges of rounded sac to be measured. *V* = vagina; B = maternal bladder; *(H)* = toward patient's head. (From Kurtz AB, Goldberg BB: *Obstetrical Measurements in Ultrasound.* Chicago, Year Book Medical Publishers, 1988, pp 3–11. Used by permission.)

MEASUREMENT OF THE GESTATIONAL SAC
BY ULTRASOUND FOR DETERMINATION
OF FETAL MATURITY

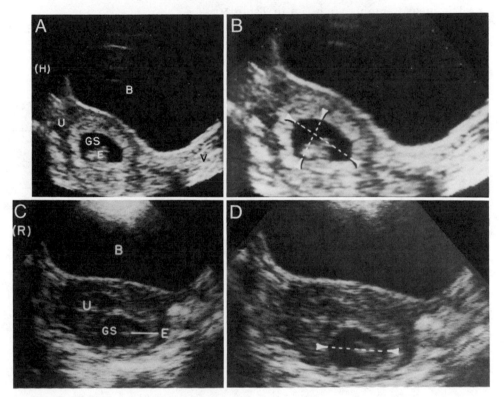

FIG 10–13.
Ultrasound images of an 8-week pregnancy within an ovoid gestational sac *(GS)*. **A,** Long-axis scan showing the uterus *(U)* with a living embryo *(E)* within the gestational sac. **B,** same image as **A** showing the length measurement *(arrowheads* and *dotted line* along the long axis of the uterus) and the AP measurement *(arrowheads* and *dotted line* perpendicular to the length). **C,** transaxial scan taken perpendicular to the point at which the AP measurement was obtained. Within the uterus *(U)* is the gestational sac *(GS)* containing the living embryo *(E)*. **D,** same image as **C** showing the width measurement *(arrowheads* and *dotted line)*. B = maternal bladder; V = vagina; (H) = toward patient's head; (R) = toward patient's right. (From Kurtz AB, Goldberg BB: *Obstetrical Measurements in Ultrasound.* Chicago, Year Book Medical Publishers, 1988, pp 3–11. Used by permission.)

MEASUREMENT OF THE GESTATIONAL SAC BY ULTRASOUND FOR DETERMINATION OF FETAL MATURITY

The measurements are given in Table 10–2.

TABLE 10–2.

Gestational Sac Measurement Table*

Mean Predicted Gestational Sac, mm	Gestational Age, wk	Mean Predicted Gestational Sac, mm	Gestational Age, wk
10.0	5.0		
11.0	5.2	36.0	8.8
12.0	5.3	37.0	8.9
13.0	5.5	38.0	9.0
14.0	5.6	39.0	9.2
15.0	5.8	40.0	9.3
16.0	5.9	41.0	9.5
17.0	6.0	42.0	9.6
18.0	6.2	43.0	9.7
19.0	6.3	44.0	9.9
20.0	6.5	45.0	10.0
21.0	6.6	46.0	10.2
22.0	6.8	47.0	10.3
23.0	6.9	48.0	10.5
24.0	7.0	49.0	10.6
25.0	7.2	50.0	10.7
26.0	7.3	51.0	10.9
27.0	7.5	52.0	11.0
28.0	7.6	53.0	11.2
29.0	7.8	54.0	11.3
30.0	7.9	55.0	11.5
31.0	8.0	56.0	11.6
32.0	8.2	57.0	11.7
33.0	8.3	58.0	11.9
34.0	8.5	59.0	12.0
35.0	8.6	60.0	12.2

Equation†: Gestational age (wk) = $\dfrac{\text{Gestational sac (mm)} + 25.43}{7.02}$

*From Hellman LM, Kobayashi M, Fillisti L, et al: *Am J Obstet Gynecol* 1969; 103:784–800. Used by permission.
†This formula was expressed in centimeters in its original form.

Source of Material
Based on a study of 25 normal pregnant women.

MEASUREMENT OF AMNIOTIC FLUID VOLUME BY ULTRASOUND*

Technique

Patients are scanned in supine position by a linear array real-time with a 3.5-MHz transducer.

The entire uterus was surveyed, and pockets of amniotic fluid were identified. The broadest dimension of fluid pockets was measured by electronic calipers on freeze-frame images.

Measurement (Table 10–3)

Normal amniotic fluid volume was judged if a pocket of fluid measured 1 cm or greater. The largest pockets are usually found in the region of fetal limbs. Abnormal fluid volume was diagnosed if pockets measured less than 1 cm.

TABLE 10–3.

Incidence of Intrauterine Growth Retardation in Patients With "Suspected" Retardation*

Method	No. Patients	% IUGR		False Positive Rate (%)	False Negative Rate (%)
		N	%		
Clinical estimate only	120	31	25.8	74.2	—
Qualitative AFV					
Normal (>1 cm)	91	5	6.6	—	6.6
Decreased (<1 cm)	29	26	89.6†	10.4	—

*From Manning FA, et al: *Am J Obstet Gynecol* 1981; 139:254. Used by permission.
†$P < 0.001$ by chi-square test.

Source of Material

One hundred twenty consecutive patients referred with a clinical diagnosis of intrauterine growth retardation based on discrepancy of at least 4 weeks between gestational age and fundal height. Patients with obviously mistaken dates were excluded from the study. At delivery, the infants were weighed and considered growth retarded if birth weight was less than the tenth percentile for gestational age and sex.

*Ref: Manning FA, et al: *Am J Obstet Gynecol* 1981; 139:254.

MEASUREMENT OF FETAL CEREBRAL VENTRICLE SIZE BY ULTRASOUND*

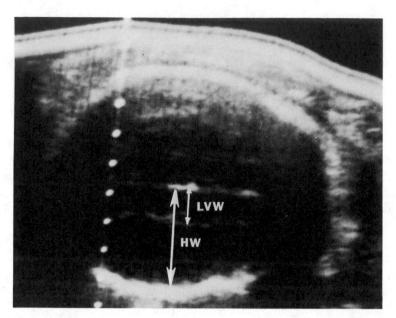

FIG 10–14.
Single-pass scan through bodies of lateral ventricles in a 31-week gestation. Lateral ventricular width *(LVW)* is measured from midline echo to first strong echo from lateral wall of lateral ventricle. Cerebral hemisphere width *(HW)* is measured from the midline echo to the first echo from the inner table of the skull. The lateral ventricular ratio is *LVW/HW*. The measurements are made at the point of maximal hemispheric dimension. (From Johnson ML, et al: *J Clin Ultrasound* 1980; 8:311. Used by permission.)

Technique

1. Both compound scanners with 3.5- and 5-MHz internally focused. Transducers and real-time are used.
2. Compound scanner images are recorded with a multi-image camera and real-time images with a Polaroid camera.
3. Image plane is transverse or axial so that anatomy is displayed similar to axial CT. Additional coronal images may be useful.

Measurement (Fig 10–14 and Table 10–4)

The lateral ventricular width *(LVW)* is measured from the middle of the midline echo to the first echo of the lateral wall of the lateral ventricle, at the point where the ventricular walls parallel the midline and the hemispheric dimension is greatest.

Cerebral hemisphere width *(HW)* is determined on the same side and in

*Ref: Johnson ML, et al: *J Clin Ultrasound* 1980; 8:311.

MEASUREMENT OF FETAL CEREBRAL VENTRICLE SIZE BY ULTRASOUND

the same planes as the LVW and is the distance from the middle of the midline echo to the inner table of the calvarium. The LVW/HW can then be calculated.

TABLE 10–4.

Dates From 196 Normal Fetuses*

Menstrual Age (wk)	Lateral Ventricular Width (cm)	Hemispheric Width (cm)	Ratio (LVW/HW) (% ± 2 SD)
15	0.75	1.4	56(40–71)
16	0.86	1.5	57(45–69)
17	0.85	1.5	52(42–62)
18	0.83	1.8	46(40–52)
19	—	—	—
20	0.82	1.9	43(29–57)
21	0.76	2.2	35(27–43)
22	0.82	2.6	32(26–38)
23	0.83	2.5	33(24–42)
24	0.83	2.7	31(23–39)
25	1.1	3.0	34(26–42)
26	0.9	3.0	30(24–36)
27	0.9	3.0	28(23–34)
28	1.1	3.3	31(18–45)
29	1.0	3.4	29(22–37)
30	1.0	3.4	30(26–34)
31	1.0	3.4	29(23–36)
32	1.1	3.6	31(26–36)
33	1.1	3.4	31(25–37)
34	1.1	3.8	28(23–33)
35	1.1	3.8	29(26–31)
36	1.1	3.9	28(23–34)
37	1.2	4.1	29(24–34)
Term	1.2	4.3	28(22–33)

*From Johnson ML, et al: *J Clin Ultrasound* 1980; 8:311. Used by permission.

Source of Material

One hundred ninety-six obstetric sonograms in which no fetal abnormalities were suspected. The gestational age ranged from 15 weeks to term.

ULTRASONIC DETERMINATION
OF FETAL MATURITY

Fetal Crown-Rump Lengths From 6 to 14 Weeks' Gestational Age*

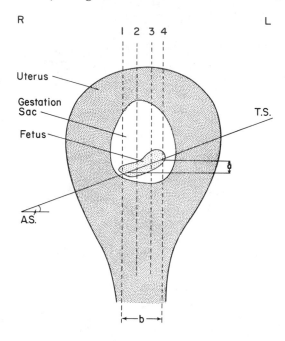

FIG 10–15.
Technique involved in determining lie of fetus in utero. Vertical lines *1–4* through uterus on lower part of figure represent longitudinal scans, and distance travelled transversely by scanning frame is *b*. Recently, Robinson and Fleming† described a simple form of the technique. The vertical scans provide serial parallel sections at small intervals from one side of the gestational sac to the other, during the course of which each end of the fetus is identified and a corresponding mark is made on the patient's abdominal wall. Further scans are then made parallel to the line defined by these two marks (line *T.S.*) until the longest length of fetal echoes is found. A measurement of this echo complex was made from a Polaroid photograph, with the screen graticule used as a rule. (From Robinson HP: *Br Med J* 1973; 4:28. Used by permission.)

Technique (Fig 10–15)

The apparatus used was the Diasonograph NE 4102 (Nuclear Enterprise). The full bladder technique was used as described by Donald.‡ Ultrasound velocity for this study equaled 1,540 m/sec.

*Ref: Robinson HP: *Br Med J* 1973; 4:28.
†Ref: Robinson HP, Fleming JEE: *Br J Obstet Gynaecol*, 1975; 82:702.
‡Ref: Donald I: *Br Med J* 1963; 2:1154.

ULTRASONIC DETERMINATION
OF FETAL MATURITY

Fetal Crown-Rump Lengths From 6 to 14 Weeks' Gestational Age

Measurements

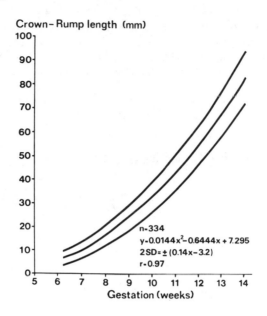

FIG 10–16.
Mean value and 2 SD limits derived from 334 crown-rump length measurements by means of a weighted nonlinear regression analysis designed to obtain the "curve of best fit." When the crown-rump length is less than 12 mm in the early stages of pregnancy the observer using this technique must remember that the fetal length may be only slightly greater than its breadth. In this situation both longitudinal and transverse scans are made, and the greater length of fetal echoes is taken as the crown-rump length. (From Robinson HP, Fleming JEE: *Br J Obstet Gynaecol* 1975; 82:702. Used by permission.)

Source of Material
Data based on a study of 80 patients, totaling 214 examinations. All patients with certain dates of their last menstrual periods, had normal menstrual cycles, and were between the sixth and fourteenth weeks of pregnancy.

ULTRASONIC DETERMINATION
OF FETAL MATURITY

Fetal Biparietal Diameters for 15–40 Weeks' Gestational Age*

Technique
Five independent studies correlating ultrasonic measurements of the fetal biparietal diameter with gestational age were used on the basis of the size of the data population and the similarity of criteria for inclusion of data. These studies represented a total of 11,645 measurements on 4,142 patients.

Ultrasound velocity for all studies equaled 1,540 m/sec.

Measurements (Fig 10–17)

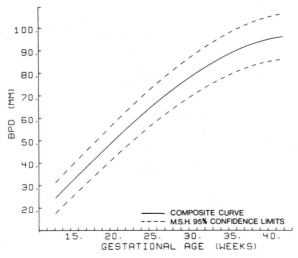

FIG 10–17.
Biparietal diameter versus gestational age. Composite curve of mean values of 5 studies *(solid line)* and 95% confidence limits *(dashed line)*. (From Wiener SN, et al: *Radiology* 1977; 122:781. Used by permission.)

Note on Measurement of Ovarian Size by Ultrasonography: Zemlyn† measured ovarian size by the methods of pelvic ultrasonography and pelvic pneumography. Normal ovary is approximately 1 cm by 2 cm by 3 cm. If the ovary is larger than 2 cm in both of the two shorter axes, enlargement should be considered.

Source of Material
This study is based upon five previously published studies of normal pregnancies and reflects 11,645 measurements done on 4,142 patients.

*Ref: Wiener, SN, et al: *Radiology* 1977; 122:781.
†Ref: Zemlyn S: *J Clin Ultrasound* 1974; 2:331.

MEASUREMENT OF BIPARIETAL DIAMETER AS AN INDICATOR OF GESTATIONAL AGE BY ULTRASOUND*

Technique

1. Kurtz et al. analyzed 17 published studies of biparietal diameter (BPD) using various sonographic techniques.
2. Techniques include two studies measuring outer-to-outer edge and 15 studies measuring outer-to-inner edge.
3. A-mode in 7 and a combination in the remaining 4 studies.
4. All measurements were corrected to an ultrasound velocity of 1,540 m/sec.

Measurement (Fig 10–18 and Table 10–5)

Measure the greatest BPD using electronic calipers or photographed graticule. Although there was no statistical difference in the studies using outer-to-inner edge and outer-to-outer edge, the former is more frequently used.

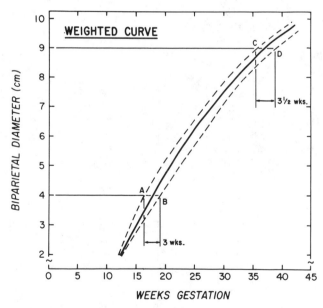

FIG 10–18.
(From Kurtz AB, et al: *J Clin Ultrasound* 1980; 8:319. Used by permission.)

Ref: Kurtz AB, et al: *J Clin Ultrasound* 1980; 8:319.

MEASUREMENT OF BIPARIETAL DIAMETER
AS AN INDICATOR OF GESTATIONAL
AGE BY ULTRASOUND

TABLE 10–5.

Composite Biparietal Diameter*

mm	Wk With Variation	mm	Wk With Variation
20	12.0	60	22.3–25.5
21	12.0	61	22.6–25.5
22	12.2–13.2	62	23.1–26.1
23	12.4–13.6	63	23.4–26.4
24	12.6–13.8	64	23.8–26.8
25	12.9–14.1	65	24.1–27.1
26	13.1–14.3	66	24.5–27.5
27	13.4–14.6	67	25.0–27.8
28	13.6–15.0	68	25.3–28.1
29	13.9–15.2	69	25.8–28.4
30	14.1–15.5	70	26.3–28.7
31	14.3–15.9	71	26.7–29.1
32	14.5–16.1	72	27.2–29.4
33	14.7–16.5	73	27.6–29.8
34	15.0–16.8	74	28.1–30.1
35	15.2–17.2	75	28.5–30.5
36	15.4–17.4	76	29.0–31.0
37	15.6–17.8	77	29.2–31.4
38	15.9–18.1	78	29.6–32.0
39	16.1–18.5	79	29.9–32.5
40	16.4–18.8	80	30.2–33.0
41	16.5–19.3	81	30.7–33.5
42	16.6–19.8	82	31.2–34.0
43	16.8–20.2	83	31.5–34.5
44	16.9–20.7	84	31.9–35.1
45	17.0–21.2	85	32.3–35.7
46	17.4–21.4	86	32.8–36.2
47	17.8–21.6	87	33.4–36.6
48	18.2–21.8	88	33.9–37.1
49	18.6–22.0	89	34.6–37.6
50	19.0–22.2	90	35.1–38.1
51	19.3–22.5	91	35.9–38.5
52	19.5–22.9	92	36.7–38.9
53	19.8–23.2	93	37.3–39.3
54	20.1–23.7	94	37.9–40.1
55	20.4–24.0	95	38.5–40.9
56	20.7–24.3	96	39.1–41.5
57	21.1–24.5	97	39.9–42.1
58	21.5–24.9	98	40.5–43.1
59	21.9–25.1		

*From Kurtz AB, et al: *J Clin Ultrasound* 1980; 8:319. Used by permission.
†Recommended BPD to gestational age, based on the calculated weighted least means square fit equation and 90% variation of the 17 studies.

MEASUREMENT OF BIPARIETAL DIAMETER AS AN INDICATOR OF GESTATIONAL AGE BY ULTRASOUND

Source of Material

More than 10,900 patients with more than 27,400 measurements in 17 published series were analyzed.

MEASUREMENT OF FETAL HEAD CIRCUMFERENCE AS AN INDICATOR OF GESTATIONAL AGE BY ULTRASOUND*

Technique

1. All studies were performed with a linear array real-time system with a 3.5-MHz single-focus transducer.
2. The cranial level was the axial plane giving the largest AP diameter. Brain settings were adjusted so that the width of the skull table nearer the transducer was 3.5 mm.
3. All measurements were made on Polaroid or transparency film along the outer perimeter of the cranium. Measurements were with a hand-held map measurer (Dietzgen) or an electronic digitizer (Numonics Corp.).

*Ref: Hadlock FP: AJR 1982; 138:649.

MEASUREMENT OF FETAL HEAD CIRCUMFERENCE AS AN INDICATOR OF GESTATIONAL AGE BY ULTRASOUND

Measurements (Tables 10–6 and 10–7)

TABLE 10–6.

Predicted Menstrual Age for Head Circumference*†

Head Circumference (cm)	Menstrual Age (wk)	Head Circumference (cm)	Menstrual Age (wk)
8.0	13.4	22.5	24.4
8.5	13.7	23.0	24.9
9.0	14.0	23.5	25.4
9.5	14.3	24.0	25.9
10.0	14.6	24.5	26.4
10.5	15.0	25.0	26.9
11.0	15.3	25.5	27.5
11.5	15.6	26.0	28.0
12.0	15.9	26.5	28.1
12.5	16.3	27.0	29.2
13.0	16.6	27.5	29.8
13.5	17.0	28.0	30.3
14.0	17.3	28.5	31.0
14.5	17.7	29.0	31.6
15.0	18.1	29.5	32.2
15.5	18.4	30.0	32.8
16.0	18.8	30.5	33.5
16.5	19.2	31.0	34.2
17.0	19.6	31.5	34.9
17.5	20.0	32.0	35.5
18.0	20.4	32.5	36.3
18.5	20.8	33.0	37.0
19.0	21.2	33.5	37.7
19.5	21.6	34.0	38.5
20.0	22.1	34.5	39.2
20.5	22.5	35.0	40.0
21.0	23.0	35.5	40.8
21.5	23.4	36.0	41.6
22.0	23.9		

*From Hadlock FP: *AJR* 1982; 138:649. Used by permission.
†Menstrual age = 8.8 + 0.55 (head circumference) + 2.8×10^{-4} (head circumference)^3; r^2 = 97.9%; 1 SD = 1.18 weeks.

MEASUREMENT OF FETAL HEAD CIRCUMFERENCE AS AN INDICATOR OF GESTATIONAL AGE BY ULTRASOUND

TABLE 10−7.

Estimate of Variability

Group No. (Menstrual Age, wk)	Method 1		Method 2
	Variability† (wk)	r^2 (%)	Variability† (wk)
1(12−18)	±1.4	57.4	±1.3
2(18−24)	±1.6	71.9	±1.6
3(24−30)	±2.1	83.0	±2.3
4(30−36)	±3.0	61.0	±2.7
5(36−42)	±2.5	33.9	±3.4

*From Hadlock FP: *AJR* 1982; 138:649. Used by permission.
†95% confidence interval.

Source of Material

Four hundred consecutive patients chosen for reliable date of last menstrual period and good correlation with clinical evaluation. Patients were excluded if they had an illness that might affect fetal growth and if there were multiple gestations.

MEASUREMENT OF FETAL ABDOMINAL CIRCUMFERENCE AS AN INDICATOR OF GESTATIONAL AGE BY ULTRASOUND*

Technique

1. All studies were performed with a linear-array real-time system and a 3.5-MHz single focus transducer.
2. The abdominal level chosen was the axial plane at the level of the umbilical vein-ductus venous complex.
3. All measurements are made on Polaroid or transparency film images around the outer perimeter of the abdomen. Measurements were by a hand-held map measurer (Dietzgen) or electronic digitizer (Numonics Corp.).

*Ref: Hadlock FP: AJR 1982; 139:367.

MEASUREMENT OF FETAL ABDOMINAL CIRCUMFERENCE AS AN INDICATOR OF GESTATIONAL AGE BY ULTRASOUND

Measurements (Tables 10−8 and 10−9)

TABLE 10−8.

Predicted Menstrual Age for Abdominal Circumference Values*†

Abdominal Circumference (cm)	Menstrual Age (wk)	Abdominal Circumference (cm)	Menstrual Age (wk)
10.0	15.6	23.5	27.7
10.5	16.1	24.0	28.2
11.0	16.5	24.5	28.7
11.5	16.9	25.0	29.2
12.0	17.3	25.5	29.7
12.5	17.8	26.0	30.1
13.0	18.2	26.5	30.6
13.5	18.6	27.0	31.1
14.0	19.1	27.5	31.6
14.5	19.5	28.0	32.1
15.0	20.0	28.5	32.6
15.5	20.4	29.0	33.1
16.0	20.8	29.5	33.6
16.5	21.3	30.0	34.1
17.0	21.7	30.5	34.6
17.5	22.2	31.0	35.1
18.0	22.6	31.5	35.6
18.5	23.1	32.0	36.1
19.0	23.6	32.5	36.6
19.5	24.0	33.0	37.1
20.0	24.5	33.5	37.6
20.5	24.9	34.0	38.1
21.0	25.4	34.5	38.7
21.5	25.9	35.0	39.2
22.0	26.3	35.5	39.7
22.5	26.8	36.0	40.2
23.0	27.3	36.5	40.8

*From Hadlock FP: *AJR* 1982; 139:367. Used by permission.
†MA = 7.6070 + 0.7645 (AC) + 0.00393 (AC)^2; r^2 = 97.8%; 1 SD = 1.2 weeks.

MEASUREMENT OF FETAL ABDOMINAL CIRCUMFERENCE AS AN INDICATOR OF GESTATIONAL AGE BY ULTRASOUND

TABLE 10–9.

Estimation of Variability in Predicting Menstrual Age From Abdominal Circumference Measurements*

Group (Menstrual Age, wk)	Variability† (wk)
1(12–18)	±1.9
2(18–24)	±2.0
3(24–30)	±2.2
4(30–36)	±3.0
5(36–42)	±2.5

*From Hadlock FP: *AJR* 1982; 139:367. Used by permission.
†95% confidence interval.

Source of Material

Four hundred consecutive patients chosen for reliable date of last menstrual period and good correlation with clinical evaluation. Patients were excluded if they had an illness that might affect fetal growth and if there were multiple gestations.

MEASUREMENT OF FETAL HEAD TO ABDOMINAL CIRCUMFERENCE RATIO BY ULTRASOUND IN THE ASSESSMENT OF GROWTH RETARDATION*

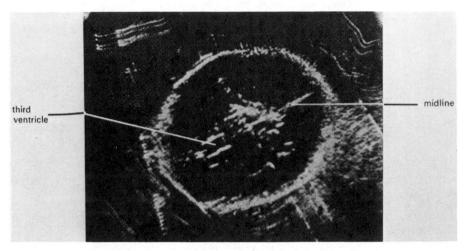

third
ventricle

midline

FIG 10–19.
Echogram showing a horizontal section of a fetal head suitable for circumference measurement. The third ventricle is clearly shown in the midline one third of the distance from the synciput. (From Campbell S: *Br J Obstet Gynaecol* 1977; 84:165. Used by permission.)

Technique

1. B-scan echograms were obtained with a 2-5-MHz transducer.
2. Head circumference was made from Polaroid photographs by means of a map measurer on images that best displayed the occipitofrontal head circumference, with the third ventricle in the midline one third of the distance from the bregma to the occiput.
3. Abdominal circumference was measured on Polaroid photographs by means of a map measurer on transverse images through the liver at the level of the umbilical vein.

Measurement (Figs 10–19 to 10–21; Table 10–10)
Corrections for minification on photographs are made if necessary.

$$\text{Head/abdominal ratios} = \frac{\text{Head circumference}}{\text{Abdominal circumference}}$$

*Ref: Campbell S: *Br J Obstet Gynaecol* 1977; 84:165.

MEASUREMENT OF FETAL HEAD TO ABDOMINAL CIRCUMFERENCE RATIO BY ULTRASOUND IN THE ASSESSMENT OF GROWTH RETARDATION

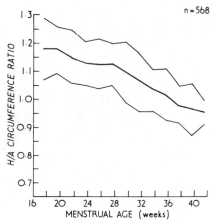

FIG 10–20.

Graphic representation of data in Table 10–10 showing mean H/A circumference ratios with 5th and 95th percentile confidence limits from 17 to 42 weeks' menstrual age. (From Campbell S: *Br J Obstet Gynaecol* 1977; 84:165. Used by permission.)

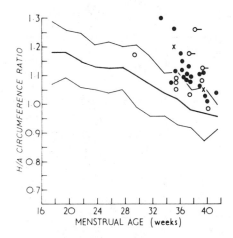

FIG 10–21.

H/A circumference ratios of 31 small-for-dates fetuses related to the normal range and classified according to the type of BPD growth curve. All measurements taken within 7 days of delivery. ● = late retardation of BPD growth; ○ = low growth profile for serial BPD measurements; ○– = low BPD growth profile with terminal arrest of growth; x = normal BPD increase. (From Campbell S: *Br J Obstet Gynaecol* 1977; 84:165. Used by permission.)

MEASUREMENT OF FETAL HEAD TO ABDOMINAL CIRCUMFERENCE RATIO BY ULTRASOUND IN THE ASSESSMENT OF GROWTH RETARDATION

TABLE 10–10.

Mean Fetal H/A Circumference Ratios*†

Menstrual Age (Wk)	Number of Measurements	H/A Circumference Ratio		
		5th Percentile	Mean	95th Percentile
13–14	18	1.14	1.23	1.31
15–16	39	1.05	1.22	1.39
17–18	77	1.07	1.18	1.29
19–20	54	1.09	1.18	1.26
21–22	41	1.06	1.15	1.25
23–24	22	1.05	1.13	1.21
25–26	18	1.04	1.13	1.22
27–28	36	1.05	1.13	1.22
29–30	23	0.99	1.10	1.21
31–32	31	0.96	1.07	1.17
33–34	42	0.96	1.04	1.11
35–36	49	0.93	1.02	1.11
37–38	67	0.92	0.98	1.05
39–40	47	0.87	0.97	1.06
41–42	4	0.93	0.96	1.00

*From Campbell S: *Br J Obstet Gynaecol* 1977; 84:165. Used by permission.
†Fifth and 95th percentile limits related to menstrual age from 13 to 42 weeks. Values combined in two-weekly groupings to smooth out fluctuations due to small numbers (568 individual measurements).

Source of Material

Five hundred sixty-eight measurements were made from 523 patients with normal singleton pregnancies. In most cases, fetal age was confirmed by crown-rump length up to 12 weeks amenorrhea or biparietal diameter between 12 and 20 weeks. Thirty patients were studied who were delivered of a total of 31 small-for-date babies as defined by being on or below the fifth percentile limit, corrected for maternal parity and sex of the child. Twenty-two infants had H/A ratios above the 95th percentile and 9 above the mean, but within the normal range (Table 10–10).

MEASUREMENT OF FETAL FEMUR LENGTH AS AN INDICATOR OF GESTATIONAL AGE BY ULTRASOUND*

Technique

1. All studies are performed with a linear-array real-time system with a 3.5-MHz focused transducer (Advanced Diagnostic Resources).
2. The transducer is aligned along the longest axis of the femur by identifying the fetal trunk, following down to the pelvis. The fetal femur is usually flexed, and the transducer usually must be rotated 30° to 45° toward the fetal abdomen to align with the femur.
3. Care must be taken to avoid tangential measurements that artificially shorten the measurement.

Measurements (Table 10–11)

Several measurements are made and the longest considered optimal.

Electronic calipers are used, but calibration must be verified in both axes using a standard test object.

*Ref: Hadlock FP, et al: AJR 1982; 138:875.

MEASUREMENT OF FETAL FEMUR LENGTH AS AN INDICATOR OF GESTATIONAL AGE BY ULTRASOUND

TABLE 10–11.

Predicted Menstrual Age for Femur Lengths*

Femur Length (mm)	Menstrual Age (wk)	Femur Length (mm)	Menstrual Age (wk)
10	12.8	45	24.5
11	13.1	46	24.9
12	13.4	47	25.3
13	13.6	48	25.7
14	13.9	49	26.1
15	14.2	50	26.5
16	14.5	51	27.0
17	14.8	52	27.4
18	15.1	53	27.8
19	15.4	54	28.2
20	15.7	55	28.7
21	16.0	56	29.1
22	16.3	57	29.6
23	16.6	58	30.0
24	16.9	59	30.5
25	17.2	60	30.9
26	17.6	61	31.4
27	17.9	62	31.9
28	18.2	63	32.3
29	18.6	64	32.8
30	18.9	65	33.3
31	19.2	66	33.8
32	19.6	67	34.2
33	19.9	68	34.7
34	20.3	69	35.2
35	20.7	70	35.7
36	21.0	71	36.2
37	21.4	72	36.7
38	21.8	73	37.2
39	22.1	74	37.7
40	22.5	75	38.3
41	22.9	76	38.8
42	23.3	77	39.3
43	23.7	78	39.8
44	24.1	79	40.4

*From Hadlock FP, et al: *AJR* 1982; 138:875. Used by permission.

MEASUREMENT OF FETAL FEMUR LENGTH AS AN INDICATOR OF GESTATIONAL AGE BY ULTRASOUND

Source of Material

The study was performed on 338 middle-class pregnant women. Menstrual age was established by reference to the last menstrual period and a correlation of ±1 week between the menstrual age and clinical evaluation. When the date of the last menstrual period was not known, or a discrepancy existed, the menstrual age was established by crown-rump length or biparietal diameter prior to 16 weeks by clinical examination. Patients with multiple gestations and illness that might affect fetal growth were excluded.

RADIOLOGIC ESTIMATION OF FETAL MATURITY*

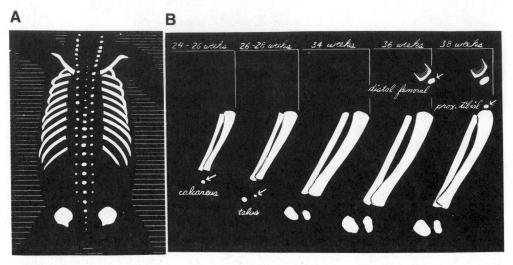

FIG 10–22.
(From Hartley JB: *Br J Radiol* 1957; 30:561. Used by permission.)

Technique

    Central ray: Anteroposterior supine: to level of iliac crest on median plane;

                  Posteroanterior prone: to level of iliac crests on median plane;

                  Oblique posteroanterior: to symphysis pubis on median plane.

      Positions: Anteroposterior supine abdomen;

                Posteroanterior prone abdomen;

                Oblique posteroanterior abdomen.

    Target-film distance: Immaterial (36 inches used by Hartley).

Measurements (Fig 10–22)

Figure 10–22,A:

        10 wk   Ossification centers appear first in the transverse arches of the cervical vertebrae, subsequently appearing in the dorsal region and lumbar region. Hartley believes that the centers are never dense enough to be identified before the end of the tenth week.

Figure 10–22,B:

    10–24 wk   Size of skull is probably the best single index of fetal age (see section on pelvimetry, p 624.) No carpal or tarsal centers are present, and no identifiable epiphyses have yet appeared.

*Ref: Hartley JB: Br J Radiol 1957; 30:561.

RADIOLOGIC ESTIMATION OF FETAL MATURITY

24–26 wk	Calcaneus appears.
26–28 wk	Talus appears.
30–36 wk	Best guide is the study of developing foot ossification centers plus overall study of skull, vertebral bodies, femora, tibiae, and soft tissues.
36 wk	Distal femoral epiphysis appears.
38 wk	Proximal tibial epiphysis appears.

Source of Material

More than 10,000 cases from a large cross-section of the population in a large industrial center in Britain were studied.

FETAL WEIGHT DETERMINATION

Skull, Spine, and Uterus Measurements to Predict Weight*

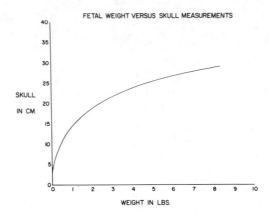

FIG 10–23.
Graph showing fetal weight versus skull measurements. (From Stockland L, Marks SA: *AJR* 1961; 86:425. Used by permission.)

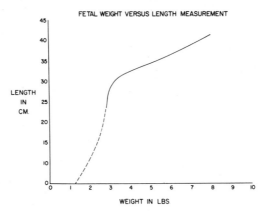

FIG 10–24.
Graph showing fetal weight versus length measurements. (From Stockland L, Marks SA: *AJR* 1961; 86:425. Used by permission.)

*Ref: Stockland L, Marks SA: *AJR* 1961; 86:425.

FETAL WEIGHT DETERMINATION

Skull, Spine, and Uterus Measurements to Predict Weight

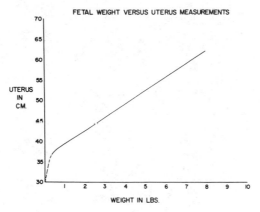

FIG 10–25.
Graph showing fetal weight versus uterus measurements. (From Stockland L, Marks SA: *AJR* 1961; 86:425. Used by permission.)

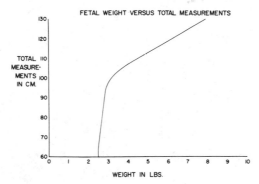

FIG 10–26.
Graph showing fetal weight versus total measurements. (From Stockland L, Marks SA: *AJR* 1961; 86:425. Used by permission.)

FETAL WEIGHT DETERMINATION

Skull, Spine, and Uterus Measurements to Predict Weight

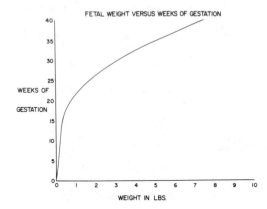

FIG 10–27.
Graph showing fetal weight versus weeks of gestation. (From Stockland L, Marks SA: *AJR* 1961; 86:425. Used by permission.)

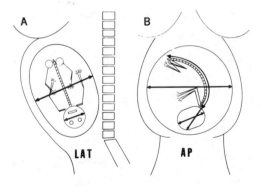

FIG 10–28.
(From Stockland L, Marks SA: *AJR* 1961; 86:425. Used by permission.)

FETAL WEIGHT DETERMINATION

Skull, Spine, and Uterus Measurements to Predict Weight

Technique

1. *Central ray:* Anteroposterior supine: midline at level of iliac crests; Lateral supine: level of iliac crest.
2. *Positions:* Anteroposterior supine and lateral supine. Wire markers made from solder wire are taped to the abdominal wall anteriorly and along both lateral abdominal walls.
3. *Target-film distance:* 40 inches.

Measurements

1. Skull measurement. Measure biparietal diameter and occipitofrontal diameter of skull. Add the two measurements (Fig 10–28). Plot total on graph (Fig 10–23).
2. Fetal length measurement. Measure length of fetal spine from coccyx to odontoid process (Fig 10–28,B).
3. Total length measurement. Add skull measurement and spine measurement. Plot total on graph (Fig 10–24).
4. Uterus measurement. Measure the greatest width of the uterus from the AP roentgenogram (Fig 10–28,B) and the greatest width of the uterus from the lateral roentgenogram (Fig 10–28,A). Add the two measurements and plot total on graph (Fig 10–25).
5. Total measurements. Add measurements of skull, total length (spine, plus skull), and uterus. Plot total on graph (Fig 10–26).
6. Average estimated weight. The weights obtained from graphs for skull, total length, uterus and total measurement are added and averaged. This is the average, or estimated weight on the day of roentgenography.
7. Gestation determination. Average weight from preceding step is plotted on graph (Fig 10–27) and weeks of gestation determined. From the graph the number of weeks necessary for the desired increase in the weight of the fetus can be read.

Source of Material

The results were obtained from the examinations of 50 patients and tested for accuracy on 179 patients.

FETAL WEIGHT DETERMINATION

Fetal Bone Measurements to Predict Weight*

Technique
  Central ray: Midline at level of iliac crest.
  Position: Anteroposterior supine.
  Target-film distance: 40 inches.

Measurements (Table 10–12)
Maximum lengths were obtained on 10 long bones; 2 femur, 2 tibia, 2 humerus, 2 radius, and 2 ulna. The smaller of each pair of measurements was discarded.

Measurements were not corrected for magnification. The measurements shown below divide fetuses into two groups, with weights above or below 2,250 gms (5 lbs). If any bone equals or exceeds the length shown, the fetus is very likely to exceed 2,250 gms.

TABLE 10–12.*

Bone	Measurement (cm)
Femur	6.6
Tibia	7.0
Humerus	7.5
Ulna	6.8
Radius	5.6

*From Howland WJ, Brandfass RT: *Invest Radiol* 1967; 2:61. Used by permission.

Source of Material
Postpartum studies were made on 60 infants within 14 days after delivery. Infant weights were between 1,500 and 3,000 gm.

Antepartum studies were done on 100 pelvimetry and maternal-abdomen roentgenograms obtained within 14 days before delivery. All infants weighed 1,500 to 3,000 gm at birth.

Ref: Howland WJ, Brandfass RT: *Invest Radiol* 1967; 2:61.

FETAL WEIGHT DETERMINATION

Ratio of Vertebral Length/Abdominal Diameter to Predict Weight*

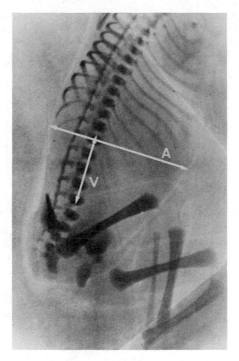

FIG 10–29.
Measurements of the fetus for weight determination. (From Ringertz HG: *Acta Radiol Diagn* 1971; 11:545. Used by permission.)

*Ref: Ringertz HG: *Acta Radiol Diagn* 1971; 11:545.

FETAL WEIGHT DETERMINATION

Ratio of Vertebral Length/Abdominal Diameter to Predict Weight

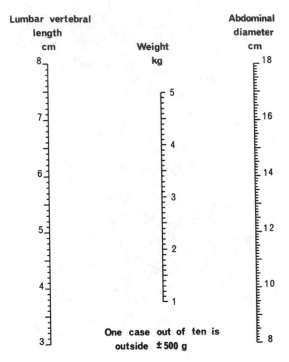

FIG 10–30.
Chart for assessment of fetal weight from the uncorrected measurement of the lumbar vertebral length and abdominal diameter. (From Ringertz HG: *Acta Radiol Diagn* 1971; 11:545. Used by permission.)

Technique
    Central ray: Perpendicular to plane of film.
    Position: Lateral with mother lying on side with compression of abdomen.
    Target-film distance: 1 meter.

Measurement (Fig 10–29)
The measurement of the lumbar vertebral length (V) lies between the middle point of the cranial surface of L1 and the middle point of the caudal surface of L5. Measurement A is the distance between the outer limits of the subcutaneous fat layers at the level of L1 and perpendicular to the spine. The nomogram (Fig 10–30) is used to determine fetal weight. These data are useful for determining fetal maturity.

Source of Material
Data derived from a study of 210 normal pregnancies.

MEASUREMENT OF TWIN AND SINGLETON FETAL GROWTH PATTERNS BY ULTRASOUND*

Technique

1. Examinations were performed using a 3.5-MHz focused transducer on mechanical sector scanners.
2. Examinations were performed at 4 to 6 week intervals once twin gestation had been established.

Measurements

Complete fetal anatomic survey was carried out for each twin and included biparietal diameter (BPD), fetal femur length (FFL), and abdominal circumference (AC).

The data for these measurements are given in Tables 10–13 to 10–17.

TABLE 10–13.

Mean Twin and Singleton BPD for 27th to 37th Week of Gestation*

Gestational Age (wk)	N	Mean Twin BPD (cm)	SD (cm)	Singleton BPD (cm) (15)	P Value†
37	6	8.5	.3	9.1	.003
36	14	8.5	.3	8.9	.005
35	18	8.4	.4	8.7	.006
34	16	8.2	.3	8.5	.002
33	24	8.1	.4	8.3	.047
32	20	7.9	.4	8.1	.028
31	18	7.8	.5	7.9	.466
30	26	7.4	.5	7.6	.028
29	22	7.4	.4	7.4	.919
28	20	7.4	.4	7.2	.057
27	20	6.9	.4	6.9	.999

*From Grumbach K, et al: *Radiology* 1986; 158:237–241. Used by permission.
†Student's *t* test.

*Ref: Grumbach K, et al: *Radiology* 1986; 158:237–241.

MEASUREMENT OF TWIN AND SINGLETON FETAL GROWTH PATTERNS BY ULTRASOUND

TABLE 10–14.

Mean Twin and Singleton FFL for 27th to 37th Week of Gestation*

Gestational Age (wk)	N	Mean Twin FFL (cm)	SD (cm)	Mean Singleton FFL (cm) (10)	P Value†
37	4	7.2	.3	7.3	.62
36	8	6.9	.3	7.1	.24
35	8	6.9	.3	6.9	.22
34	10	6.6	.3	6.7	.62
33	10	6.4	.5	6.5	.68
32	10	6.3	.5	6.3	.99
31	8	5.9	.6	6.0	.44
30	16	5.9	.4	5.8	.12
29	4	5.2	.3	5.6	.60
28	8	5.7	.2	5.4	.60
27	10	5.1	.3	5.1	.99

*From Grumbach K, et al: *Radiology* 1986; 158:237–241. Used by permission.
†Student's *t* test.

TABLE 10–15.

Mean Twin and Singleton AC for 27th to 37th Week of Gestation*

Gestational Age (wk)	N	Mean Twin AC (cm)	SD (cm)	Mean Singleton AC (cm) (11)	P Value†
37	8	29.2	2.6	33.7	.009
36	10	29.8	1.6	32.6	.001
35	14	29.6	1.7	31.5	.001
34	14	28.9	1.9	30.4	.012
33	14	27.1	2.1	29.3	.002
32	18	27.2	1.8	28.2	.035
31	12	26.9	1.9	27.1	.68
30	18	25.3	1.9	26.0	.11
29	12	24.9	2.5	24.9	.56
28	19	23.9	2.7	23.8	.68
27	12	23.6	1.7	22.7	.07

*From Grumbach K, et al: *Radiology* 1986; 158:237–241. Used by permission.
†Student's *t* test.

MEASUREMENT OF TWIN AND SINGLETON FETAL GROWTH PATTERNS BY ULTRASOUND

TABLE 10–16.

Predicted BPDs of Twin Fetuses Between 20 and 37 Weeks of Gestation*

Week of Gestation	Mean BPD (cm)	10th Percentile (cm)	90th Percentile (cm)
20	5.1	4.9	5.3
21	5.1	4.9	5.7
22	5.4	5.0	6.5
23	5.7	4.5	5.9
24	6.0	5.3	7.4
25	6.3	5.5	7.5
26	6.6	5.9	7.8
27	6.8	6.5	7.5
28	7.1	6.9	8.2
29	7.3	6.8	7.9
30	7.5	6.8	8.1
31	7.7	6.9	8.6
32	7.9	7.3	8.4
33	8.0	7.4	8.6
34	8.2	7.9	8.5
35	8.3	7.9	8.9
36	8.5	8.0	9.0
37	8.6	8.2	8.8

*From Grumbach K, et al: *Radiology* 1986; 158:237–241. Used by permission.

MEASUREMENT OF TWIN AND SINGLETON
FETAL GROWTH PATTERNS BY ULTRASOUND

TABLE 10-17.

Predicted ACs of Twin Fetuses Between 20 and 37 Weeks of Gestation*

Week of Gestation	Mean AC (cm)	10th Percentile (cm)	90th Percentile (cm)
20	16.8	14.9	17.1
21	17.5	15.7	19.0
22	18.6	15.8	20.9
23	19.4	16.3	19.6
24	20.2	16.7	23.9
25	21.1	18.8	23.9
26	21.9	18.9	26.2
27	22.7	21.5	25.9
28	23.6	19.9	27.7
29	24.4	21.6	27.4
30	25.2	22.4	26.6
31	26.0	24.5	28.9
32	26.7	24.7	29.6
33	27.4	23.2	29.0
34	28.3	25.9	30.3
35	29.1	26.9	31.1
36	29.8	27.5	31.5
37	30.5	23.9	32.1

*From Grumbach K, et al: *Radiology* 1986; 158:237–241. Used by permission.

Source of Material

Data are based on a study of 103 twin gestations.

SUMMARY OF FETAL GROWTH PARAMETER*

Seeds and Cefalo have prepared a composite of measurements for determination of fetal maturation. Their data are derived from a number of sources. The summary is presented in Table 10−18. The interested reader should consult this reference for more detailed information.

*Ref: Seeds JW, Cefalo RC: *Practical Obstetrical Ultrasound*. Rockville, Md, Aspen Publishers, Inc, 1986, p 52.

SUMMARY OF FETAL GROWTH PARAMETER

TABLE 10–18.

Fetal Growth Parameters (mm)*

Gestational Age	Biparietal Diameter	Femur Length	Humerus Length	Head Circumference	Average Head Diameter	Abdominal Circumference	Average Abdominal Diameter
14	28	15	15	101	32	84	27
15	32	18	18	114	36	95	30
16	36	20	21	128	41	106	34
17	39	23	23	141	45	117	37
18	42	26	26	154	49	128	41
19	45	29	28	167	53	139	44
20	48	32	31	179	57	150	48
21	51	35	33	192	61	161	51
22	54	37	35	204	65	172	55
23	58	40	37	215	68	183	58
24	61	42	39	227	72	194	62
25	64	45	41	238	76	205	65
26	67	48	44	249	79	216	69
27	70	50	46	259	82	227	72
28	72	53	48	269	86	238	76
29	75	55	49	279	89	249	79
30	78	57	51	288	92	260	83
31	80	60	53	297	95	271	86
32	82	62	55	306	97	282	90
33	85	64	57	314	100	293	93
34	87	67	59	322	102	304	97
35	88	69	60	329	105	315	100
36	90	71	62	336	107	326	104
37	92	73	64	342	109	337	107
38	93	76	66	348	111	348	111
39	94	78	67	354	113	359	114
40	95	80	69	359	114	370	118

95% confidence intervals

Biparietal diameter	14–20 weeks ± 7 days
	20–30 weeks ± 10 days
	30–40 weeks ± 21 days
Femur or humerus length	14–20 weeks ± 7 days
	20–30 weeks ± 10 days
	30–40 weeks ± 12 days
Head circumference (diameter)	14–28 weeks ± 1.5 cm
	28–40 weeks ± 2.5 cm
Abdominal circumference (diameter)	14–40 weeks ± 13%

*From Seeds JW, Cefalo RC: *Practical Obstetrical Ultrasound*. Rockville, Md, Aspen Publishers, Inc, 1986, p 52. Used by permission.

MEASUREMENT OF THE FETAL RENAL PELVIS BY ULTRASOUND FOR THE DETECTION OF UPPER URINARY TRACT ABNORMALITY*

Technique
Unstated.

Measurement (Figs 10–31 and 10–32)

RP = Maximal renal pelvic diameter.
RD = Renal diameter.

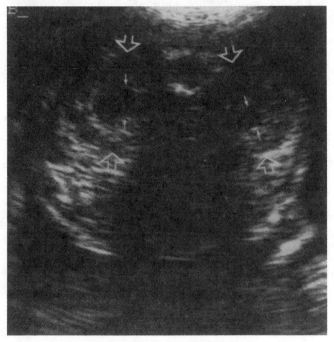

FIG 10–31.
Normal kidney. Transverse section through both fetal kidneys shows bilateral prominence of renal pelvis (right, 8 mm; left, 6 mm) *(small arrows)*. Transverse AP renal width (right, 21 mm; left, 20 mm) *(open arrows)*. RP/RD ratio: right, 38%; left, 30%. Both kidneys were normal with extrarenal pelvis on post-delivery follow-up. (From Arger PH, et al: *Radiology* 1985; 156:485–489. Used by permission.)

Ref: Arger PH, et al: *Radiology* 1985; 156:485–489.

MEASUREMENT OF THE FETAL RENAL PELVIS BY ULTRASOUND FOR THE DETECTION OF UPPER URINARY TRACT ABNORMALITY

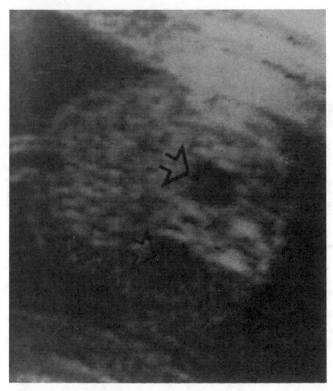

FIG 10–32.
Normal kidney. Renal pelvis prominence bilaterally (right, 9 mm; left, 8 mm) *(open arrows)* in fetus at 22 weeks of gestation. Four subsequent examinations showed less prominence of the renal pelvis. At 32 weeks' gestation and 3 days after delivery, no renal pelvis dilatation was present. (From Arger PH, et al: *Radiology* 1985; 156:485–489. Used by permission.)

The authors conclude that any renal pelvis that measures 5 mm or greater on the initial examination should be monitored in utero for the first few days after birth. When a renal pelvis reaches 1 cm or more and the RP/RD ratio exceeds 50%, the observer should be alerted to the highly likely fact that significant renal hydronephrosis is present. Additionally, loculated cystic areas indicate an important renal abnormality.

Source of Material
Data are based on a study of 4,832 routine fetal genitourinary obstetrical ultrasound examinations.

CHAPTER 11

The Metric System*

The metric system had its origin in France in the year 1670. It was proposed by Gabriel Mouton, a Lyons vicar, who saw the need for a decimal system, using Latin prefixes for multiples or fractions, based upon a measurement of the earth. However, 129 years passed before official recognition was given to this system, and it was 170 years later that the metric system was adopted as the only allowable system of weights and measures in France.

In the United States, 26 more years were to pass before the Law of 1866 was passed by Congress allowing use of the metric system. In 1893 the meter and the kilogram gained recognition as the standards of length and mass by the Office of Standard Weights and Measures.

International standardization began in 1870 in Paris and led to the acceptance of the International System of Units (SI). This system has six base units, which are of defined magnitude.

Quantity	Unit	SI Symbol
Length	Meter	m
Mass	Kilogram	kg
Time	Second	s
Electric current	Ampere	A
Thermodynamic temperature	Degree Kelvin	°K
Luminous intensity	Candela	cd

*Reprinted from *The Journal of Bone and Joint Surgery* with permission of the editor and the publisher. The material was prepared by Albert H. Burstein, Ph.D.

METRIC SYSTEM

All other quantities are derived from these six using, when desired, the following prefixes or multipliers:

Multiplication Factor†		Prefix‡	SI Symbol
1,000,000	$= 10^6$	Mega	M
1,000	$= 10^3$	Kilo	k
100	$= 10^2$	Hecto	h
10	$= 10^1$	Deka	da
0.1	$= 10^{-1}$	Deci	d
0.01	$= 10^{-2}$	Centi	c
0.001	$= 10^{-3}$	Milli	m
0.000001	$= 10^{-6}$	Micro	μ
0.000000001	$= 10^{-9}$	Nano	n
0.000000000001	$= 10^{-12}$	Pico	p

†Abbreviated list.

‡When these prefixes are used to form new unit designations, only one prefix is used at a time. Thus, instead of a millimicrogram (mμg), nanogram (ng) would be used, and micromicron ($\mu\mu$) would become picometer (pm). Unit designations should consist of a single prefix to designate a multiplier and a single suffix to describe the physical quantity to which the multiplier is applied. Thus micrometers (μm) is preferred to microns (μ).

The unit of *force* in the SI system is the *newton* (N), which is the force required to give one kilogram of mass an acceleration of one meter per second per second. However, in engineering and the physical sciences in this country the accepted practice is to use the kilogram-force (kgf), which is defined as the force required to accelerate one kilogram of mass (kg) 9.80665 meters per second per second. A kilogram-force is approximately equal to the weight of a kilogram of mass. (The gravitational acceleration varies 0.5% over the surface of the earth.)

A modified system that differs from the SI system in that it uses kilogram-force instead of newtons may be useful as a transition system. It is suggested that if this modified system is used, a footnote of the following form appear in the publications in which the unit kilogram-force (kgf) appears:

A kilogram-force (kgf) is exactly equal to 9.80665 newtons (N) and approximately equal to the weight of a kilogram (kg) of mass.

The use of the newton as the unit of force is certainly preferable, but the use of the kilogram-force can be accepted to allow an easier transition to the SI system.

The old centimeter-gram-second (CGS) system, because it is one of the most familiar metric systems, is compared with the SI system and the modified metric system just described in Table A-1. Subsequent tables give the conversion factors for the commonly used units of measure.

METRIC SYSTEM

TABLE A–1.

Comparison of Basic Units

	CGS	SI*	Modified Metric†
Mass	Gram (gm)	Kilogram (kg)	Kilogram (kg)
Length	Centimeter (cm)	Meter (m)	Meter (m)
Time	Second (s)	Second (s)	Second (s)
Force	Dyne‡	Newton (N)§	Kilogram-force (kgf)#

*Le Systeme International d'Unites, which is called the SI system, is used by most countries of the world as the official system of weights and measures and is the preferred system.

†The Modified Metric system is acceptable as an interim or transitional system.

‡A dyne is the force required to give a free mass of one gram an acceleration of one centimeter per second per second.

§A newton is the force required to give a free mass of one kilogram an acceleration of one meter per second per second.

#A kilogram-force is the force required to give a free mass of one kilogram an acceleration of 9.80665 meters per second per second (exact conversion, i.e., all subsequent digits are zeros). This acceleration is the international standard gravity value ("standard acceleration"). Therefore, 1 *kilogram-force* (kgf) is *approximately* equivalent to the *weight* of a 1 *kilogram* (kg) *mass*, since the value of gravity varies 0.5% over the earth's surface.

$$1 \text{ kilogram-force} = 9.80665 \text{ newtons}$$
$$1 \text{ kilogram-force} = 9.80665 \times 10^5 \text{ dynes}$$

The term kilopond has been used to mean kilogram-force.

A gram-force (gmf) is defined by: 1000 gmf = 1 kgf.

METRIC SYSTEM

TABLE A–2.

Conversion Factors

LENGTH

Equivalences:

Angstrom	$= 1 \times 10^{-10}$ meter (0.0000000001 m)	
Millimicron*	$= 1 \times 10^{-9}$ meter (0.000000001 m)	
Micron (micrometer)	$= 1 \times 10^{-6}$ meter (0.000001 m)	

To convert from	To	Multiply by
Inches	Meters	0.0254†
Feet	Meters	0.30480†
Yards	Meters	0.91440†
Miles	Kilometers	1.6093

AREA

To convert from	To	Multiply by
Square inches	Square meters	0.00064516†
Square feet	Square meters	0.092903

VOLUME

Definition:

1 liter $= 0.001$† cubic meter or 1 cubic decimeter (dm^3)
(1 milliliter $= 1$† cubic centimeter)

To convert from	To	Multiply by
Cubic inches	Cubic centimeters	16.387
Ounces (U.S. fluid)	Cubic centimeters	29.574
Ounces (Brit. fluid)	Cubic centimeters	28.413
Pints (U.S. fluid)	Cubic centimeters	473.18
Pints (Brit. fluid)	Cubic centimeters	568.26
Cubic feet	Cubic meters	0.028317

MASS

To convert from	To	Multiply by
Pounds (avdp.)	Kilograms	0.45359
Slugs‡	Kilograms	14.594

FORCE

To convert from	To	Multiply by
Ounces-force (ozf)	Newtons	0.27802
Ounces-force (ozf)	Kilogram-force	0.028350
Pounds-force (lbf)	Newtons	4.4732
Pounds-force (lbf)	Kilogram-force	0.45359

*This double-prefix usage is not desirable. This unit is actually a nanometer (10^{-9} meter $= 10^{-7}$ centimeter).
†Exact conversion; all subsequent digits are zeros.
‡A slug is a unit of mass that if acted on by a force of 1 pound will have an acceleration of 1 foot per second per second.

METRIC SYSTEM

STRESS (OR PRESSURE)

To convert from	To	Multiply by
Pounds-force/square inch (psi)	Newton/square meter	6894.8
Pounds-force/square inch (psi)	Newton/square centimeter	0.68948
Pounds-force/square inch (psi)	Kilogram-force/square centimeter	0.070307

TORQUE (OR MOMENT)

To convert from	To	Multiply by
Pound-force · feet	Newton meter	1.3559
Pound-force · feet	Kilogram-force · meters	0.13826

ENERGY (OR WORK)

Definition:

1 joule (J) is the work done by a one-newton force moving through a displacement of 1 meter in the direction of the force.

(1 cal (gm) = 4.1840 joules)

To convert from	To	Multiply by
Foot · pounds-force	Joules	1.3559
Foot · pounds-force	Meter · kilogram-force	0.13826
Ergs	Joules	1×10^{-7}†
BTU	Cal (gm)	252.00
Foot · pounds-force	Cal (gm)	0.32405

†Exact conversion; all subsequent digits are zero.

TABLE A–3.

Temperature Conversion Table

$$°C = \frac{°F - 32}{1.8}$$

°F	°C
98.6	37
99	37.2
99.5	37.5
100	37.8
100.5	38.1
101	38.3
101.5	38.6
102	38.9
102.5	39.2
103	39.4
103.5	39.7
104	40.0

References

U.S. Department of Commerce, National Bureau of Standards: *Units of Weights and Measures*, Pub 286, May 1967; *National Bureau of Standards Handbook 102, ASTM Metric Practice Guide*, ed 2, March 1967.

Ritchie-Calder PR: *Sci Am* 1970; 223:17. (Overview of the problem of metric conversion.)

Index

H

Hand
  left
    female, 276
    male, 275
  measurements in gonadal dysgenesis
      detection, 169–171
  right
    female, 275
    male, 274
Head
  circumference (see Fetus, head
      circumference)
  mean areas and normal ranges, CT of,
      80–81
  midventricular slice, CT of, 78
Heart, 393–477
  anteroposterior projection,
      406
  in children, 394–405
    first 6 years, 395
    first year, 394
    7 to 12 years, 395
  left, by MRI, 424–428
    measurements, 424–428
    source of material, 428
    techniques, 424
  structures, by CT, 420–423
    measurements, 421
    normal measurements, 422
    source of material, 423
    technique, 421
  transverse cardiac diameter (see
      Transverse cardiac diameter)
  volume, 409–416
    in adolescents, 410
    body surface predicting, 411
    body weight predicting, 411
    in children, 410
    in infant, 413
    measurements, 415
    normal, upper limits of, 415
    source of material, 416
    technique, 415
Heel pad (see Acromegaly, heel pad in)
Hemispheric sulci
  measurement by CT, 16–19
  width, maximum, 18
Hepatic duct: common, 515
Hepatitis: serum, 515
Hilar
  height ratio in displacement, 385
    measurements, 385
    source of material, 385
    technique, 385
  outlines, 383–384
    measurements, 383–384

source of material, 384
  technique, 383
Hinck's measurement: in skull base for
    basilar invagination, 98
Hindfoot: relationships of, 349
Hip, 287–310
  acetabular angle (see Acetabular
      angle in growing hip)
  bone mineral, normal, 285
  dislocation (see Dislocation of hip)
  dysplasia, beta angle of acetabulum
      in, 306
  growing
    abnormality detection, 302–305
    abnormality detection
        measurements, 303–305
    abnormality detection, source of
        material, 305
    abnormality detection technique,
        303
    acetabular angle (see Acetabular
        angle in growing hip)
    iliac angle and index (see Iliac
        angle and index in growing hip)
  joint, axial relationships, 289
    measurements, 289
    source of material, 289
    technique, 289
  joint space width, 290–291
    measurements, 290
    source of material, 291
    technique, 290
Hirschsprung's disease (see
    Rectosigmoid index in
    Hirschsprung's disease)
Holmquist nomogram, 3
  with Ball method, 628
Horn
  anterior
    quotient of, 13
    width of, 13
    width, as function of age, 17
  frontal, 9, 78
  occipital, 9
Humerus
  female, 281
  fracture (see Fracture, humerus)
  head ossification in newborn for
      gestational age assessment,
      164
  and metacarpal thickness (see
      Metacarpal and humerus
      thickness)
Hyoid bone: position as tracheal
    transection sign, 62
Hypertrophic
  cardiomyopathy, 457, 458, 459
  pyloric stenosis, 483–484

698